DATE DUE

4353361	SEP 1 1 1998

Hormonal Carcinogenesis

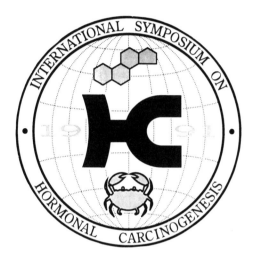

Jonathan J. Li   Satyabrata Nandi
Sara Antonia Li
Editors

Hormonal Carcinogenesis

Proceedings of the
First International Symposium

With 81 Illustrations

Springer-Verlag

New York Berlin Heidelberg London Paris
Tokyo Hong Kong Barcelona Budapest

Jonathan J. Li, Ph.D.
Hormonal Carcinogenesis Laboratory and
Department of Pharmaceutical Sciences
College of Pharmacy
Washington State University
Pullman, WA 99164-6510
USA

Satyabrata Nandi, Ph.D.
Department of Molecular and
  Cell Biology
Cancer Research Laboratory
University of California
Berkeley, CA 94720
USA

Sara Antonia Li, Ph.D.
Hormonal Carcinogenesis Laboratory and
Department of Pharmaceutical Sciences
College of Pharmacy
Washington State University
Pullman, WA 99164-6510
USA

Library of Congress Cataloging-in-Publication Data
International Symposium on Hormonal Carcinogenesis (1st   1991
   Cancun, Mexico)
     Hormonal carcinogenesis: proceedings of the First International
   Symposium on Hormonal Carcinogenesis, March 19-21, 1991, Cancun,
   Mexico/editors, Jonathan J. Li, Satyabrata Nandi, Sara Antonia Li.
       p.   cm.
     Includes bibliographical references and index.
     ISBN 0-387-97797-X. − ISBN 3-540-97797-X
     1. Steroid hormones − Carcinogenecity − Congresses.   2. Hormones −
   Carcinogenicity − Congresses.   3. Carcinogenesis − Congresses.
   I. Li, Jonathan J.   II. Nandi, Satyabrata.   III. Li, Sara Antonia.
   IV. Title.
     [DNLM. 1. Hormones − adverse effects − congresses.   2. Neoplasms −
   chemically induced − congresses.   WK 102 I6093h 1991]
   RC268.7S7I58   1991
   616.99′4071 − dc20
   DNLM/DLC   92-220

Printed on acid-free paper.

Production managed by Natalie Johnson; manufacturing supervised by Jacqui Ashri.
Camera-ready copy prepared using the editors' WordPerfect files.
Printed and bound by Edwards Brothers, Inc., Ann Arbor, MI.
Printed in the United States of America.

9 8 7 6 5 4 3 2 1

ISBN 0-387-97797-X Springer-Verlag New York Berlin Heidelberg
ISBN 3-540-97797-X Springer-Verlag Berlin Heidelberg New York

This volume is dedicated to five pioneers in hormonal carcinogenesis and hormone action whose contributions laid much of the foundation for these fields.

Howard A. Bern

Cancer Research Laboratory
University of California, Berkeley

Roy Hertz

George Washington University

Charles B. Huggins

Ben May Laboratory for Cancer Research
University of Chicago

Hadley Kirkman

Stanford University

Gerald C. Mueller

McArdle Laboratory for Cancer Research
University of Wisconsin

List of Supporters

Sustaining Members

National Institute of Environmental Health Sciences
National Cancer Institute
National Institute of Child Health & Human Development
Nitta Gelatin, Inc.
Farmos Group Ltd.
Orion Corporation
Schering AG
Adria Laboratories

Affiliating Members

National Institute of Diabetes & Digestive & Kidney Diseases
R.W. Johnson Pharmaceutical Research Institute
Ortho Pharmaceutical
CIBA-Geigy Pharmaceutical Division
Syntex Laboratories
The Upjohn Company
Wyeth-Ayerst Research
Berlex Laboratories
IVAX Corporation

Executive and Scientific Advisory Boards

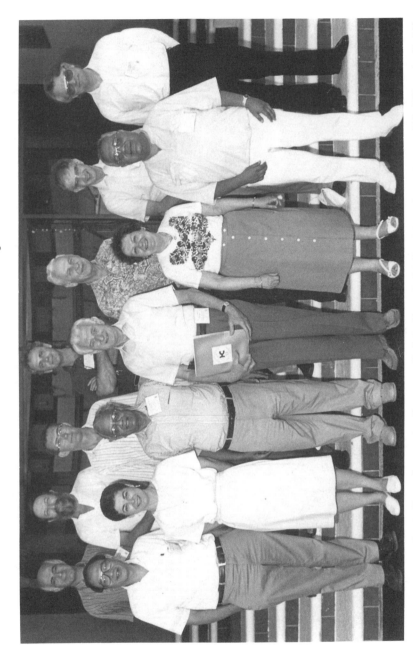

Top Row, R to L: J. Gustafsson, A. Conney, G. Mueller, J. McLachlan, M. Metzler, M. Pike, A. Baldi
Bottom Row, R to L: G. Palacios, L.Sekely, L. Lerner, Executive Board: S. Nandi, S.A. Li, and J.J. Li

Participants of the First Hormonal Carcinogenesis Symposium

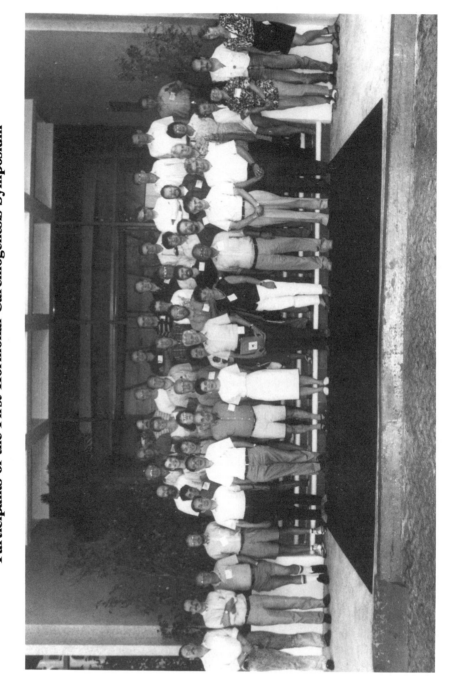

Preface

In the past decade there has been a growing public interest and resurgence in research in the field of hormonal carcinogenesis. This is due to the widespread use of therapeutic hormonal agents worldwide and to the increasing awareness of the causal association of hormones, both endogenous and exogenously administered, and a variety of human cancers. These associations include estrogens in uterine, cervical, vaginal, liver, testicular, prostatic, and possible breast cancers; progesterone and progestational hormones in breast cancer; androgens and anabolic steroids in hepatic and prostatic cancers. Additionally, gonadotrophins play a role in the etiology of ovarian and testicular cancers and thyroid-stimulating hormones in thyroid cancers. Therefore, hormonal carcinogenesis encompasses the study of both natural and synthetic hormonal agents, including growth factors and other peptide and protein factors, which contribute substantially to the *etiology* of both human and animal neoplasms, benign or malignant. Hormones may be involved in all aspects of neoplastic transformation, including initiation, promotion, and progression, and the inhibition of these processes.

There are a number of important issues in women's health that need to be addressed. More than 40 million U.S. women are menopausal, and these women have a life expectancy of over 30 years after the menopause. When these figures are multiplied worldwide, the numbers become staggering. After the menopause, estrogen replacement therapy (ERT) is the choice of most women in industrialized countries. Still unresolved is whether or not concomitant progestational hormone treatment, now commonly given with ERT, will increase the risk for breast cancer in women.

The benefits of ERT for hot flashes, osteoporosis, cardiovascular disease, genitourinary dysfunction, nervous, psychological, and sexual functions are well established. Recently, the beneficial use of estrogens in relation to heart disease has been publicized in a Boston study. While there is concern regarding the widespread and recent rise in the use of oral contraceptives (OCs), among OC users there is evidence for a significant reduction in the incidence of benign breast disease, ovarian cysts, iron deficiency anemia, pelvic inflammatory disease, and ectopic pregnancy.

Despite the evident and substantial benefits derived from these hormonal agents, safer preparations appear mandatory in light of their carcinogenic potential. It is also essential that we have a greater understanding of the normal physiologic, biochemical, and molecular processes by which hormones affect cell proliferation, differentiation, and ultimately, neoplastic processes. Many fundamental questions remain unresolved. Although it seems clear that hormones can result in tumor promotion by virtue of their ability to affect cell proliferation and differentiation, there is as yet no concensus on whether or not hormones can act as nongenotoxic or genotoxic carcinogens. Even in the absence of other chemical or physical agents, it is not known whether hormone-induced tumor formation is a result of some intrinsic property of the parent hormone molecule operating through a specific receptor mechanism, or whether a metabolite(s) interacts directly with the genetic apparatus of target cells. It is also not known whether such events bring about specific chromosomal alterations or abnormalities, mutations, translocations, or permanent gene reiterations that would lead to hormonally induced neoplastic transformation.

Because of the high relative human risk, understanding the endocrine involvement in the etiology of breast and prostate cancer should be given a high priority. There is no agreement, for example, whether or not ERT should be given to women who have been previously treated for breast cancer or other endocrine-associated malignancies. A related issue of equal urgency is determining whether DES daughters and their progeny are at higher risk for endocrine-related neoplasms.

In an effort to respond to the growing interest in hormonal carcinogenesis, and to address these timely questions, the First International Symposium on Hormonal Carcinogenesis was convened in Cancun, Mexico. This symposium brought together scientists from a wide variety of disciplines. They included clinicians, epidemiologists, pathologists, endocrinologists, reproductive toxicologists, cell and molecular biologists, biochemists, pharmacologists, and chemists, who presented and discussed their individual approaches and identified fruitful lines of research to elucidate the involvement of hormones in neoplastic processes.

We would like to express our deep gratitude to members of the Scientific Advisory Board for their suggestions, advice, and support in the formation of the scientific program. The editors thank Drs. A.H Conney, G.W. Lucier, G.C. Mueller, and J.S. Norris for their assistance in critically reviewing the chapters in this volume. We are grateful to Ms. Jan Dennie and her staff at Travel Concern, Minneapolis, for their expert assistance in the arrangement of this symposium. We also thank Ms. Cheri Yost for her dedication and great care in the preparation of the manuscripts for publication. Finally, we wish to thank Ms. Esther Gumpert and the Springer-Verlag staff for their support and for the high quality of this first volume in the field.

Pullman	Jonathan J. Li
Berkeley	Satyabrata Nandi
Pullman	Sara Antonia Li

Contents

Participants

ALBERTO BALDI* Instituto de Biologia y Medicina Experimental, 1428 Buenos Aires, Argentina

J. CARL BARRETT Molecular Carcinogenesis, Laboratory, NIEHS, NIH, Research Triangle Park, NC 27709, USA

CRAIG W. BEATTIE Division of Surgical Oncology, University of Illinois, School of Medicine, Chicago, IL 60612, USA

FORD BELL Department of Small Animal Clinical Sciences, College of Veterinary Medicine, University of Minnesota, St. Paul, MN 55413, USA

HOWARD A. BERN Cancer Research Laboratory and Department of Integrative Biology, University of California-Berkeley, Berkeley, CA 94720, USA

AGNETA BLANCK Department of Medical Nutrition, Karolinska Institutet, Huddinge University Hospital, S141 86 Huddinge, Sweden

MAARTEN C. BOSLAND Institute of Environmental Medicine, New York University Medical Center, New York, NY, USA

H. LEON BRADLOW Institute for Hormone Research, New York, NY 10016, USA

ROBERT W. BRUEGGEMEIER College of Pharmacy, The Ohio State University, Columbus, OH 43210, USA

BERTIL G. CASSLÉN Department of Obstetrics and Gynecology, University of Lund, S-221 85 Lund, Sweden

EDUARDO H. CHARREAU Instituto de Biologia y Medicina Experimental, 1428 Buenos Aires, Argentina

PAT CODY DES Action, Oakland, CA 04612, USA

---

*Member, 1991 Hormonal Carcinogenesis Symposium Scientific Advisory Board.

ALLAN H. CONNEY Laboratory for Cancer Research, Department of Chemical Biology and Pharmacognosy, College of Pharmacy, Rutgers University, Piscataway, NJ 08855-0789, USA

GISELA H. DEGEN Institute of Toxicology, University of Wuerzburg, D-8700 Wuerzburg, Germany

BRUNO DE LIGNIERES Endocrinologie et Medecine de la Reproduction, Hospital Necker-Enfant Malades, Paris Cedex 15, France

RICHARD P. DIAUGUSTINE Hormones and Cancer Group, Laboratory of Biochemical Risk Assessment, NIEHS, NIH, Research Triangle Park, NC 27709, USA

JACK FISHMAN IVAX Corporation, Miami, FL 33178-2404, USA

F. PETER GUENGERICH Department of Biochemistry, Vanderbilt University, School of Medicine, Nashville, TN 37232, USA

JAN-ÅKE GUSTAFSSON* Department of Medical Nutrition, Karolinska Institutet, Huddinge University Hospital, S14186 Huddinge, Sweden

RAPHAEL C. GUZMAN Cancer Research Laboratory, University of California-Berkeley, Berkeley, CA 94720, USA

INGER P. HÄLLSTRÖM Department of Medical Nutrition, Karolinska Institutet, Huddinge University Hospital, S14186 Huddinge, Sweden

STEPHEN E. HARRIS Department of Medicine, Division of Endocrinology, University of Texas Health Sciences Center, San Antonio, TX 78284, USA

SHUK-MEI HO Department of Biology, Tufts University, Medford, MA 02155, USA

HOWARD L. HOSICK Department of Genetics and Cell Biology, Washington State University, Pullman, WA 99164-4236, USA

NANCY E. HYNES Friedrich Miescher Institute, CH-4002 Basel, Switzerland

KUMIKO IWAMOTO Department of Epidemiology, Division of Cancer Etiology, NCI, NIH, Bethedsa, MD 20892, USA

PETER H. JELLINCK Department of Biochemistry, Queen's University, Kingston, Ontario K7L 3N6, Canada

ELWOOD V. JENSEN   New York Hospital, Cornell Medical Center, Cornell University, New York, NY   10021, USA

MARTINA KLOESS   Department of Food Chemistry and Environmental Toxicology, University of Kaiserslautern, D-6570 Kaiserslautern, Germany

DAVID KUPFER   Worcester Foundation for Experimental Biology, Shrewsbury, MA   01545, USA

FREDERIQUE KUTTENN   Service d'Endocrinologie et de Medecine de la Reproduction, Faculte de Medecine Necker-Enfants Malades, Universite Rene Descartes, 75743 Paris Cedex 15, France

CORAL A. LAMARTINIERE   Department of Environmental Health Sciences, University of Alabama at Birmingham, Birmingham, AL   35294, USA

LEONARD J. LERNER*   Department of Pharmacology, Jefferson Medical College, Thomas Jefferson University, Philadelphia, PA   19107, USA

JONATHAN J. LI   Hormonal Carcinogenesis Laboratory, College of Pharmacy, Washington State University, Pullman, WA   99163-6410, USA

SARA ANTONIA LI   Hormonal Carcinogenesis Laboratory, College of Pharmacy, Washington State University, Pullman, WA   99163-6410, USA

SHUTSUNG LIAO   Biochemistry/Molecular Biology, Ben May Laboratory for Cancer Research, University of Chicago, Chicago, IL   60637, USA

GEORGE W. LUCIER*   Laboratory of Biochemical Risk Assessment, NIEHS, NIH, Research Triangle Park, NC   27709, USA

JOHN A. MCLACHLAN*   Laboratory of Reproductive and Developmental Toxicology, NIEHS, NIH, Research Triangle Park, NC   27709, USA

MANFRED METZLER*   Department of Food Chemistry and Environmental Toxicology, University of Kaiserslautern, D-6570 Kaiserslautern, Germany

GERALD C. MUELLER*   McArdle Laboratory for Cancer Research, University of Wisconsin Medical School, Madison, WI   53706, USA

SATYABRATA NANDI   Department of Molecular and Cell Biology and Cancer Research Laboratory, University of California-Berkeley, Berkeley, CA   94720, USA

JAMES S. NORRIS   Department of Med/Cell Biology, University of South Carolina, Medical School, Charleston, SC 29425, USA

GREGORIO PÉREZ-PALACIOS*   Department of Reproduction, Instituto Nacional de la Natruton, 14000 Mexico City DF, Mexico

ERICKA PFEIFFER   Department of Food Chemistry and Environmental Toxicology, University of Kaiserslautern, D-6750 Kaiserslautern, Germany

JAMES H. PICKAR   Clinical Research and Development, Wyeth-Ayerst Research, Philadelphia, PA 19101-1245, USA

MALCOLM C.PIKE   Department of Preventive Medicine, University of California, School of Medicine, Los Angeles, CA 90033, USA

JOHN POLLOCK   Wyeth-Ayerst Research, Chazy, NY 12921, USA

ROBERT SCHNITZLER   Department of Food Chemistry and Environmental Toxicology, University of Kaiserslautern, D-6750 Kaiserslautern, Germany

LEA I. SEKELY*   Chemical & Physical Carcinogenesis Branch, Division of Cancer Etiology, NCI, NIH, Bethesda, MD 20205, USA

TOMOYUKI SHIRAI   First Department of Pathology, Nagoya City University, Medical School, Mizuho-cho, Mizuho-ku, Nagoya 467, Japan

GEORGE M. STANCEL   Department of Pharmacology, University of Texas Medical School, Houston, TX 77025, USA

LISA A. SUCHAR   Laboratory for Cancer Research, Department of Chemical Biology and Pharmacognosy, College of Pharmacy, Rutgers University, Piscataway, NJ 08855-0789, USA

ANNI WARRI   Orion Corporation, Farmos, 20101 Turku, Finland

JAMES D. YAGER   Department of Environmental Health Sciences, Johns Hopkins University, School of Hygiene and Public Health, Baltimore, MD 21205-2179, USA.

Contributors

CONWELL H. ANDERSON Division of Surgical Oncology, University of Illinois, School of Medicine, Chicago, IL, USA

NESTOR V. ANNIBALI Instituto de Biologia y Medicina Experimental, Buenos Aires, Argentina

ALBERTO BALDI Instituto de Biologia y Medicina Experimental, Buenos Aires, Argentina

ROLAND BALL Friedrich Miescher Institute, Switzerland

SNIGDHA BANERJEE Hormonal Carcinogenesis Laboratory, College of Pharmacy, Washington State University, Pullman, WA, USA

SUSHANTA K. BANERGEE Hormonal Carcinogenesis Laboratory, College of Pharmacy, Washington State University, Pullman, WA, USA

JACQUE BARRAT Endocrinologie et Medecine de la Reproduction, Hospital Necker-Enfant Malades, Paris, France

J. CARL BARRETT Molecular Carcinogenesis Laboratory, NIEHS, NIH, Research Triangle Park, NC, USA

NICOLE BAUDOT Service d'Endocrinologie et de Medecine de la Reproduction, Faculte de Medecine Necker-Enfant Malades, Universite Rene Descartes, Paris, France

CRAIG W. BEATTIE Division of Surgical Oncology, University of Illinois, School of Medicine, Chicago, IL, USA

MUSTAPHA A. BELEH Graduate School Administration, Ohio State University, Columbus, OH, USA

HOWARD A. BERN   Cancer Research Laboratory and Department of Integrative Biology, University of California-Berkeley, Berkeley, CA, USA

AGNETA BLANCK   Department of Medical Nutrition, Karolinska Institutet, Huddinge University Hospital, Huddinge, Sweden

MAARTEN C. BOSLAND   Institute of Environmental Medicine, New York University Medical Center, New York, NY, USA

DENNIS M. BOYLE   Instituto de Biologia y Medicina Experimental, Buenos Aires, Argentina

H. LEON BRADLOW   Institute for Hormone Research, New York, NY, USA

ROBERT W. BRUEGGEMEIER   College of Pharmacy, Ohio State University, Columbus, OH, USA

BILL C. BULLOCK   Laboratory of Reproductive and Developmental Toxicology, NIEHS, NIH, Research Triangle Park, NC, USA

BERTIL G. CASSLÉN   Department of Obstetrics and Gynocology, University of Lund, Lund, Sweden

RICHARD L. CHANG   Laboratory for Cancer Research, Department of Chemical Biology and Pharmacognosy, College of Pharmacy, Rutgers University, Piscataway, NJ, USA

EDUARDO H. CHARREAU   Instituto de Biologia y Medicina Experimental, Buenos Aires, Argentina

CONNIE CHIAPPETTA   Department of Pharmacology, University of Texas Medical School, Houston, TX, USA

GEORGE C. CLARK   Laboratory of Biochemical Risk Assessment, NIEHS, NIH, Research Triangle Park, NC, USA

PAT CODY   DES Action, Oakland, CA, USA

ALLAN H. CONNEY   Laboratory for Cancer Research, Department of Chemical Biology and Pharmacognosy, College of Pharmacy, Rutgers University, Piscataway, NJ, USA

GENEVIEVE CONTESSO   Endocrinologie et Medecine de la Reproduction, Hospital Necker-Enfant Malades, Paris, France

ΓINA COOPER   Department of Medicine and Cell Biology, University of South Carolina Medical School, Charleston, SC, USA

GISELA H. DEGEN   Institute of Toxicology, University of Wuerzburg, Wuerzburg, Germany

BRUNO DE LIGNIERES   Endocrinologie et Medecine de la Reproduction, Hospital Necker-Enfant Malades, Paris, France

RICHARD P. DIAUGUSTINE   Hormones and Cancer Group, Laboratory of Biochemical Risk Assessment, NIEHS, NIH, Research Triangle Park, NC, USA

DENISE L. DONLEY   College of Pharmacy, Ohio State University, Columbus, OH, USA

PATRICIA ELIZALDE   Instituto de Biologia y Medicina Experimental, Buenos Aires, Argentina

WEIMIN FAN   Department of Medicine and Cell Biology, University of South Carolina Medical School, Charleston, SC, USA

JACK FISHMAN   IVAX Corporation, Miami, FL, USA

JURGEN FOTH   Institute of Toxicology, University of Wuerzburg, Wuerzburg, Germany

SABINE FOURNIER   Endocrinologie et Medecine de la Reproduction, Hospital Necker-Enfant Malades, Paris, France

FRANK S. FRENCH   Department of Pediatrics, Laboratories for Reproductive Biology, University of North Carolina Medical School, Chapel Hill, NC, USA

ANNE GOMPEL   Service D-Endocrinologie et de Medecine de la Reproduction, Faculte de Medecine Necker-Enfant Malades, Universite Rene Descartes, Paris, France

BERND GRONER   Friedrich Miescher Institute, Basel, Switzerland

F. PETER GUENGERICH   Department of Biochemistry, Vanderbilt University, School of Medicine, Nashville, TN, USA

FABIANA GUERRA   Instituto de Biologia y Medicina Experimental, Buenos Aires, Argentina

JAN-ÅKE GUSTAFSSON   Department of Medical Nutrition, Karolinska Institutet, Huddinge University Hospital, Huddinge, Sweden

RAPHAEL C. GUZMAN   Cancer Research Laboratory, University of California, Berkeley, CA, USA

JEFFREY A. HALL   W. Alton Jones Cell Science Center, Lake Placid, NY, USA

INGER P. HÄLLSTRÖM   Department of Medical Nurtition, Karolinska Institutet, Huddinge University Hospital, Huddinge, Sweden

BRIGITTE HAPP   Friedrich Miescher Institute, Basel, Switzerland

MURRAY A. HARRIS   Department of Medicine, Division of Endocrinology, University of Texas Health Sciences Center, San Antonio, TX, USA

STEPHEN E. HARRIS   Department of Medicine, Division of Endocrinology, University of Texas Health Sciences Center, San Antonio, TX, USA

SHUK-MEI HO   Department of Biology, Tufts University, Medford, MA, USA

MICHAEL B. HOLLAND   Department of Environmental Health Sciences, University of Alabama at Birmingham, Birmingham, AL, USA

HOWARD L. HOSICK   Department of Genetics and Cell Biology, Washington State University, Pullman, WA, USA

SOO-IN HWANG   Cancer Research Laboratory, University of California, Berkeley, CA, USA

SALMAN M. HYDER   Department of Biochemistry, Hormone Research Laboratory, University of Louisville, James Graham Brown Cancer Center, Louisville, KY, USA

NANCY E. HYNES   Friedrich Miescher Institute, Basel, Switzerland

NOBUYUKI ITO   First Department of Pathology, Nagoya City University Medical School, Mizuho-cho, Mizuho-ku, Nagoya, Japan

SHOGO IWASAKI   First Department of Pathology, Nagoya City University Medical School, Mizuho-cho, Mizuho-ku, Nagoya, Japan

GLORIA D. JAHNKE   Hormones and Cancer Group, Laboratory of Biochemical Risk Assessment, NIEHS, NIH, Research Triangle Park, NC, USA

PETER H. JELLINCK   Department of Biochemistry, Queen's University, Kingston, Ontario, Canada

ELWOOD V. JENSEN   New York Hospital, Cornell Medical Center, Cornell University, New York, NY, USA

TAKUYA KANAZAWA   Department of Genetics and Cell Biology, Washington State University, Pullman, WA, USA

JOHN L. KIRKLAND   Department of Pediatrics, Baylor College of Medicine, Houston, TX, USA

HADLEY KIRKMAN   Department of Anatomy, Stanford University, Stanford, CA, USA

WERNER KÖHL   Department of Food Chemistry and Environmental Toxicology, University of Kaiserslautern, Kaiserslautern, Germany

KENNETH S. KORACH   Laboratory of Reproductive and Developmental Toxicology, NIEHS, NIH, Research Triangle Park, NC, USA

EDITH KORDON   Instituto de Biologia y Medicina Experimental, Buenos Aires, Argentina

DAVID KUPFER   Worcester Foundation for Experimental Biology, Shrewsbury, MA, USA

FREDERIQUE KUTTENN   Service d'Endocrinologie et de Medecine de la Reproduction, Faculte de Medecine Necker-Enfant Malades, Universite Rene Descartes, Paris, France

CORAL A. LAMARTINIERE   Department of Environmental Health Sciences, University of Alabama at Birmingham, Birmingham, AL, USA

CLAUDIA LANARI   Instituto de Biologia y Medicina Experimental, Buenos Aires, Argentina

IRWIN LEAV   Department of Biology, Tufts University, Medford, MA, USA

CATHERINE LEGRAVEREND   Department of Medical Nutrition, Karolinska Institutet, Huddinge University Hospital, Huddinge, Sweden

LEONARD J. LERNER   Department of Pharmacology, Jefferson Medical College, Thomas Jefferson University, Philadelphia, PA, USA

ETIENNE LEYGUE Service d'Endocrinologie et de Medecine de la Reproduction, Faculte de Medecine Necker-Enfant Malades, Universite Rene Descartes, Paris, France

JONATHAN J. LI Hormonal Carcinogenesis Laboratory, College of Pharmacy, Washington State University, Pullman, WA, USA

SARA ANTONIA LI Hormonal Carcinogenesis Laboratory, College of Pharmacy, Washington State University, Pullman, WA, USA

SHUTSUNG LIAO Department of Biochemistry and Molecular Biology, Ben May Laboratory for Cancer Research, University of Chicago, Chicago, IL, USA

CHRISTOPHER LIDDLE Department of Medical Nutrition, Karolinska Institutet, Huddinge University Hospital, Huddinge, Sweden

FU-HSIUNG LIN Laboratory of Biochemical Risk Assessment, NIEHS, NIH, Research Triangle Park, NC, USA

TSU-HUI LIN Department of Pediatric Endocrinology, Baylor College of Medicine, Houston, TX, USA

YOUNG C. LIN Department of Veterinary Physiology and Pharmacology, Ohio State University, College of Veterinary Medicine, Columbus, OH, USA

GUSTAVO LINARES Endocrinologie et Medecine de la Reproduction, Hospital Necker-Enfant Malades, Paris, France

DAVID S. LOOSE-MITCHELL Department of Pharmacology, University of Texas Medical School, Houston, TX, USA

DENNIS B. LUBAHN Department of Pediatrics, University of North Carolina, Chapel Hill, NC, USA

GEORGE W. LUCIER Laboratory of Biochemical Risk Assessment, NIEHS, NIH, Research Triangle Park, NC, USA

CATHERINE MALET Service d'Endocrinologie et de Medecine de la Reproduction, Faculte de Medecine Necker-Enfant Malades, Universite Rene Descartes, Paris, France

CHITRA MANI Worcester Foundation for Experimental Biology, Shrewsbury, MA, USA

PIERRE MAUVAIS-JARVIS Service d'Endocrinologie et de Medecine de la Reproduction, Faculte de Medecine Necker-Enfant Malades, Universite Rene Descartes, Paris, France

JOHN A. MCLACHLAN Laboratory of Reproductive and Developmental Toxicology, NIEHS, NIH, Research Triangle Park, NC, USA

MANFRED METZLER Department of Food Chemistry and Environmental Toxicology, University of Kaiserslautern, Kaiserslautern, Germany

JON J. MICHNOVICZ Institute for Hormone Research, New York, NY, USA

SHIGEKI MIYAMOTO Department of Molecular and Cell Biology and Cancer Research Laboratory, University of California, Berkeley, CA, USA

AGNETA MODE Department of Medical Nutrition, Karolinska Institutet, Huddinge University Hospital, Huddinge, Sweden

GERALD C. MUELLER McArdle Laboratory for Cancer Research, University of Wisconsin Medical School, Madison, WI, USA

LATA MURTHY Department of Pharmacology, University of Texas Medical School, Houston, TX, USA

KAHIL NAHOUL Endocrinologie et Medecine de la Reproduction, Hospital Necker-Enfant Malades, Paris, France

SATYABRATA NANDI Department of Molecular and Cell Biology and Cancer Research Laboratory, University of California, Berkeley, CA, USA

KAREN G. NELSON Laboratory of Reproductive and Developmental Toxicology, NIEHS, NIH, Research Triangle Park, NC, USA

RETHA R. NEWBOLD Laboratory of Reproductive and Developmental Toxicology, NIEHS, NIH, Research Triangle Park, NC, USA

M. CAITRIONA NICMHUIRIS Friedrich Miescher Institute, Basel, Switzerland

JAMES S. NORRIS Department of Medicine and Cell Biology, University of South Carolina Medical School, Charleston, SC, USA

SHUZO OKUMURA Laboratory for Cancer Research, Department of Chemical Biology and Pharmacognosy, College of Pharmacy, Rutgers University, Piscataway, NJ, USA

SYLVIA A. OLIVER   Department of Genetics and Cell Biology, Washington State University, Pullman, WA, USA

CLAUDIA A. ORENGO   Department of Pharmacology, University of Texas Medical School, Houston, TX, USA

MICHAEL OSBORNE   Institute for Hormone Research, New York, NY, USA

REBECCA C. OSBORN   Department of Molecular and Cell Biology and Cancer Research Laboratory, University of California, Berkeley, Berkeley, CA, USA

CHRISTIANE DOSNE PASQUALINI   Instituto de Biologia y Medicina Experimental, Buenos Aires, Argentina

GREGORIO PÉREZ-PALACIOS   Department of Reproduction, Instituto Nacional de la Natruton, Mexico City, Mexico

ERIKA PFEIFFER   Department of Food Chemistry and Environmental Toxicology, University of Kaiserslautern, Kaiserlautern, Germany

MALCOLM C. PIKE   Department of Preventive Medicine, University of California School of Medicine, Los Angeles, CA, USA

GENEVIERE PLU   Service d'Endocrinologie et de Medecine de la Reproduction, Faculte de Medecine Necker-Enfant Malades, Universite Rene Descartes, Paris,

INGER PORSCH-HÄLLSTRÖM   Department of Medical Nutrition, Karolinska Institutet, Huddinge University Hospital, Huddinge, Sweden
France

TRACY G. RAM   Department of Genetics and Cell Biology, Washington State University, Pullman, WA, USA

ZENG X. RONG   W. Alton Jones Cell Science Center, Lake Placid, NY, USA

RAMASAMY SAKTHIVEL   Department of Molecular and Cell Biology and Cancer Research Laboratory, University of California, Berkeley, CA, USA

MICHAEL SCHMITT-NEY   Friedrich Miescher Institute, Basel, Switzerland

ROBERT SCHNITZLER   Department of Food Chemistry and Environmental Toxicology, University of Kaiserslautern, Kaiserslautern, Germany

DAVID A SCHWARTZ   Department of Medicine and Cell Biology, University of South Carolina Medical School, Charleston, SC, USA

TOMOYUKI SHIRAI First Department of Pathology, Nagoya City University Medical School, Mizuho-cho, Mizuho-ku, Nagoya, Japan

ROY G. SMITH Department of Urology, Baylor College of Medicine, Houston, TX, USA

SUZANNE M. SNEDEKER Hormones and Cancer Group, Laboratory of Biochemical Risk Assessment, NIEHS, NIH, Research Triangle Park, NC, USA

DARCY V. SPICER Department of Preventive Medicine, University of California School of Medicine, Los Angeles, CA, USA

GEORGE M. STANCEL Department of Pharmacology, University of Texas Medical School, Houston, TX, USA

URS STIEFEL Friedrich Miescher Institute, Basel, Switzerland

LISA A. SUCHAR Laboratory for Cancer Research, Department of Chemical Biology and Pharmacognosy, College of Pharmacy, Rutgers University, Piscataway, NJ, USA

GEORGE SWANECK IVAX Corporation, Miami, FL, USA

SEIKO TAMANO First Department of Pathology, Nagoya City University Medical School, Mizuho-cho, Mizuho-ku, Nagoya, Japan

DANIELA TAVERNA Friedrich Miescher Institute, Basel, Switzerland

NITIN T. TELANG Institute for Hormone Research, New York, NY, USA

JEAN-CHRISTOPHE THALABARD Service d'Endocrinologie et de Medecine de la Reproduction, Faculte de Medecine Necker-Enfant Malades, Universite Rene Descartes, Paris, France

ULKA TIPNIS Department of Pathology, University of Texas Medical Branch, Galveston, TX, USA

ANGELIKA M. TRITSCHER Laboratory of Biochemical Risk Assessment, NIEHS, NIH, Research Triangle Park, NC, USA

VASUNDARA VENKATESWARAN Department of Genetics and Cell Biology, Washington State University, Pullman, WA, USA

TODD VICCIONE Department of Biology, Tufts University, Medford, MA, USA

MICHAEL WALKER Hormones and Cancer Group, Laboratory of Biochemical Risk Assessment, NIEHS, NIH, Research Triangle Park, NC, USA

ELIZABETH M. WILSON Department of Pediatrics and Biochemistry, University of North Carolina, Chapel Hill, NC, USA

JAMES L. WITTLIFF Hormone Receptor Laboratory, James Graham Brown Cancer Center, University of Louisville, Louisville, KY, USA

JAMES D. YAGER Department of Environmental Health Sciences, Johns Hopkins University, School of Hygiene and Public Health, Baltimore, MD, USA

MARGARET YU Department of Biology, Tufts University, Medford, MA, USA

Opening Remarks

Gregorio Pérez-Palacios

Ladies and Gentlemen:

On behalf of the Executive Council of the Mexican Endocrine Society, it gives me pleasure to welcome all of you to Cancun, in the Mexican Caribbean, on this most important occassion. We are glad that the Yucatán peninsula was selected as the scenario to house this first symposium on hormonal carcinogenesis, that represents indeed the starting point of a large road in the search for a better understanding on the manner by which natural and synthetic hormones contribute to the etiology of benign or malignant neoplasia.

It must be stressed that elucidation of the underlying molecular events involved in hormone-induced neoplastic transformation requires a multi-disciplinary, world-wide effort of scientists and a wide variety of research strategies and experimental approaches. It is needless to say that recent advances on the molecular biology of hormone receptors, growth factors, and oncogenes have contributed in a most impressive way to strengthening our current knowledge of hormonal carcinogenesis. The Program Organizers and particularly the Executive Board of this symposium had the capability to blend all these ingredients together including a series of relevant issues in the field, highlights on human and animal research, and a group of distinguished speakers from all over the world. As a result, we have now in front of us a superb scientific program that in the course of the next three days will provide us with a most comprehensive overview of hormonal carcinogenesis. Drs. Jonathan Li, Satyabrata Nandi, and Sara Antonia Li deserve to be congratulated for their effort and success in doing this job.

Even though there is a long tradition in endocrinological research in Mexico, particularly in the area of synthetic steroid hormones, most of the emphasis has been given to the field of reproductive biology, mainly because of the problems on population growth our country has experienced and faced over the last years.

However, the Mexican endocrine and scientific communities have realized that hormonal carcinogenesis is a novel, top-priority area of research of the contemporary biomedical sciences. Therefore we are looking at this first symposium for seeding scientific and intellectual stimulus, and we do hope to have Mexican contributions in the subsequent symposia on hormonal carcinogenesis.

Our Society is proud in cosponsoring this event, and to me, it is a privilege to wish you all a most successful and productive meeting and scientific exchange as well as a pleasant stay at Cancun, the land of ancient Mayans. For those of you who are in Mexico for the first time, let me wish you have a pleasant experience visiting this part of Mexico's ancient past, which always seems to be beneath the surface. Enjoy the pyramids and temples of the nearby Mayan cities, the cuisine and the arts, and also the wonderful varieties of blues and greens of the Caribbean Sea.

Finally, I would like to underline a most interesting coincidence. This symposia will occur simultaneously with an ancient Mayan festivity. Every year on March 21 at the spring equinox, the god Kukulkan is supposed to return to his people bringing prosperity. This happens at a pyramid in Chichen-Itzá. As the sun sets a series of triangles of light and shadow are formed gradually on the pyramid stairway running down and ending at the head of a stone snake. The image created is that of a great snake coming down the pyramid, representing Kukulkan, the feathered serpent god.

I anticipate that both the Mayan spring equinox and the symposium on hormonal carcinogenesis will be of great benefit to all of us.

SYMPOSIUM PRESENTATION

Diethylstilbestrol (DES) Syndrome: Present Status of Animal and Human Studies

Howard A. Bern

Introduction

Two decades ago, Arthur Herbst and colleagues recognized the clinical syndrome of cervicovaginal clear-cell carcinoma arising in daughters exposed *in utero* to diethylstilbestrol (DES) ingested by their mothers during the first trimester of pregnancy. Although this relationship is generally accepted for patients in the U.S. as well as in several other countries (1), the epidemiological basis is still occasionally questioned and defended (2,3). Other factors associated with "problem pregnancy" may alter the consequences of DES exposure (4,5). Ovarian cancer has recently been linked to DES exposure (6).

Three decades ago, two laboratories independently recognized that early (perinatal) exposure of female mice to sex hormones, including DES, led to pathological changes, including neoplasia, in the cervicovaginal region (7). Thus, there was a preexisting model for the human DES syndrome when the latter was delineated (7). The clinical reports on the long-term effects of intrauterine exposure to DES have become considerably fewer in recent years. On the other hand, the experimentalists using the prenatal/neonatal mouse model continue to contribute at a fairly active level new information that may prove of value when extrapolated to the clinical problem. The experimental studies include reports of changes in a variety of genital (and nongenital) structures.

At the present time, it may be particularly useful to assess the status of the human situation in both females and males and to reconsider the relevance of animal data to "DES daughters and sons." Women exposed *in utero* in the early years of DES usage to avoid premature births are now approaching the postmenopausal period, and vaginal clear-cell carcinoma was once considered to be essentially confined to postmenopausal women. Similarly, men are approaching the period when prostatic disorders can be expected, and animal data indicate male genital pathologies potentially relevant to the human condition (8).

1

Extensive surveys of the long-term effects of exposure to sex hormones in humans and rodents have been published in the past decade (7,9), and most recently, in a valuable, multiauthored CRC Review edited by Mori and Nagasawa (8). Therefore, this brief essay will not reiterate the data available in these collations, but will focus on aspects that may not have been adequately recognized to date.

Mode of Action of DES

The role of early exposure to DES (and presumably any estrogen) in the development of cervicovaginal cancer in humans and rodents suggests a direct carcinogenic action of these sex hormones. However, the incidence of this cancer is low in both humans and rodents, suggesting that other agent(s) may intervene in the neoplastic transformation. What these agents may be is unknown, although certainly the postnatal hormonal milieu seems to be supportive of the ultimate emergence of neoplasia. It is possible that DES acts as a transforming agent early in development (10). On the other hand, the initial pathological changes in both human and rodent cervicovaginal tracts may be essentially teratogenic, resulting in the maintenance of cell populations that may otherwise disappear and thus providing a "bed" from which neoplastic cell populations may eventually emerge.

For many years, the bulk of the data obtained with the mouse model has been histopathological in nature, reporting major changes in all segments of the female and male genital tracts. The pathological consequences of perinatal estrogen exposure may arise indirectly, from permanent alteration of the hypothalamo-hypophysio-gonadal axis and persistent estrogen secretion, or directly, from permanent histogenetic alterations of the genital tract itself (epithelial, stromal, or both), or from a combination of both direct and indirect effects (7).

Utility of the Mouse Model for the DES Syndrome

The mouse model has served excellently as a predictor of some of the changes that have been encountered in humans, both female and male. It is questionable whether the clinician has made adequate use of the model, however, as a basis for searching for human changes parallel to those seen in mice after early DES exposure. Although there has been past emphasis on a variety of parallels in genital tract changes between rodent and human species (7,8), indications of other involvements, such as changes in the immune system (7,8), were rather belatedly recognized.

Limits to the applicability of the model must also be recognized. To date, for example, there is essentially no linkage between human DES exposure and breast dysplasia and neoplasia. On the other hand, mice expressing the mammary tumor virus (MTV) early manifested a major increase in incidence and an accelerated time of onset of mammary tumors, accompanied by a variety of dysplastic and preneoplastic alterations, as a consequence of early exposure to sex hormones. The roles of MTV and of prolactin in the observed murine changes delineate a biology that differs in part from the biology of human breast cancer. Similarly, the frequency of occurrence of polyovular follicles in the ovaries of neonatally DES-exposed mice (11) suggests that a similar phenomenon might occur in DES daughters. Although there is no direct evidence that this is the case, polyovular follicles do occur in the female human, and an activated gonadotropin-estrogen axis, such as occurs in neonatally DES-exposed mice, could increase their incidence (12).

Among the more recent work in which our laboratory has participated is the examination of various target organs in both female and male mice for the occurrence of subtle or occult changes that may have occurred. As a consequence of such alterations—as opposed to the obvious gross and histopathological features of prenatally and neonatally DES-exposed animals—the biology of target tissues may be irreversibly changed. Thus, their sensitivity to hormones, to growth factors, to carcinogens and cancer-enhancing agents (13-15), etc., may be increased or decreased, leading to a greater or lesser cancer risk.

Examples of the alterations resulting from neonatal DES exposure that we have observed in mice include changes in steroid receptor levels in the vagina, uterus, mammary gland (16), and male sex accessories (17), in epidermal growth factor (EGF) receptor levels in the vagina (18), and in prolactin receptor levels in the male genital tract (19). In the vagina, Eiger (20) examined the specific binding of estrogen and progestin by epithelial and fibromuscular components separately, noting independent variations in the two tissues. Although steroid receptor levels are generally decreased by DES exposure (21), this is not always the case.

Thus, whereas both estrogen and androgen receptors decreased in most male sex accessories after neonatal DES exposure, estrogen receptor levels were higher in the seminal vesicle (17). In the vagina, DES exposure resulted in increased progestin binding (16,20), although estrogen receptors decreased after exposure to higher doses of DES. Male sex accessories showed decreased prolactin binding after DES exposure (19); the vagina showed decreased EGF receptor levels after DES exposure, but other female structures were not affected (18). The relation between receptor levels and sensitivity of the target is uncertain, and DES may result in increased sensitivity (as in the mammary gland hyperplastic response to adult estrogen treatment—Bern, Mills, Hatch, Ostrander, and Iguchi, unpublished) or decreased sensitivity (as in the mammary response to prolactin as judged by casein production) (22).

Vaginal (23,24), mammary (25), and prostatic (26) epithelial cells isolated from neonatally DES-exposed mice show different behaviors when cultured in a serum-free defined medium in collagen gel. An initial time lag in proliferation of genital cells from DES-exposed mice is encountered, and cell colonies from these mice include rounded types along with the usual stellate types.

Protein patterns in the female genital tract of mice exposed to DES may vary from the control when examined by two-dimensional gel electrophoresis (27), and changes in protein and in RNA profiles occur in the genital tract of neonatally estradiol-exposed male mice (28). The DES-exposed vaginal epithelium and fibromuscular wall both differ from their unexposed counterparts in protein patterns (29).

In view of the occurrence of long-term subtle changes in various rodent organs exposed early to DES, it is regrettable that similar studies, especially of receptors, were not conducted on biopsy and autopsy specimens from human DES offspring when such were available. A similar comment can be made about circulating hormone levels and about immunological characteristics after intrauterine DES exposure (30), where only limited information is available. The rodent model early indicated significant immunological changes (7,8), but it was belatedly recognized that changes in the immune system also occurred in DES offspring (31,32). Neurological and phychological changes also may occur in DES-exposed humans (33), as is certainly indicated in rodents and in the rhesus monkey (8).

Early Exposure to Agents Other than DES

The basic phenomenology associated with early DES exposure is applicable to other agents that may be present in high levels during critical periods of intrauterine development in humans. Plant estrogens, such as coumestrol or zearalenone, could be ingested in sufficient quantities at critical times to play a DES-like role, and "environmental estrogens" of other kinds are also present. Neonatal exposure of mice to coumestrol or zearalenone results in changes paralleling those seen after exposure to DES and steroidal estrogens (34-36). Increased levels of endogenous estrogens during embryonic and fetal development as a consequence of maternal dysfunction might not ordinarily be detected as a pathological condition and yet be adequate to affect genital tract differentiation. Trichopoulos (37) has recently raised this possibility in regard to breast cancer. In the rat, intrauterine hormone titers may affect sexual development (38).

Progestins, the "logical" agents for maintaining pregnancy when its premature termination is threatened, need to be carefully considered. The mouse model indicates long-term histopathological consequences from the neonatal administration of progesterone (39,40), although other studies with progestin (41,42) indicate no teratogenic potential (based largely on examination of fetuses, however). To date, data from clinical studies have not indicated comparable effects. Major effects on sexual differentiation of prenatal exposure to androgens (or proandrogens) have long been recognized. Reproduction-related drugs continued into early pregnancy: clomiphene, tamoxifen (43), "the pill," could also result in undesirable consequences during early intrauterine development. Other drugs, such as barbiturates (44) and glucocorticoids, could also have developmental effects on steroidogenic organs, steroid-catabolizing organs (especially the liver), as well as the usual targets of sex hormones and other organs. "The central point is that the developing organism is subject to a variety of stimuli, some of which are still undefined, the influence of which during a critical period in development may result not only in teratological alterations that are readily discernible, but also in subtle changes expressed much later in life. One expression of these delayed effects could be an alteration in tumor risk in tissues affected directly or indirectly by the initial stimulus." (8)

Conclusions

Concern with the possible consequences of intrauterine exposure of humans to DES must be sustained. The populations at risk are approaching menopause and the male climacteric, marking the onset of the time when reproductive disorders may arise. The nongenital effects of early DES exposure, especially on the immune system, require attention, and possible dangers of exposure to other hormones and to drugs during development are indicated. The prenatal and neonatal mouse models, when judiciously employed, continue to provide indicators of possible significance to DES-exposed human offspring.

Acknowledgments

I am indebted to generations of students and associates, beginning with Noboru Takasugi in 1960 and including most recently my colleagues, Taisen Iguchi, Takao Mori, Karen T. Mills, Francis-Dean Uchima, Marc Edery, the late Diane Russell, Brett Levay-Young, Steven Eiger, and Judy Turiel, and students, Timothy Turner, Cynthia Burroughs, Pei-San Tsai, Tomàs Magaña, Brian Williams, and Satoshi Ozawa. They and many others have contributed importantly to "the mouse model for the DES syndrome." Our research program was long supported by NIH through grants CA-05388 and CA-09041.

References

1. Herbst AL (1988) The effects in the human of diethylstilbestrol (DES) use during pregnancy. In: Miller, RW, et al., (eds). Unusual occurrences as clues to cancer etiology, Japan Sci Soc Press, Tokyo pp 67-75.
2. Forsberg J-G (1987) Diethylstilbestrol, clear cell adenocarcinoma, and striking discoveries in Norway. Am J Med 84:184.
3. Edelman DA (1989) Diethylstilbestrol exposure and the risk of clear cell cervical and vaginal adenocarcinoma. Int J Fertil 34:251-255.
4. Horwitz RI, Viscoli CM, Merino M, Brennan TA, Flannery JT, Robboy SJ (1988) Clear cell adenocarcinoma of the vagina and cervix: incidence, undetected disease, and diethylstilbestrol. J Clin Epidemiol 41:593-597.
5. Sharp GB, Cole P (1990) Vaginal bleeding and diethylstilbestrol exposure during pregnancy: relationship to genital tract clear cell adenocarcinoma and vaginal adenosis in daughters. Am J Obstet Gynecol 162:994-1001.

6. Walker AH, Ross RK, Haile RWC, Henderson BE (1988) Hormonal factors and risk of ovarian germ cell cancer in young women. Br J Cancer 57:418-422.

7. Herbst AL, Bern HA, eds. (1981) Developmental effects of diethylstilbestrol (DES) in pregnancy. New York: Thieme-Stratton.

8. Mori T, Nagasawa H (1988) Toxicity of hormones in perinatal life. Boca Raton, FL: CRC Press.

9. Edelman DA (1986) DES/Diethylstilbestrol—new perspectives. Boston: MTP Press.

10. Newbold RR, Bullock BC, McLachlan JA (1990) Uterine adenocarcinoma in mice following developmental treatment with estrogens: a model for hormonal carcinogenesis. Cancer Res 50:7677-7681.

11. Iguchi T, Fukazawa Y, Uesugi Y, Takasugi N (1990) Polyovular follicles in mouse ovaries exposed neonatally to diethylstilbestrol *in vivo* and *in vitro*. Biol Reprod 45:478-485.

12. Dandekar PV, Martin MC, Glass RH (1988) Polyovular follicles associated with human *in vitro* fertilization. Fertil Steril 49:483-486.

13. Taguchi O, Michael SD, Nishizuka Y (1988) Rapid induction of ovarian granulosa cell tumors by 7,12-dimethylbenz(a)anthracene in neonatally estrogenized mice. Cancer Res 48:425-429.

14. Walker BE (1988) Vaginal tumors in mice from methylcholanthrene and prenatal exposure to diethylstilbestrol. Cancer Lett 39:227-231.

15. Walker BE (1990) Tumors in female offspring of control and diethylstilbestrol-exposed mice fed high-fat diets. J Nat Cancer Inst 82:50-54.

16. Bern HA, Edery M, Mills KT, Kohrman AF, Mori T, Larson L (1987) Long-term alterations in histology and steroid receptor levels of the genital tract and mammary gland following neonatal exposure of female BALB/cCrgl mice to various doses of diethylstilbestrol. Cancer Res 47:4165-4172.

17. Turner T, Edery M, Mills KT, Bern HA (1989) Influence of neonatal diethylstilbestrol treatment on androgen and estrogen receptor levels in the mouse anterior prostate, ventral prostate and seminal vesicle. J Steroid Biochem 32:559-564.

18. Iguchi T, Edery M, Tsai P-S, Ozawa S, Bern HA Epidermal growth factor receptor levels in reproductive organs of female mice exposed neonatally to diethylstilbestrol (unpublished data).

19. Edery M, Turner T, Dauder S, Young G, Bern HA (1990) Influence of neonatal diethylstilbestrol treatment on prolactin receptor levels in the mouse male reproductive system. Proc Soc Exper Biol Med 194:289-292.

20. Eiger S, Mills KT, Bern HA (1990) Steroid binding alterations in tissue compartments of the vagina of control and neonatally diethylstilbestrol-treated adult mice. J Steroid Biochem 35:617-621.

21. Csaba G, Inczefi-Gonda A, Dobozy O (1986) Hormonal imprinting by steroids: a single neonatal treatment with diethylstilbestrol or allylestrenol gives rise to a lasting decrease in the number of rat uterine receptors. Acta Physiol Hung 64:207-212.

22. Levay-Young BK, Bern HA (1989) Prolactin sensitivity of mammary epithelial cells from mice exposed neonatally to diethylstilbestrol. Proc Soc Exper Biol Med 192:187-191.

23. Uchima F-D A, Iguchi T, Pattamakom S, Mills KT, Bern HA (1991) Effects of neonatal diethylstilbestrol exposure on the growth of mouse vaginal epithelial cells in serum-free collagen gel culture. Zool Sci 8:713-719.

24. Ozawa S, Iguchi T, Takemura KK, Bern HA (1991) Effect of certain growth factors on proliferation in serum-free collagen gel culture of vaginal epithelial cells from prepuberal mice exposed neonatally to diethylstilbestrol. Proc Soc Exper Biol Med 198:760-763.

25. Tomooka Y, Bern HA, Nandi S (1983) Growth of mammary epithelial cells from neonatally sex hormone-exposed mouse in serum-free collagen gel culture. Cancer Lett 20:255-261.

26. Turner T, Bern HA (1990) Growth responses of prostatic epithelial cells from male mice neonatally exposed to diethylstilbestrol (DES) in serum-free collagen gel culture. Cancer Lett 52:209-218.

27. Newbold RR, Carter DB, Harris SE, McLachlan JA (1984) Molecular differentiation of the mouse genital tract: altered protein synthesis following prenatal exposure to diethylstilbestrol. Biol Reprod 30:459-470.

28. Normand T, Jean-Faucher C, Jean C (1990) Neonatal exposure to oestrogens alters the protein profiles and gene expression in the genital tract of adult male mice. J Steroid Biochem 36:415-423.

29. Uchima F-D A, Vallerga AK, Firestone GL, Bern HA (1990) Effects of early exposure to diethylstilbestrol on cellular protein expression by mouse vaginal epithelium and fibromuscular wall. Proc Soc Exper Biol Med 195-:218-224.

30. Wingard DL, Turiel J (1988) Long-term effects of exposure to diethylstilbestrol. West J Med 149:551-554.

31. Ways SC, Mortola JF, Zwaifler NJ, et al. (1987) Alterations in immune responsiveness of women exposed to diethylstilbestrol *in utero*. Fertil Steril 48:193-197.

32. Noller KL, Blair PB, O'Brien P, et al. (1988) Increased occurrence of autoimmune disease among women exposed *in utero* to diethylstilbestrol. Fertil Steril 49:1080-1082.

33. Ehrhardt AA, Meyer-Bahlburg HFL, Rosen LR, et al. (1989) The development of gender-related behavior in females following prenatal exposure to diethylstilbestrol (DES). Hormones Behavior 23:526-541.

34. Burroughs CD, Mills KT, Bern HA (1990) Long-term genital tract changes in female mice treated neonatally with coumestrol. Reprod Toxicol 4:127-135.

35. Burroughs CD, Mills KT, Bern HA (1990) Reproductive abnormalities in female mice exposed neonatally to various doses of coumestrol. J Toxicol Environ Health 30:105-122.

36. Williams BA, Mills KT, Burroughs CD, Bern HA (1989) Reproductive alterations in female C57BL/Crgl mice exposed neonatally to zearalenone, an estrogenic mycotoxin. Cancer Lett 46:225-230.

37. Trichopoulos D (1990) Hypothesis: does breast cancer originate *in utero*? Lancet 335:939-940.

38. Houtsmuller EJ, Slob AK (1990) Masculinization and defeminization of female rats by male located caudally in the uterus. Physiol Behav 48:555-561.

39. Jones LA, Bern HA (1977) Long-term effects of neonatal treatment with progesterone, alone and in combination with estrogen, on the mammary gland and reproductive tract of female BALB/cfC3H mice. Cancer Res 37:67-75.

40. Jones LA, Bern HA (1979) Cervicovaginal and mammary gland abnormalities in BALB/cCrgl mice treated neonatally with progesterone and estrogen, alone or in combination. Cancer Res 39:2560-2567.

41. Seegmiller RE, Nelson GW, Johnson CK (1983) Evaluation of the teratogenic potential of delalutin (17α-hydroxyprogesterone caproate) in mice. Teratology 28:201-208.

42. Varma SK, Bloch E (1987) Effects of prenatal administration of mestranol and two progestins on testosterone synthesis and reproductive tract development in male rats. Acta Endocrinol 116:193-199.

43. Irisawa S, Iguchi T, Takasugi N (1990) Critical period of induction by tamoxifen of genital organ abnormalities in male mice. Zool Sci 7:541-545.

44. Goldhaber MK, Selby JV, Hiatt RA, Quesenberry CP (1990) Exposure to barbiturates *in utero* and during childhood and risk of intracrania and spinal cord tumors. Cancer Res 50:4600-4603.

PART 1. SEX HORMONES AND CARCINOGENESIS

INTRODUCTION

Androgen Receptors and Regulation of Androgen Action in Normal and Abnormal Cells

Shutsung Liao

Joseph Needham, a distinguished British biochemist, has remarked that the greatest achievement in the prenatal history of biochemistry was the use of crystals, obtained by sublimation of extracts of sexual (and accessory) organs, in the treatment of patients in China during the 11th to 17th centuries. Most of these crystals were apparently sex hormones whose chemical structures were determined during the 1920s to 1930s. By the end of the 1930s, pure androgenic steroids were used in the treatment of some patients, and Huggins demonstrated that metastatic prostatic cancer could be treated by castration (1).

Studies since the late 1960s have shown that, in the prostate, testosterone (T), the major testicular androgen circulating in blood, acts mainly after its conversion to 5α-dihydrotestosterone (DHT) by a 3-keto-5α-steroid reductase (5α-reductase). DHT then forms a complex with a specific receptor that interacts with an androgen response element (ARE) within target genes. Certain aspects of embryonic male urogenital tract differentiation, growth of kidney and muscle, testicular functions, and sexual behavior, however, appear to utilize T (or its aromatized product, estradiol); whereas DHT is the active form of androgens in many peripheral androgen-sensitive cells, including skin cells and hair follicles.

DHT-binding androgen receptors (ARs) obtained from different organs or prepared from AR cDNAs can bind T to some extent. There is no evidence for separate ARs for T and DHT encoded by different genes. The reason for differential response of different tissues to T and DHT is not clearly understood, but if different ARs are involved, they may be produced from the same AR gene by alternative splicing, editing, or other posttranscriptional processes. If the same AR is involved, T-R and DHT-R complexes may function differently because of differences in: the conformation of these complexes, the intracellular AR recycling kinetics and anchoring mechanism, the threshold concentration of ARs and other factors needed for regulation of specific genes, the interaction of AR with other steroid receptors or oncoproteins, and the cellular concentrations and metabolism of T and DHT. DHT produced by 5α-reductase in target cells may be more effective than circulating DHT that is bound to blood proteins in promoting specific gene transactivation. Also, the intracellular localization of 5α-reductase, DHT metabolizing enzymes, and AR may favor the utilization of intracellularly produced DHT over extracellular DHT.

Excessive formation and/or retention of DHT in target cells have been implicated in certain androgen-dependent pathological conditions including benign prostatic hyperplasia (BPH), acne, male-pattern baldness, and female idiopathic hirsutism. Appropriate 5α-reductase inhibitors, therefore, should be very useful in the selective treatment of these DHT-dependent abnormalities without affecting T-dependent organs. One such 5α-reductase inhibitor, finasteride or Proscar (Merck), has been shown to be effective in the treatment of benign prostatic hyperplasia and prostatic cancer.

The primary structure of 5α-reductases, elucidated from cDNA sequences, can provide new information essential in analyzing reductase gene regulation and mutation at the molecular level. 5α-reductase activity can be regulated by various cellular substances (including polyunsaturated fatty acids and phospholipids) that interact with the hydrophobic enzyme and/or affect the membrane localization of the reductase (2).

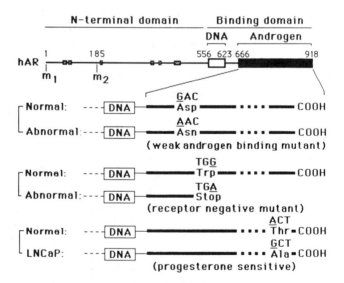

Fig. 1. Overall structures of hAR. The first and second methionines in the N-terminal domains are indicated by m_1 and m_2. The positions of amino acids are indicated by amino acid numbers started from m_1. Point mutations in nucleotides (underlined) can change the coded amino acid to make truncated AR (see text).

An androgenic steroid is bound by the AR as though the steroid molecule is being enveloped. The concept of "steroid enveloping by SR" implies that a steroid hormone can substantially alter the conformation of its receptor protein especially at the hormone-binding domain (3). Classical steroidal antiandrogens, such as cyproterone and its 17α-acetate, appear to act by competing with androgens for binding to AR. Flutamide, a nonsteroidal antiandrogen, acts after a conversion to hydroxyflutamide.

Cloning and sequencing of AR cDNA have made it possible to analyze the roles of different AR domains in eliciting androgenic responses (4-6). Studies of other steroid receptors (SRs) have also provided important information on how ARs may function and be regulated. The open reading frames present in human (h) and rat (r) AR cDNAs, starting from the first ATG at the 5' end, can code for proteins with 918 and 902 amino acids, which have a molecular mass of about 100 kDa (Figure 1). If the second ATG is used as the initiator, the encoded hAR and rAR are 80 kDa proteins with 734 and 733 amino acids, respectively. It is possible that both the 100 kDa and the 80 kDa ARs are produced and function differently in target cells. Progestin receptor (PR) has been shown to exist in cells in two forms possibly due to differential translational or transcriptional initiation. These forms of PR function differently with HREs in different target genes.

Among SRs, hAR and rAR are unique in that they have many oligo or poly (amino acid) sequences in the amino terminal domain (4). Some of these sequences may be important in the specific regulation of AR function. The amino acid sequences in the DNA-binding and androgen-binding domains (excluding the hinge region between the two domains) are 100% identical among hAR, rAR, and mouse AR. There is also a high homology (75-80%) among ARs and hPR, hGR, hMR in the DNA-binding domain. In fact, AR, GR, and PR can recognize the same HRE or ARE.

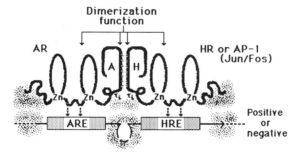

Fig. 2. A hypothetical model indicating the roles of AR domains and a regulatory zipper structure at the hormone-binding domain that may be important in forming a dimer with another AR, another hormone receptor, or an oncoprotein to exert positive or negative regulation of gene transcription. The target gene has (ARE) and/or other hormone-response elements (HRE).

Like other SRs, the androgen-binding domain may have a region that can function as a transcriptional inhibitor (TI) (Figure 2). This domain may inhibit the interaction of the DNA-binding domain with ARE or HRE. Binding of the androgen to the domain may result in the removal of this interference. In the androgen-binding domain there are at least nine amino acid heptads that contain Leu or other hydrophobic amino acids at positions 1 and 8. These repeats may behave like a leucine zipper motif (7) and provide a site for dimerization of ARs or AR and other SRs, transcription factors, or oncoproteins. Homo- or heterodimerization of GRs or other transcriptional factors has been shown to play a key role in promoting positive or negative regulation of gene transcription.

Androgen insensitivity can be caused by a mutation or abnormal expression of the genes for the AR or 5α-reductase or defects in other cellular components that are needed to exert normal androgen responses in AR- and 5α-reductase-positive cells. A deficiency in 5α-reductase has been related to abnormal male sexual differentiation; whereas a defect in the X-chromosome-linked AR has been considered to be responsible for syndromes of androgen resistance, such as testicular feminization (TFM). Mutations in AR genes have been observed in more than 20 individuals with abnormal androgen responses. So far, the abnormalities in AR genes are due to point mutations (Figure 1) rather than gross structural alterations of the AR gene. Mutations in the androgen-binding domain have resulted in changes in one amino acid, introduction of a premature stop codon, deletion of part or all of a domain, or alternative splicing (5,8,9).

When androgen-insensitive and AR-deficient human prostate cancer cells (PC-3) were transfected with an expression vector encoding AR (pSG5-AR), the cells were able to transactivate a MMTV-CAT reporter gene, but the growth of PC-3 cells was not stimulated by androgens. One possiblity for the lack of an androgenic effect in these transfected PC-3 cells is that defects in factors other than AR production are responsible for the androgen-insensitivity. Since treatment of PC-3 cells with androgens after cotransfection with MMTV-CAT-stimulated CAT gene expression, PC-3 cells have the factors that are necessary for transactivation of the transfected gene, but not for the expression of genes that are needed for the proliferation of the prostate cells. Alternatively, these proliferation-linked genes may be expressed without AR and are androgen-insensitive.

Veldscholte et al. (10) and our group (11) have found that the AR gene in the androgen-sensitive prostate cancer cell, LNCaP, has a G to A mutation that changes amino acid 876 in the androgen-binding domain from Thr to Ala (Figure 1). The mutated AR (LNCaP AR) was more efficient than normal AR in utilizing progesterone as a ligand in the transactivation of a CAT gene cotransfected into PC-3 cells. In the same system, we have found that, with cells transfected with LNCaP AR, hydroxyflutamide at 1 to 10 nM can effectively stimulate transactivation in the absence of an androgen, whereas with cells transfected with normal hAR, the amount of stimulation was insignificant even at 100 nM of hydroxyflutamide (11). The usefulness of antiandrogens as therapeutic agents for prostate cancer has been questioned because antiandrogens can stimulate proliferation of LNCaP cells (12). This effect has been attributed to an AR-independent neutralization of growth inhibitors. However, our finding suggests that, under certain conditions, hydroxyflutamide and other nonsteroidal compounds may act as *nonsteroidal androgens* and transactivate certain genes (Figure 3). The action of an androgen on AR function, therefore, is not absolutely dependent on the presence of a steroidal carbonyl or hydroxyl group on the ligand.

In the rat prostate, androgens autoregulate the production of AR mRNA by down regulation. In the presence of 2,4-dinitrophenol, AR is rapidly deactivated (half-life, 2 min) to an inactive form (R°) that does not bind androgen unless it is reactivated by an energy-dependent process to the androgen-binding form (R). A majority of the A-R complexes formed may not bind to DNA/chromatin unless they are "transformed" by a temperature-dependent process. It is not clear whether this is due to a chemical modification of the A-R complexes or to the association/dissociation of other cellular factors, such as a heat shock protein. Besides their effect on transcription, androgens have significant effects on the stabilization of certain mRNAs. Although AR and other SRs can bind RNA, the role of SR in the posttranscriptional process is not clear.

To regulate the growth of target organs, androgens can stimulate the expression of certain genes but also repress the expression of some genes simultaneously. In the rat ventral prostate, genes for a nonreceptor steroid-binding protein (α-protein) and a spermine-binding protein are positively regulated, whereas genes for glutathione S-transferase and sulfated glycoprotein-2 are negatively regulated (13). Dr. Chung Lee and his co-workers (14) have shown that, in normal rats, cell proliferation occurred in distal segments while sulfated glycoprotein-2 and cathepsin D (two marker proteins for cells undergoing programmed death) were actively produced by cells in the proximal region of the prostatic ductal system. After castration, the level of these two proteins decreased in the proximal region and increased in the distal region, indicating that the cell degeneration pattern shifted from the proximal region to the distal region. This interesting phenomenon may be related to mechanisms controlling prostatic cell homeostasis.

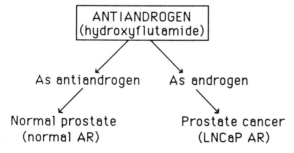

Fig. 3. Nonsteroidal androgen and antiandrogen.

Neuroendocrine systems may have a regulatory role in normal and diseased prostate function. Dr. Leland Chung and his co-workers (15) have used rat ventral prostate fragments implanted under the renal capsules of syngeneic rats to study the production of secretory protein in the denervated prostate. The denervated prostate had a reduced level of α-protein production, but this decrease was restored by the administration of exogenous androgen and/or the β-adrenergic agonist, isoproterenol. This observation suggested that androgens can also act through β-adrenergic receptor pathways.

Acknowledgments

The work described in this article was supported by the U.S. National Institutes of Health, Grants DK 37694 and DK41670. Unpublished studies in our laboratory on the AR functions in human prostate cancer cells were carried out by Drs. John Kokontis, Kiyoshi Ito, and Richard Hiipakka.

References

1. Bettuzzi S, Hiipakka RA, Gilna P, Liao S (1989) Identification of the androgen-repressed mRNA for a 48-kilodalton prostate protein as sulfated glycoprotein-2 by cDNA cloning and sequence analysis. Biochem J 257:293-296.
2. Forman BM, Samuels HH (1990) Interactions among a subfamily of nuclear hormone receptors: the regulatory zipper model. Mol Endocrinol 4:1293-1301.
3. Guthrie PD, Freeman MR, Liao S, Chung LWK (1990) Regulation of gene expression in rat prostate by androgen and β-adrenergic receptor pathways. Mol Endocrinol 4:1343-1353.
4. He WW, Fischer LM, Sun S, Bilhartz DL, Zhu X, Charles Y-F, Kelley DB, Tindall DJ 1990. Molecular cloning of androgen receptors from divergent species with a polymerase chain reaction technique: complete cDNA sequence of the mouse androgen receptor and isolation of androgen receptor cDNA probes from frog, guinea pig, and clawed frog. Biochem Biophys Res Commun 171:697-704.
5. Huggins C, Hodges CV (1941) Studies on prostatic cancer. I. The effect of castration, of estrogen and of androgen injection on serum phosphatases in metastatic carcinoma of the prostate. Cancer Res 1:293-297.
6. Kokontis J, Ito K, Hiipakka RA, Liao S (1991) Expression of normal and LNCaP androgen receptors in androgen-insensitive human prostatic cancer cells: altered hormone and antihormone specificity in gene transactivation. Receptor 1:271-279.
7. Lee C, Sensibar JA, Dudek SM, Hipakka RA, Liao S (1990) Prostatic ductal system in rats: regional variation in morphological and functional activities, Biol Reprod 43:1079-1086.

8. Liang T, Liao S (1992) Inhibition of steriod 5α-reductase by specific aliphatic unsaturated fatty acids. Biochem J, in press.
9. Liao S, Liang T, Fang S, Casteneda E, Shao T (1973) Steriod structure and androgenic activity: specificities involved in the receptor binding and nuclear retention of various androgens. J Biol Chem 248:6154-6162.
10. Liao S, Kokontis J, Sai T, Hiipakka RA (1989) Androgen receptor structures, mutations, antibodies and cellular dynamics. J Steroid Biochem 34:41-51.
11. Olea N, Sakabe K, Soto AM, Sonnenschein C (1990) The proliferative effect of antiandrogens on the androgen-sensitive human prostate tumor cell line LNCaP. Endocrinology 126:145-1463.
12. Ris-Stalpers C, Trifiro MA, Kuiper GGJM, Jenster G, Romalo G, Sai T, van Rooij HCJ, Kaufman M, Rosenfield RL, Liao S, Schweikert H-U, Trapman J, Pinsky, L, Brinkmann AO (1991) Substitution of aspartic acid 686 by histidine of asparagine in the human androgen receptor leads to a functionally inactive protein with altered hormone-binding characteristics. Mol Endrocrinol 5:1562-1569.
13. Sai T, Seino S, Chang C, Trifiro M, Pinsky L, Mhatre A, Kaufman M, Lambert B, Trapman J, Brinkmann AO, Rosenfield RL, Liao S (1990) An exonic point mutation of the androgen receptor gene in a family with complete androgen insensitivity. Am J Human Genetics 46:1095-1100.
14. Simental A, Madhabananda S, Lane MV, French FS, Wilson EM (1991) Transcriptional activation and nuclear targeting signals of the human androgen receptor. J Biol Chem 266:510-518.
15. Veldscholte J, Ris-Stalpers C, Kuiper GGJM, Jenster G, Berrevoets C, Claassen E, van Rooij HCJ, Trapman J, Brinkmann AO, Mulder E (1990) A mutation in the ligand binding domain of the androgen receptor of human LNCaP cells affects steroid binding characteristics and response to anti-androgens. Biochem Biophys Res Commun 173:534-540.

1

The Conjoint Actions of Androgens and Estrogens in the Induction of Proliferative Lesions in the Rat Prostate

Shuk-Mei Ho, Margaret Yu, Irwin Leav, and Todd Viccione

Sex Hormones and Prostatic Carcinogenesis

Age-Associated Damages in the Sex Hormone Milieu May Be the Underlying Cause of Human Prostatic Cancer

Despite extensive past investigations, the etiology of human prostatic carcinoma remains largely undefined. It has been suggested that age-associated changes in the sex hormone milieu may be the common cause of prostatic cancer development in man. Several lines of evidence furnish support for this credence. First, circulating levels of free testosterone (T) in men decline with age while those of free 17ß-estradiol (E_2) remain unchanged, thus resulting in a much higher ratio of free E_2 to T in older men (1,2). Second, it has been reported that among black Americans who have the highest incidence of prostatic cancer in the world, both plasma free T and estrone levels are elevated at young age (3). Taken together, these findings suggest that changing levels of circulating androgens and/or estrogens or an altered ratio of the two classes of steroids in plasma are important determinants of prostatic carcinogenesis in the human male. Moreover, the influence of sex hormones could begin in the early decades of a man's life and have a long-lasting impact on the prostate.

Androgens Alone Are Not the Causative Factors of Aberrant Growth in the Prostate

Although androgens have long been recognized as the principal regulatory hormones for the growth and development of the normal prostate, it is uncertain whether androgens alone are the causative factors of aberrant growth in the gland. Although some human studies have indicated higher levels of circulating T in patients with prostate cancers when compared with healthy subjects of the same age, others have failed to demonstrate significant differences in plasma androgen levels between the two groups (4). Experiments in rodents have provided insightful information on the role of androgens in prostate cancer induction. Long-term treatment of Noble (NBL) rats (5) or Lobund-Wistar (L-W) rats (6) with T induces prostatic carcinoma in these animals. However, when T is replaced with 5α-dihydrotestosterone (DHT), an androgen, prostatic carcinomas are not found in the treated rats (6). Since T can be aromatized to (E_2) *in vivo*, a definitive conclusion that only androgenic action is involved in prostatic carcinogenesis cannot be drawn from these studies. Furthermore, Bruchovsky and co-workers (7) have put forth an intrinsic homeostatic constraint theory to explain the regulation of the growth response of the prostate to androgens. Basically, they envision the initial wave of androgen-induced cell proliferation in a regenerating prostate to terminate once the normal gland size is restored. Continued stimulation of a normal-sized gland with T fails to bring about further growth of the tissue.

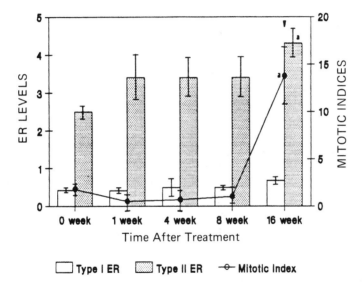

Fig. 1. Kinetics of alterations in nuclear type I and type II ER levels and mitotic activity in the DLP following T + E_2 treatment. NBL rats were implanted with two T (2.0 cm)- and one E_2 (1.0 cm)-filled capsules (Silastic™ tubing : 1.6 mm i.d. x 3.2 mm o.d.) and sacrificed at various time points following hormone treatment. [^{3}H-E_2] binding to DLP nuclei were measured by saturation analyses and expressed as pmol per mg nuclear DNA. Cell division in DLP was quantitated by a demecolcine-metaphase-arrest technique followed by counting mitoses on histological sections. Mitotic index is the number of mitoses per 1,000 cells. Each datum point represents the mean ($\pm$ SEM) of values found in at least four animals. a = significant difference ($p < 0.05$) between the mean of the treated group and that of the untreated controls. v indicates the appearance of dysplasia in the DLPs.

The Combined Action of an Estrogen and an Androgen Brings About Proliferation and Aberrant Growth of the Prostate

Contrary to pure androgenic action, estrogens *per se* can cause both atrophy and proliferative changes in the canine prostate (8). When synergized with androgens, estrogens are effective growth promoters of the rat gland (9). In view of the strong association of endometrial cancer and breast cancer with cumulative estrogen exposure (10), we therefore hypothesize that chronic estrogenic stimulation of an androgen-supported prostate is the underlying cause of prostatic carcinogenesis. Protracted androgen-supported estrogenic action is needed to overcome intrinsic constraints that normally operate to limit excessive growth of the gland.

To test this possibility, we have utilized the NBL rat as an experimental model of study. Simultaneous long-term ($>$ 52 weeks) treatment of NBL rats with T and E_2 induced a high frequency of carcinoma in the dorsolateral lobe (DLP) but not in the ventral lobe (VP) of the rat prostate (11). Shorter-term (16 weeks) treatment of NBL rats with the combined hormonal regimen consistently generated prostatic dysplasia (100%), a form of preneoplastic proliferative lesion, exclusively within the enlarged DLPs. Dysplastic foci appeared throughout the DLPs, but were not found in the VPs of the treated animals. The proliferative lesion was characterized by a layering of piled-up acinar epithelial cells, exhibiting varying degrees of anisokaryosis. Mitotic index in the tissue was dramatically increased, with mitoses restricted almost entirely to the areas of dysplasia. Close morphological similarities exist between this proliferative lesion found in the rat gland and a form of preneoplastic lesion found in the human disease (12). Since the separate administration of either androgens (T or DHT) or E_2 suppressed epithelial proliferation (see B III for details) and induce no dysplasia in rat DLP, we conclude that the combined androgenic-estrogenic action is the necessary factor in the genesis of this proliferative lesion. This paper aims at revealing the mechanism of action of estrogen in the androgen-supported DLP.

Mechanism of Estrogen Action in an Androgen-Supported Prostate

Presence of Two Types of Nuclear Estrogen Receptors in the DLP

It is commonly accepted that an estrogen exerts its effects on a target tissue primarily through interaction with the classical, nuclear, high-affinity, low-capacity receptor (type I ER) in the cell nucleus (13). However, a second, lower affinity, nuclear, estrogen-binding protein, termed type II ER, was also found in estrogen target tissues and tumors derived from them (14). It has been suggested that this latter receptor species plays a key role in the regulation of proliferation and long-term growth of estrogen target tissues. Saturation analyses revealed two types of estrogen binding sites in the DLP nuclei of NBL rats (15). Type I estrogen binding sites bind estrogen with high-affinity ($K_d \approx$ 1-2 nM) and low capacity ($B_{max} = 421 \pm 51$ fmol/mgDNA, n = 17), while type II binding sites have moderate affinity ($K_d \approx$ 15-20 nM) and higher capacity ($B_{max} = 2.46 \pm 0.17$ pmol/mg DNA, $n = 17$). VP nuclei, on the contrary, contain only the high-affinity type I sites and no detectable amount of type II sites. This finding supports the concept that basic biological differences exist between the two major lobes of the rat gland, and the presence of type II ER in rat DLP, but not in the VP, may explain the apparent susceptibility of DLP to T + E_2 stimulation and the refractoriness of VP to this hormonal challenge.

T + E_2 Treatment of NBL Rats Induced Dysplasia and Nuclear Type II ER Elevation Exclusively in the DLP

We have examined the kinetics of dysplasia induction and of the alterations of type I and type II nuclear ER levels in rat DLP (Fig. 1). Following treatment of NBL rats with T +E_2, a gradual enlargement of DLP to twofold the normal gland size was observed (data not shown). Dysplasia, however, did not develop until after 16 weeks of hormone treatment. The proliferative lesion was characterized by a significant increase in mitotic index (from 1.8 ± 0.2 to 13.8 ± 3.1 mitoses per 1,000 cells) in the tissue. Concomitant with the appearance of dysplasia at the 16th week of hormonal exposure was a twofold increase in the type II ER level in DLP nuclei. Parallel increases in type I ER and androgen receptor (data not shown) levels were not observed. Inferred from the work of Markaverich and co-workers (16) who found that induction of uterine type II ER in E_2-treated ovariectomized rats closely parallels long-term growth in the uterus, we conclude that elevations in nuclear type II ER are causally linked to enhanced cell proliferation and dysplastic development in the DLP.

Induction of Proliferative Dysplasia and Type II ER Elevation in Rat DLP Require the Conjoint Action of an Androgen and E_2

While E_2 is the sole inducer of growth and modulation of type II ER levels in the rat uterus (16), the hormonal requirements for the induction of type II ER elevation in the DLP is unknown. We recently demonstrated that T, DHT, or E_2 administered separately causes neither dysplasia development nor a significant elevation of type II ER in the DLPs of intact NBL rats (Fig. 2). While T and DHT were able to maintain DLP tissue weight, despite reduced mitotic indices observed in the tissue, E_2-treatment caused massive atrophy of the gland along with no observable mitotic activity.

In contrast to the single-hormone treatments, the combined administration of an androgen (T or DHT) and E_2 induced a twofold increase in tissue weight and type II ER levels. In all instances, these increases were accompanied by dysplasia (Fig. 2). These findings clearly indicate that dysplasia induction and type II ER elevation in the DLP require both androgenic and estrogenic action.

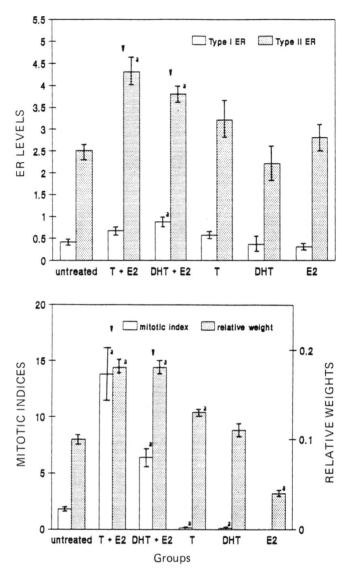

Fig. 2. Hormonal requirement for the induction of proliferative dysplasia and type I and type II ER elevations in the DLP. Rats were treated with E_2, DHT, T, DHT + E_2, and T + E_2. Androgen capsules were 2.0 cm long, and E_2 capsules were 1.0 cm long. Captions are similar to those described in Fig. 1. The relative weight of a DLP is expressed as a percentage of body weight of the animal.

The fact that the two cellular processes have the same hormonal requirements suggests that they may be intimately linked. It is tempting to speculate that E_2 acting in concert with an androgen elevates type II ER levels that directly confer a higher proliferative potential to this prostatic lobe.

Do Ligands of Type II ER Have Antiproliferative Activity in Rat DLP?

Since we believe nuclear type II ERs are involved in growth-regulatory processes of the prostate, we postulate that compounds capable of interacting with this receptor species may have antiproliferative activity in the gland. Previous research of Markaverich and co-workers demonstrated the unique ability of bioflavonoids and related compounds to interact with type II ER and inhibit growth in the rat uterus and in several tumor tissues (17). In a recently completed study we have evaluated the abilities of several bioflavonoids (quercetin, rutin, and hesperidin), methyl p-hydroxyphenyllactate (MeHPLA), 4,4'-dihydroxylbenzylidene acetophenone (DHBA) to interact with nuclear type II ERs in the DLP nuclei. Data in Fig. 3 show that MeHPLA, a possible bioflavonoid metabolite, competes as effectively as E_2 for nuclear type II ER

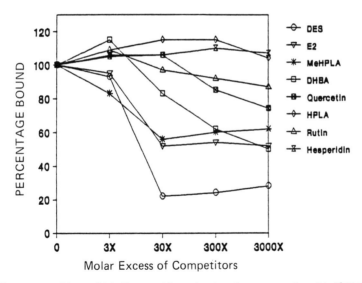

Fig. 3. Competition of bioflavonoids and related compounds with [³H-E₂] for nuclear type II estrogen binding sites in rat DLP. Aliquots of DLP nuclei were incubated with 40 nM of [³H-E₂] in the presence of 3-, 30-, 300-, and 3,000-fold molar excess of the competitors. Incubations were performed at 35°C. At the end of incubation, free and bound steroids were separated by 30-min hydroxylapatite procedure. [³H-E₂] in each incubation with competitors was normalized against the one without competitor and expressed as % bound.

binding, whereas its demethylated product, HPLA, is completely ineffective. DHBA, a chalone or a known bioflavonoid precursor, and quercetin, a bioflavonoid, are both effective in binding nuclear type II ER, but only when present at molar concentrations higher than those of E_2. Two other bioflavonoidal compounds, rutin and hesperidin, demonstrate no binding affinities for nuclear type II ER in rat DLP. Current experiments in our laboratory focus on assessing the *in vivo* effectiveness of these compounds in suppressing dysplasia development in $T + E_2$ treated rats. Results from these *in vitro* and *in vivo* studies should enhance our understanding of type II ER-mediated proliferation and help determine whether these compounds can be developed into antitumor agents.

Conclusion

Carcinogenesis is a complex process involving sequential accumulation of genetic errors in susceptible cell populations resulting in altered growth behavior of the transformed cells and subsequent clonal expansion of these cells into malignant tumors (6). Genetic errors, including mutations, translocations, amplification of growth regulating genes (e.g., protooncogenes) and loss of tumor suppressor genes, can be induced by exogenous genotoxic agents as well as by endogenous oxidative metabolites. Several of these events require cell division for their occurrence, and all of them need proliferation for fixation into the cell population. Thus rapidly dividing tissues are at greater risk for undergoing malignant transformation than quiescent ones. Agents that cause cell proliferation in a susceptible tissue are likely to be carcinogenic in that tissue. In our rat prostatic carcinogenesis model, E_2 acting in concert with an androgen is able to increase cell proliferation and induce neoplastic changes in the normal DLP. The unique sensitivity of DLP to E_2 stimulation appears to be conferred by the expression of type II ER in this prostatic lobe. Protracted androgenic-estrogenic action elevates the level of this receptor, an event we believe to be crucial to the induction of proliferative lesions, and ultimately, carcinomas in the DLP. In short, we have suggested a possible mechanism to explain androgen-estrogen synergism in rat prostatic carcinogenesis.

Acknowledgments

DHBA was a generous gift of Dr. Barry Markaverich; MeHPLA and HPLA were synthesized by Sean Collins in Dr. Edward Brush's laboratory. This work was supported in part by a National Cancer Institute grant (CA-15776) and an American Cancer Society grant (CN-5). We thank Ms. Valerie Ricciardone for her superior secretarial assistance.

References

1. Reubens R, Dohnt M, and Vermeulen A (1974) Further studies on Leydig cell function in old age. J Clin Endocrinol Metab 39:40-45.
2. Levell MJ, Row E, Glashan RW, Picock NB, and Siddall JK (1985) Free testosterone in carcinoma of prostate. Prostate 7:363-368.
3. Ross R, Bernstein L, Judd H, Hanisch R, Pike M, Henderson B (1986) Serum testosterone levels in healthy young black and white men. J Natl Cancer Inst 75:45-48.
4. Voight KD and Krieg M (1978) Biochemical endocrinology of prostatic tumors. Curr Top Exp Endocrinol 3:173-199.
5. Noble RL (1982) Prostate carcinoma of the Nb rat in relation to hormones. Int Rev Exp Pathol 23:113-159.
6. Pollard M, Snyder DL, and Luckert PH (1987) Dihydrotestosterone does not induce prostate adenocarcinoma in L-W rats. The Prostate 10: 325-331.
7. Bruchovsky N and Lesser B (1976) Control of proliferative growth in androgen responsive organs and neoplasms. Adv Sex Hormone Res 2:1-55.
8. Leav I, Merk FB, Ofner P, Goodrich G, Kwan PW-L, Stein BM, Sar M, Stumpf WE (1978) Bipotentiality of response to sex hormones by the prostate of castrated or hypophysectomized dogs: direct effects of estrogen. Am J Pathol 93:69-92.
9. Drago JR (1984) The induction of Nb rat prostatic carcinomas. Anti Cancer Res 4:255-256.
10. Preston-Martin S, Pike MC, Ross RK, Jones PA, and Henderson BE (1990) Increased cell division as a cause of human cancer. Cancer Res 50:7415-7421.
11. Leav I, Merk FB, Kwan PW-L, and Ho S-M (1989) Androgen-supported estrogen-enhanced epithelial proliferation in the prostates of intact Noble rats. The Prostate 15:23-40.
12. McNeal JE and Bostwich DG (1986) Intraductal dysplasia: a premalignant lesion of the prostate. Human Pathol 17:64-71.
13. Gorski J, Welshons WV, Sakai D, Hansen J, Walent J, Kassis J, Shull J, Stack G and Campen C (1986) Evolution of a model of estrogen action. Recent Prog Horm Res 42:297-329.
14. Markaverich BM, Roberts RR, Alejandro MA, and Clark JH (1984) An endogenous inhibitor of [^{3}H]-estradiol binding to nuclear type II estrogen binding sites in normal and malignant tissues. Cancer Res 44:1575-1579.
15. Yu M, Cates J, Leav I, and Ho S-M (1979) Heterogeneity of [^{3}H]-estradiol binding sites in the rat prostate: properties and distribution of type I and type II sites. J Steroid Biochem 33:449-457.

16. Markaverich BM, Roberts RR, Alejandro M, and Clark JH (1984) The effects of low dose continuous exposure to estradiol on the estrogen receptor (type I) and nuclear type II sites. Endocrinology 114:814-820.
17. Markaverich BM, Roberts RR, Alejandro MA, Johnson GA, Middleditch BS, and Clark JH (1988) Bioflavonoid interaction with rat uterine type II binding sites and cell growth inhibition. J Steroid Biochem 30:71-78.

2

Enhancement of Prostate Carcinogenesis in Rats by Testosterone and Prolactin

Tomoyuki Shirai, Seiko Tamano, Shogo Iwasaki, and Nobuyuki Ito

Introduction

The development and differentiation of normal male accessory sex organs depend on endogenous androgen. Much evidence indicates that androgen is also essential for the development of prostate carcinomas, and since Noble (1) first reported grossly recognizable prostate adenocarcinomas after a prolonged administration of testosterone propionate (TP) to Nb rats, there are sufficient data to indicate that exogenous testosterone enhances naturally occurring or chemically induced prostate carcinomas in rodents (2). Invasive and desmoplastic rat prostatic tumors associated with TP have been reported to occur in the dorsolateral lobes. Prolactin has been also shown to play an important role in regulating the growth and function of the prostate gland.

The carcinogen 3,2'-dimethyl-4-aminobiphenyl (DMAB) has been revealed to induce *in situ* carcinomas of the ventral prostate in rats (3). The present experiments were carried out to evaluate the effects of TP and prolactin on the development of lesions in the accessory sex organs of rats exposed to DMAB. Enhancing effects of TP were also evaluated in N-methylnitrosourea (MNU)-treated animals.

Experiment I (Promotion of DMAB Prostate Carcinogenesis by Testosterone)(4)

Male F344 rats, 6-weeks-old, were used. Animals in groups 1 and 3 received subcutaneous (sc) implantation of 40 mg TP-containing silastic tubes (one per rat), replaced at 6-week intervals. Starting one week after the first implantation, all animals were given DMAB subcutaneously at a dose of 50 mg/kg b.w. 10 times at 2-week intervals. Groups 2 and 4 were given DMAB at the same dose and times as groups 1 and 3, but each carcinogen application was preceded daily by 3 consecutive sc injections of TP at a dose of 100 mg/kg b.w. After the last DMAB injection, animals in groups 1 and 2 received TP implants until the end of the experiment. Group 5 served as a carcinogen control and was given only

Table 1. Incidences of carcinomas in the dorsolateral prostate and seminal vesicles of rats treated with DMAB and TP.

Group Treatment[a]	No. of prostates	No. (%) of rats with lesions			
		Dorso lateral glands	Seminal vesicle	Coagu- lating	Totals
1 TP(p)+DMAB-TP(p)	19	9(47.4)[b]	7(36.8)[b]	2(10.5)	16(84.2)[b]
2 TP(i)+DMAB-TP(p)	18	6(33.3)[c]	6(33.3)[b]	3(16.7)	12(66.7)[b]
3 TP(p)+DMAB	19	0 -	0 -	0 -	0 -
4 TP(i)+DMAB	20	0 -	0 -	1 (5.0)	1 (5.0)
5 DMAB	20	0 -	0 -	0 -	0 -
6 TP(i) -TP(p)	10	0 -	0 -	0 -	0 -

[a] TP(p), TP by silastic tube; TP(i), TP by sc injection.
[b,c] $P < 0.01$, $P < 0.05$, respectively.

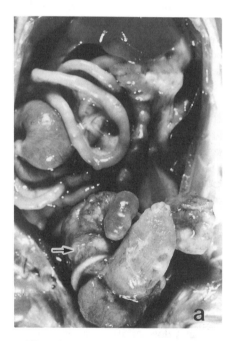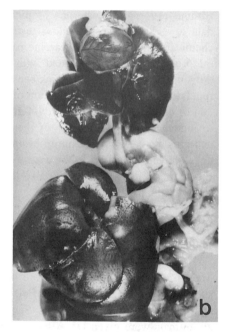

Fig. 1. Macroscopic appearances of gross prostate tumors. (a) Tumors are present in the lateral prostate (arrow). (b) Note metastatic lesions on the peritoneum and in the liver and lung.

DMAB. Group 6 was given TP implants throughout the experiment without DMAB administration. At week 56, all surviving animals were subjected to complete autopsy. Rats receiving TP-implants had 10 to 20 times the serum levels of testosterone as controls: averages for groups given DMAB alone, DMAB and then TP, or TP alone were 0.94, 21.00, and 11.21 ng/ml, respectively. Prolonged administration of TP increased the weights of prostate and seminal vesicles about twofold. Macroscopical as well as microscopical adenocarcinomas in the dorsolateral prostate, seminal vesicles, and coagulating glands were induced in the groups given TP plus DMAB and subsequent long-term administration of TP. Gross lesions were pale and firm, ranging from 0.5 to 3 cm in diameter (Fig. 1[a]), and found in 7 out of 19 rats (36.8%) in group 1 and 6 out of 18 (33.3%) in group 2. Eight cases demonstrated metastasis to the abdominal cavity, liver, or lung (Fig. 1[b]). Histological assessment revealed well- to poorly differentiated adenocarcinomas forming varying-sized glandular or ductal structures accompanied by abundant fibrous connective tissue (Fig. 2). No cribriform patterns were noted. The overall incidences of carcinomas found in the dorsolateral prostate, seminal vesicle, and coagulating glands were 84.2, 66.7, and 5.0% in groups 1, 2, and 4, respectively. None of the group 3, 5, 6 or 7 animals had equivalent tumors (Table 1). Development of carcinomas of cribriform morphology in the ventral prostate was not increased by subsequent treatment with TP, the incidences in groups 1 to 5 were 10.5, 5.6, 15.8, 20.0, and 35.0%, respectively.

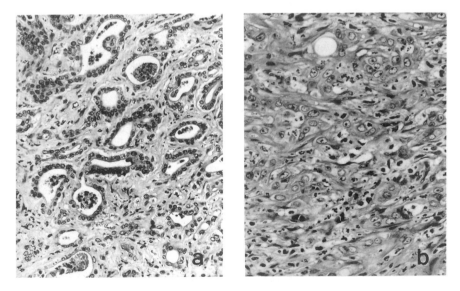

Fig. 2. Microscopic appearances of prostate tumors. (a) Well-differentiated adenocarcinoma. (b) Poorly differentiated adenocarcinoma.

Table 2. Incidences (%) of atypical hyperplasias and carcinomas of the prostate and seminal vesicles of rats.

Group	Treatment after DMAB[a]	No. of rats	Prostate Ventral AH[b]	Prostate Ventral Carci- noma	Prostate Lateral AH	Seminal vesicles AH
1	Mt	9	8(89)***	1(11)	4(44)*	4(44)
2	Mt, CB154	14	9(64)	1(7)	5(36)	6(43)
3	CB154	23	4(17)	0	1(4)*	7(30)
4	None	15	7(47)	3(20)	1(7)	9(60)

[a] Mt, MtT/F84
[b] AH, Atypical hyperplasia
* $p < 0.05$, *** $p < 0.001$

Experiment II (Promotion of MNU Prostate Carcinogenesis by Testosterone)

Rats, 6-weeks-old, were alternately given a 0.75 ppm ethynyl estradiol(EE)-containing diet for 2 weeks and a basal diet not supplemented with EE for two weeks, five times. Three days after each change to basal diet, a single iv 15 mg/kg bw injection of MNU or vehicle was given. Intermittent administration of EE induced atrophy and repeated regenerative cell proliferation of prostate epithelium after transfer to basal diet (3). The carcinogen administration was synchronized with the peak of DNA synthesis. From week 20, the carcinogen group received TP implants for 40 weeks. Animals given MNU and then TP developed tumors localized in the seminal vesicles (6/18, 33%) and coagulating glands (1/18, 6%), but not in the ventral and dorsolateral prostate (Table 2). One of them had multiple metastatic foci in the abdominal cavity. MNU or TP alone did not induce tumors (0/20 and 0/19, respectively).

Experiment III (Promotion of DMAB Prostate Carcinogenesis by Prolactin)(5)

Rats, 6-weeks-old, received 5 dietary cycles composed of 3 weeks on ethynyl estradiol followed by 2 weeks on the basal diet accompanied by a single sc 50 mg/kg injection of DMAB on the third day after each change to basal diet. After completion of the carcinogen administration stage, rats received repeated sc transplantation of a prolactin-producing pituitary tumor, MtT/F84, for induction

Table 3. Cytosolic androgen and estrogen receptors in male rat accesory sex glands.

	Androgen receptors[a]		Estrogen receptors[a]	
Ventral prostate	17.1 ± 5.1	(4)	0.9	(1)
Dorsolateral prostate	13.8 ± 3.8	(4)	2.0 ± 0.4	(3)
Coagulating glands	3.9 ± 4.8	(4)	1.5 ± 1.0	(3)
Seminal vesicles	44.9 ± 7.6	(4)	4.4 ± 0.4	(3)

[a] fmol/mg cytosol protein, Mean ± SE. ( ), Number of samples.

of hyperprolactinemia until sacrifice at week 51. Effects of a prolactin-suppressing agent, bromocriptine (CB154, Sandoz Ltd., Basel, Switzerland), were also investigated.

Slight elevation of prolactin level in the serum was associated with the transplantation of MtT/F84 at week 32. CB154 alone slightly depressed the prolactin level (5). More marked effects of MtT/F84 and CB154 were evident at week 51. Carcinoma of the prostate only developed sporadically, and the incidence was not affected by the observed hyperprolactinemia. However, incidences of atypical hyperplasia in the ventral and lateral prostate but not the seminal vesicles were significantly increased.

Discussion

The present data clearly demonstrate testosterone to have strong enhancing effects on tumor development in the dorsolateral prostate, seminal vesicles, and coagulating glands, but not in the ventral prostate. The fact that the simultaneous administration of DMAB and TP for 20 weeks without further TP exposure was not effective for induction of a high yield of prostate tumors suggests that postinitiation enhancing factors are involved. Such enhancing potential of TP on prostate tumor development has earlier been shown in Noble, Lobund-Wistar, and ACI rats. All reported neoplasms were located in the dorsolateral prostate and associated structures and, in terms of histological and growth patterns, seemed comparable to those in the present work. With regard to mechanisms, TP itself does not induce a significant increase in DNA synthesis in the epithelial cells of the accessory sex glands (4). Whether selective enhancing effects on growth of preneoplastic lesions might be involved remains to be clarified.

The lack of promotion of ventral prostate lesions by TP is in agreement with earlier findings for spontaneous ventral prostate carcinomas in ACI/seg rats (6). No difference in response to exogenous testosterone regarding either cell proliferation or organ weight increases in the ventral prostate, dorsolateral prostate, and seminal vesicles was observed (4). Differences in cytosolic androgen receptors did not correlate with selective enhancement by TP (Table 3).

Promoting effects of hyperprolactinemia noted for atypical hyperplasias, which are considered to be precancerous lesions of the prostate but not seminal vesicles, require further investigation in terms of organ-specific mechanisms. The recent finding that MtT/F84 also secretes growth hormone indicates the need for another experimental system for investigation of the effects of prolactin alone.

Concluding Remarks

Exogenous testosterone can exert strong enhancing effects on chemically induced carcinogenesis of the dorsolateral prostate as well as the seminal vesicles and coagulating glands, indicating that this hormone may play an important role in the development of similar types of cancer prevalent in man.

Acknowledgments

This work was supported in part by Grants-in-aid for Cancer Research from the Ministry of Education, Science, and Culture, and from the Ministry of Health and Welfare of Japan, by a Grant-in-aid from the Ministry of Health and Welfare for the Comprehensive 10 years Strategy for Cancer Control, Japan, and by a grant from the Society for Promotion of Cancer Research of Aichi Prefecture.

References

1. Noble RL (1977) The development of prostatic adenocarcinoma in Nb rats following prolonged sex hormone administration. Cancer Res 37:1929-1933.
2. Pollard M Luckert PH and Snyder DL (1989) The promotional effect of testosterone on induction of prostate-cancer in MNU-sensitized L-W rats. Cancer Lett 45:209-212.
3. Shirai T, Fukushima S, Ikawa E, et al (1986) Induction of prostate carcinoma in situ at high incidence in F344 rats by a combination of 3,2'-dimethyl-4-aminobiphenyl and ethinyl estradiol. Cancer Res 46:6423-6426.
4. Shirai T, Tamano S, Kato T, et al (1991) Induction of invasive carcinomas in the accessory sex organs other than the ventral prostate of rats given 3,2'-dimethyl-4-aminobiphenyl and testosterone propionate. Cancer Res 51:1264-1269.
5. Nakamura A, Shirai T, Ogawa K, et al (1990) Promoting action of prolactin released from a grafted transplantable pituitary tumor (MtT/F84) on rat prostate carcinogenesis. Cancer Lett 53:151-157.
6. Isaacs JT (1984) The aging ACI/Seg vs. Copenhagen male rat as a model system for the study of prostatic carcinogenesis. Cancer Res 44:5784-5796.

3

Hormonal Carcinogenesis in Syrian Hamsters: A Hypothesis Involving Glutathione S-Transferase Regulation

James S. Norris, David A. Schwartz, Tina Cooper, and Weimin Fan

Introduction

In Syrian hamsters, a special case of hormonal carcinogenesis exists where the obligatory combined action of androgens and estrogens results in the development of leiomyosarcomas in the vas deferens or uterus. Both of these tissues are derived from the mesonephric ridge during development. The following hypothesis has been put forth to explain this type of hormonal carcinogenesis.

In the normal vas deferens, smooth muscle cells are in a differentiated status characterized by a lack of cell division (Go), and these noncycling cells express a glutathione S-transferase (GST). However, in androgen-treated animals one observes a limited hyperplasia in the vas deferens smooth musculature, and we have shown that during cell growth expression of a Mu class, GST is repressed. This GST is active in the cytoplasmic and nuclear compartments as a DNA hydroperoxidase and perhaps more importantly is able to couple glutathione to the genotoxic quinone metabolites of estrogen. Thus, the lack of GST in cycling cells might permit the genotoxic action of estrogen-quinones and could lead to smooth muscle cell transformation. Therefore, our hypothesis predicts that androgens increase cell growth in the vas deferens resulting in reduced GST expression, thus allowing estrogen metabolites to act genotoxically as DNA damaging agents whose cumulative action results in neoplasia. Because we already understand that expression of GST is regulated as a secondary response to glucocorticoids and is dependent on the growth status of the tumor cells (see below), we believe that the Syrian hamster model provides the opportunity to test the above hypothesis and also to understand how the regulation of a specific gene might control neoplastic transformation. On the following pages we present evidence to support our proposed pathway of hormonal carcinogenesis.

Table 1. Tumor induction was carried out as previously described (3).

Incidence of Leiomyosarcoma Induction (Male) (600 days)	
Treatment	**% Incidence**
Diethylstilbestrol (DES)	1.30 ($n=95$)
Testosterone propionate (TP)	0.96 ($n=104$)
DES/TP	100.00 ($n=41$)
Estradiol/TP	94.70 ($n=19$)
Progesterone (P)	0.00 ($n=7$)
Deoxycorticosterone acetate (DOCA)	0.00 ($n=3$)
DES/TP/P	100.00 ($n=7$)
Triamcinolone acetonide	0.00 ($n=4$)

n=number of animals in the sample group

Induction of Leiomyosarcomas

The procedure used to induce this class of mesenchymal tumor involves prolonged administration of pelleted testosterone propionate and estrogen. Male animals typically receive the steroids at 40-60 days of age, and the first tumors are seen around 260 days with 100% incidence at 450 days. The histology, pathology, and hormone dependence of the tumors have been described in detail elsewhere (1).

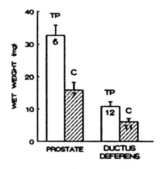

Fig. 1. Animals were castrated under ketamine anesthesia. Ten days later a 30 mg pellet of testosterone propionate (TP) or a control pellet (C, cholesterol) was implanted subpannicularly. Animals were sacrificed 72 hours later and organ wet weight determined. Number of animals per group is indicated within the bars. Both groups were statistically significant at $p < 0.01$ by Student's t test.

The spontaneous incidence of this tumor is essentially zero, and when either androgen or estrogen alone is administered to the animals, no tumor formation is observed, nor have we found any other single steroid protocol that proved positive for tumor induction (Table 1). However, androgens when administered alone do cause a thickening of the vas deferens. Histologically, this thickening appears to be a mild hyperplastic response. This is not a surprising result, since we have now demonstrated that a hamster vas deferens is an androgen-target organ (Fig. 1).

Estrogens will also cause mild disruption of tissue organization in the vas deferens, but this effect is much more pronounced in the epididymis. The role of estrogens in the smooth musculature of the vas deferens is uncertain because there is no evidence by immunological or biochemical criteria for estrogen receptors (unpublished). Estrogens have been shown to effectively compete for the androgen receptor in hamster tissues (2) and to be mitogenic for DDTl tumor cells (3).

Vas Deferens Derived Tumor Cell Line DDT1 MF2

The DDT1 MF2 smooth muscle cell line was derived from an androgen-estrogen induced leiomyosarcoma arising in the hamster ductus deferens. This cell line contains receptors for both androgens and glucocorticoids, and its proliferation is differentially sensitive to these classes of steroids (3,4). Androgens dramatically stimulate wild-type cell growth and augment the level of intracellular androgen receptors, whereas glucocorticoids inhibit growth and prevent androgen receptor level augmentation. A glucocorticoid-resistant variant, DDT1 GR has been developed (5). A number of genes linked to growth regulation in DDT1 cells and shown to be modulated by steroids have been studied. These include the α1 and β2 adrenergic receptors that have been cloned (6,7). The β2 adrenergic receptor is regulated by glucocorticoids (8) and is at least suggested to be involved in growth regulation because DDT1 cells blocked in Go/Gl by glucocorticoids are released from the block by dibutyryl cAMP.

Growth factor genes have also been studied in relationship to steroid modulation of DDT1 cell growth. For example, we have shown the v-*sis* oncogene product is downregulated by glucocorticoids and upregulated by androgens (9). We have further demonstrated that platelet-derived growth factor (PDGF) overcomes glucocorticoid-induced Go/Gl arrest (10). More recently, our collaborators (11,12) have cloned from DDTl cells the cDNA and gene for acidic fibroblast growth factor (aFGF) and demonstrated its role in cell growth, specifically demonstrating that androgens increase its expression. aFGF is a potent mitogen for DDT1 cells and will also overcome glucocorticoid-induced Go/Gl block at ng levels.

Other DDT1 cell growth regulatory pathways involve ornithine decarboxylase and protein kinase c. Ornithine decarboxylase activity is downregulated in DDT1 cells by glucocorticoids, and spermidine will partially overcome glucocorticoid-induced Go/Gl block (13). Protein kinase c activity is increased in DDT1 cells by glucocorticoids (14), and diacylglycerol analogs are inhibitory to DDT1 cell growth.

Recently, a Mu class GST cDNA and gene (hGSTYBX) have been cloned in our laboratory and have been shown to be regulated as a secondary response by glucocorticoids (15).

Metabolism and Genotoxicity of Estrogens

Very little is known about the metabolism of estrogen in either the seminal vesicle, fat pad, or vas deferens of Syrian hamsters. However, in other hamster tissues it is established that estrogens can be metabolized by estrogen hydroxylases to semiquinone intermediates and subsequently to quinones (16,17). The latter compounds are believed to be genotoxic agents. How these agents exert their genotoxic effect is not clear. Several groups believe that the quinone metabolites are able to form DNA adducts, at a low frequency, that are hypothesized to be responsible for mutations in DNA. Another postulated mechanism for quinone genotoxicity is that steroid metabolites disrupt microtubular assembly, resulting in diverse chromosome changes including micronuclei formation (18). Because in the vas deferens there is no evidence that estrogens induce damage at the DNA level, the microtubule disruption during mitosis is a more appealing hypothesis. Disruptions of this type can result in nondisjunction and might lead to aneuploidy and eventually cell transformation. If a population of smooth muscle cells gained a growth advantage through this mechanism, then a subset of more rapidly growing cells would arise and one would predict they would be aneuploid. The DDT1 tumor cell line when first characterized was in fact aneuploid with a $2N$ chromosome number of 41 with no clear-cut chromosomal abnormalities (Fig. 2). This is consistent with the findings of Tsutsui et al. (19) who reported that DES induced transformation of SHE cells resulting primarily in aneuploidy. As seen below, this might lead to genetic instability mediated by the estrogen metabolites. These changes might then be fixed by androgen-induced cell cycling. A similar progression that parallels this hypothesis is found in colon cancer development (20).

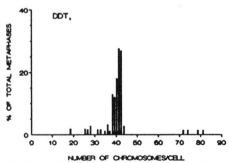

Fig. 2. Cells were blocked with colcemid and processed by standard procedures.

Specific Expression of Xenobiotic Drug Metabolizing Enzymes

Much effort has gone into studies on genes that regulate entry of cells into or out of the cell cycle. Conversely, little is known about genes that are expressed in noncycling or Go stage mesenchyme-derived cells except that one expects to see expression of genes associated with the differentiated stage, for example, as seen in adipocytes differentiated from 10T 1/2 mouse fibroblasts.

Our interest in hormonal carcinogenesis has led to the cloning of a glutathione S-transferase which is expressed at a high level in response to glucocorticoids and is also constitutively expressed at a lower level in confluent noncycling cells (Fig. 3). The precise activity of this enzyme against genotoxic agents such as the quinone metabolites of estrogens is under study. Little is known about the regulation of this class of enzymes; we were the first to describe the glucocorticoid regulation of its gene as a secondary response (15).

Another enzyme with activity against quinones, quinone reductase, has been observed to be expressed in mouse 3T3 cells arrested in Go by serum starvation (21). Confirmation of the expression of this gene in DDTl cells is under way. If it is also regulated by growth status and perhaps by glucocorticoids, then it raises to two the number of detoxifying enzymes that are expressed only in Go or in response to glucocorticoids.

Cellular Distribution of Glutathione S-Transferases

hGSTYBX protein is found in both the cytoplasmic and nuclear fractions of DDTl cells. Traditionally, the cytoplasmic enzymes have been thought to be responsible for metabolism of xenobiotics. The nuclear enzymes are not well studied but seem to include mu 4-4 and 5-5 class enzymes, both of which have activity against DNA hydroperoxides, thus implicating them in DNA repair (22). In addition, other studies have localized a GST enzyme to splicesomes (23) and

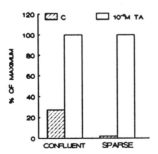

Fig. 3. Cells were plated at the indicated density and treated for 12 hours with 1×10^{-7} *M* triamcinolone acetonide (TA) or ethanol vehicle (C). RNA was harvested, Northern blotted, and probed with an RNA probe prepared from hGSTYBX or with hamster β actin. Blot densities were measured and plotted as percent of maximum.

demonstrated that nuclear uptake of the enzyme occurs (24). Binding of this enzyme to DNA has also been reported (25). We have carried out studies to localize the hamster mu GST and from these data we conclude that most of the enzyme is cytoplasmic, although a small fraction is in the nucleus (unpublished).

Conclusion

There is little question that instability of the genome coupled with the selective growth advantage that tumor cells seem to acquire ultimately results in neoplasia. We propose to understand and interrelate both series of events. With respect to androgen-estrogen carcinogenesis, we have developed a hypothesis to describe leiomyosarcoma induction in the Syrian hamster (Fig. 4). The three key elements to our hypothesis are: (1) androgen induction of smooth muscle cell growth (hyperplasia); (2) the concomitant reduction in glutathione S-transferase activity; and (3) subsequent induction of genomic instability by estrogen metabolites and development of neoplasia. With respect to growth we have clearly demonstrated that androgens are mitogenic for vas deferens smooth muscle cells (Fig. 1 and [4]) and that glutathione S-transferase expression is very low in cycling cells (Fig. 3). Furthermore, in all tumors examined, the initial isolates were aneuploid (Fig. 2) suggesting that genomic alteration parallels or precedes tumor formation. Each of these parameters is now being examined in detail to gain a better understanding of which normal cellular pathways perturbed by steroids lead to neoplasia. With respect to specific events occurring during genomic instability we are now investigating the role of retrotransposons and/or retroviral infection in the steroid-mediated neoplastic process, since new data from our laboratory have demonstrated that over 30 retroviral RNAs are expressed in normal hamster vas deferens and epididymis

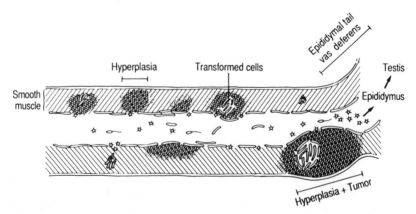

Fig. 4. Depiction of events occurring in vas deferens around 450 days post-androgen-estrogen treatment.

(submitted). It is our intent to further define and characterize these events to develop an inclusive understanding of the cellular and molecular events defining androgen-estrogen carcinogenesis in the Syrian hamster vas deferens.

Acknowledgments

A special thanks to Carol Devoll and Ann Donaldson for manuscript preparation. Supported by NIH CA 49949 and CA 52085.

References

1. Kirkman H, Kempson RL (1982) Tumors of the testis and accessory male sex glands. IARC Sci Publ 34:175-90.
2. Norris JS, Kohler PO (1977) The coexistence of androgen and glucocorticoid receptors in the DDT1 cloned cell line. Endocrinology 100:613-18.
3. Norris JS (1989) Tumors of the accessory sex glands of male Syrian hamsters and hormone action. In: Hafex ESE, Spring-Mills E, eds., Human Reproductive Medicine, Vol. 4, Amsterdam: Elsevier/North Holland Biomedical Press 609-616.
4. Syms AJ, Norris JS, Smith RG (1983) Proliferation of a highly androgen-sensitive cloned cell line (DDT1 MF-2) is regulated by glucocorticoids and modulated by growth on collagen. In Vitro 19:929-36.
5. Smith RG, Nag A, Syms AJ, Norris JS (1986) Steroid regulation of receptor concentrations and oncogene expression. J Steroid Biochem 24:51-5.
6. Cotecchia S, Schwinn DA, Randall RR, et al (1988) Molecular cloning and expression of the cDNA for the hamster αl-adrenergic receptor. Proc Natl Acad Sci USA 85:7159-63.
7. Kobilka BK, Frielle T, Dohlman HG, et al (1987) Delineation of the intronless nature of the gene for the human and hamster β2-adrenergic receptor and their putative promoter regions. J Biol Chem 262:7321-27.
8. Norris JS, Cohen J, Cornett LE, et al (1987) Glucocorticoid induction of β-adrenergic receptors in the DDT1 MF-2 smooth muscle cell line involves synthesis of new receptor. Mol Cell Biochem 74:21-7.
9. Norris JS, Cornett LE, Hardin JW, et al (1984) Autocrine regulation of growth: II. Glucocorticoids inhibit transcription of c-*sis* oncogene-specific RNA transcripts. Biochem Biophys Res Commun 122:124-8.
10. Syms AJ, Norris JS, Smith RG (1989) Autocrine regulation of growth: I: glucocorticoid receptor forms to sulfhydryl reactive agent. Biochem 28:7373-79.
11. Harris SE, Smith RG, Zhou H, et al (1989) Androgens and glucocorticoids modulate heparin-binding growth factor I *mRNA* accumulation in DDT1 cells as analyzed by *in situ* hybridization. Mol Endo 3:1839-44.

12. Hall JA, Harris MA, Malark M, et al (199) Characterization of the hamster DDT1 cell aFGF/HGBF-1 gene cDNA and its modulation by steroids. J Cell Biochem 43:17-26.

13. Lamb D. Personal communication.

14. Harris S. Personal communication.

15. Norris JS, Schwartz DA, MacLeod SL, Fan W, et al (1991) Cloning of a mu class glutathione S-transferase cDNA and characterization of its glucocorticoid inducibility in a smooth muscle tumor cell line. Mol Endo, accepted.

16. Li JJ, Li SA (199) Estrogen carcinogenesis in hamster tissues: a critical review. Endocrin Rev 11:524-31.

17. Liehr JG (1990) Genotoxic effects of estrogens. Mutation Res 238:269-76.

18. Epe B, Harttig UH, Schiffmann D, et al (1989) Microtubular proteins as cellular targets for carcinogenic estrogens and other carcinogens. Prog Clin Biol Res 318:345-51.

19. Tsutsui T, Maizumi H, McLachlan JA, et al (1983) Aneuploidy induction and cell transformation by diethylstilbestrol: a possible chromosomal mechanism in carcinogenesis. Cancer Res 43:3814-21.

20. Fearon E, Cho KR, Nigro JM, et al (1990) Identification of a chromosomal 18q gene that is altered in colorectal cancer. Science 247:49-56.

21. Manfioletti G, Ruaro ME, Del Sal G, et al (1990) A growth arrest-specific (gas) gene codes for a membrane protein. Mol Cell Biol 10:2924-30.

22. Tan KH, Meyer DJ, Gillies N, et al (1988) Detoxification of DNA hydroperoxides by glutathione transferases and the purification and characterization of glutathione transferases of the rat liver nucleus. Biochem J 254:841-5.

23. Bennett FC, Yeoman LC (1985) Co-localization of nonhistone protein BA with U-snRNPs to the same regions of the cell nucleus. Exp Cell Res 157:379-86.

24. Bennett FC, Yeoman LC (1987) Microinjected glutathione S-transferase YB subunits translocate to the cell nucleus. Biochem J 247:109-112.

25. Bennett FC, Rosenfeld BI, Huang C-H, et al (1982) Evidence for two conformational forms of nonhistone protein BA which differ in their affinity for DNA. BBRC 104:649-56.

PART 2. HORMONES, CELL PROLIFERATION, AND CARCINOGENESIS

INTRODUCTION

Current Concepts of Sex Hormone Action (An Overview)

Elwood V. Jensen

For three decades it has been known that steroid sex hormones exert their principal biological actions in combination with specific receptor proteins. As first shown with estrogens, the steroid binds to an intracellular receptor and induces hormonal response without itself undergoing chemical change. Studies in many laboratories established that an early event in hormone action is the enhanced expression of genes that are somehow restricted in hormone-dependent cells (for early references see 1,2). Two forms of the receptor were identified, including a native form, with little affinity for nuclei, and an activated or transformed modification, which binds tightly to chromatin and is produced by the action of the hormone on the native receptor. With the demonstration that only the transformed receptor has the ability to influence RNA synthesis in isolated target cell nuclei, there emerged a general concept of steroid hormone action, in which the role of the steroid is to convert the native receptor protein to a modulator of transcription (3).

But though the overall pattern was established, the structure of the receptor, the chemical nature of the transformation process, and the mechanism by which the transformed hormone-receptor complex enhances RNA synthesis remained unclear.

During the past few years, the techniques of molecular biology and immunology have complemented biochemical approaches in providing insight into the nature of receptor proteins and their function in hormone action. This overview will summarize briefly some major recent advances and point out some areas where present understanding is still deficient. More detailed descriptions of the current state of knowledge can be found in recent reviews and monographs (4-7).

Receptor Structure

With the isolation of receptor proteins in pure form and the preparation of specific antibodies to them, it has been possible to clone the cDNAs and deduce the primary structures for the principal intracellular receptors. With the aid of deletion mutants, individual domains in the receptor molecule have been identified and correlated with different aspects of receptor function. As shown in Figure 1, the sex hormone receptors belong to a general family of intracellular proteins that mediate the actions of many important cell regulators in the nuclei of their target cells (6-9). Though they vary in length from 427 amino acids for vitamin D receptors to 984 for mineralocorticoid (corresponding to molecular weights shown in Table 1), they are composed of comparable units. Each receptor contains a DNA-binding domain of 66-68 amino acids (C), which show a high degree of homology with other members of the family, a ligand-binding region (E) showing some homology, a small "hinge" region (D) joining these two domains, and variable regions (A/B, F) with little homology. The

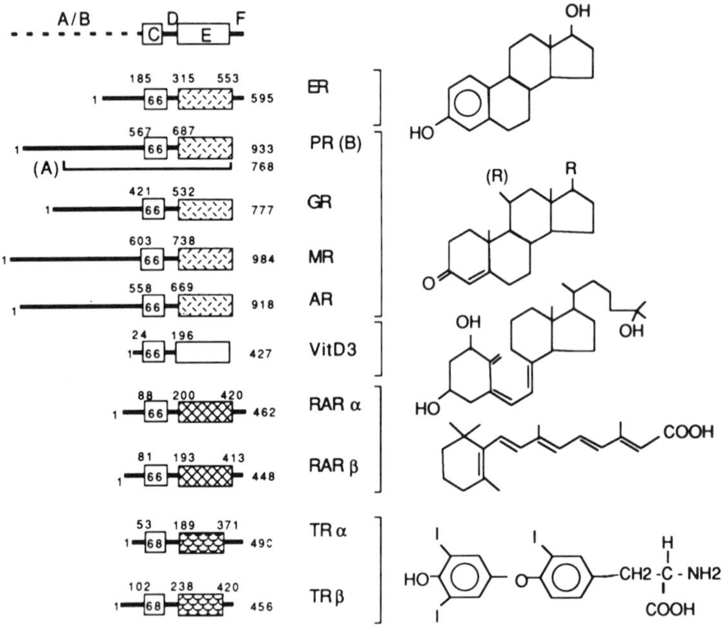

Fig. 1. The human intracellular family and its ligands. The top diagram shows functional domains; boxes indicate conserved areas while thin black lines are regions of low homology. The position of each domain boundary is given as the number of amino acids from the N-terminus; figures in the C boxes indicate the number of amino acids in the DNA-binding domain. Receptors are ER, estrogen; PR, progestin [(R) = H, R = CH$_3$CO]; GR, glucocorticoid [(R) = OH, R = CH$_2$OHCO, OH]; MR, mineralocorticoid [(R) = OH, R = CH$_2$OHCO, plus =O at C$_{18}$]; AR, androgen [(R) = H, R = OH]; VitD$_3$, vitamin D; RAR, retinoic acid; TR, thyroid hormone. (Courtesy of Professor Pierre Chambon).

Table 1. Molecular weights of receptors calculated from amino acid composition (kDa).

Receptor	Human	Avian
Estrogen	66	66
Progestin (B)	99	86
Progestin (A)	81	72
Androgen	99	
Glucocorticoid	94	
Mineralocorticoid	107	
Vitamin D	47.5	55

latter are not essential for function, but they appear to contribute to optimal activity. The DNA-binding domain contains two "zinc fingers," looped structures involving chelated metal ions that are responsible for reaction with DNA in the hormone-response elements of target genes. Chicken and human (but not rabbit) progesterone receptors come in two sizes, A and B; the B form consists of the A protein plus an additional unit at the N-terminus and appears to arise by alternate initiation of transcription of receptor mRNA.

Intracellular Localization and Interaction

Because untransformed receptors for most steroid hormones usually appear in the cytosol fraction of tissue homogenates, it was originally assumed that the native, unoccupied receptor is a cytoplasmic protein and that its hormone-induced conversion to the transformed state was accompanied by translocation to the nucleus. But subsequent observations suggested that much of the native receptor may already be in the nucleus before exposure to hormones. As described and documented more completely elsewhere (7,10), unfilled and presumably untransformed receptors for many steroid hormones were sometimes found in the nuclear fraction of tissue homogenates, and autoradiographic studies of rat uteri, exposed to estradiol or progesterone in the cold to inhibit transformation, showed most but not all the radioactive steroid in the nucleus. Most immunocytochemical studies with monoclonal antibodies to estrogen, androgen, and progestin receptors have shown only nuclear staining in target tissue sections, whereas on enucleation of cultured rat pituitary cells essentially all the estrogen, progestin, and glucocorticoid receptors were found to be associated with the karyoblast fraction. These results led some investigators to conclude that native receptors for the sex hormones reside exclusively within the nucleus of the target cell and to proclaim that the so-called two-step mechanism for hormone-receptor interaction is no longer valid.

While the foregoing observations clearly show that, contrary to earlier belief, much of the untransformed receptor for gonadal hormones is associated with the nuclear compartment, they by no means establish that the native receptor is exclusively nuclear or that the two-step mechanism is invalid. As discussed in more detail elsewhere (7), immunocytochemical and autoradiographic techniques measure concentrations rather than amounts; in target cells where the cytoplasmic volume greatly exceeds the nuclear volume, more than 25% of the receptor could be in the cytoplasm and still be undetected. Enucleation experiments that find 90% of the glucocorticoid receptor in the nucleus are suspect inasmuch as many investigators have demonstrated that receptors for glucocorticoids, as well as for mineralocorticoids and vitamin D, are in both the cytoplasm and the nucleus, often with the extranuclear receptor predominating. One cannot rule out the possibility that, for gonadal hormones as well, a significant amount of the native receptor is present in the extranuclear region, perhaps in equilibrium with a nuclear pool.

The presence of much or even all of the untransformed receptor within the nucleus has no bearing on the validity of the two-step mechanism. If there is equilibrium between the nuclear and extranuclear receptor, as there appears to be with glucocorticoids, the concentration of the cytoplasmic receptor would be less than originally considered, but it would be continually replenished from the nuclear pool (Fig. 2[A]). However, if it can be established that the native receptor actually is confined to the nucleus, one must explain how the steroid makes its way so rapidly *in vivo* from the blood transport proteins to the cell

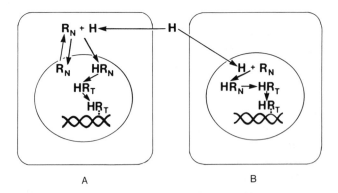

Fig. 2. Schematic representation of hormone-receptor interaction in target cell. H, hormone; R_N, native (untransformed) receptor; R_T, transformed receptor. (A) Extranuclear receptor in equilibrium with nuclear pool of loosely bound native receptor. (B) Native receptor confined entirely to the nucleus.

nucleus. But once it is in the nucleus, the two-step mechanism of receptor transformation followed by genomic binding would operate as previously conceived (Fig 2[B]).

Receptor Transformation

The ability of a steroid hormone to convert the native receptor to its nuclear binding form was first demonstrated for estrogens, making use of the finding that the nuclear receptor sediments more rapidly in salt-containing gradients than does the cytosol form. This situation results from the tendency of the transformed receptor to form a dimer. Although transformed receptors for other steroid hormones do not sediment more rapidly than their native counterparts, it was shown by other criteria that glucocorticoid and progesterone receptors exist as less stable dimers, and that all these transformed receptors interact in dimeric form with the palindromic response elements in target genes.

The nature of the transformation reaction has been extensively investigated, for the induction of this process represents a key biochemical role for the steroid. As documented more completely elsewhere (7,11-14), much has been learned about receptor transformation, but precise understanding is still not complete. Under physiological conditions this reaction requires the presence of hormone and temperatures of 25-35°C, but it can be effected in the cold in the absence of hormones by ammonium sulfate precipitation, gel filtration, dialysis, or prolonged exposure to salt. Hormone-induced receptor transformation is blocked by molybdate and other transition metal oxyanions (11), which has provided a useful way to stabilize the native form of the receptor.

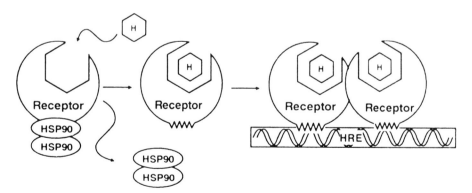

Fig. 3. Schematic representation of hormone-induced receptor transformation and interaction of dimeric transformed receptor with target gene. H, steroid hormone; HSP90, heat shock protein; HRE, hormone response element. From Carson-Jurica et al. (5)

Early experiments on the kinetics of the transformation of estrogen and glucocorticoid receptors suggested that a rate-limiting step is the dissociation from other components present in the native receptor. A major advance in understanding transformation came with the discovery that the native receptors for several classes of steriod hormones consist of a steroid-binding subunit associated with another protein of molecular weight 90,000 that is present as a dimer and is lost on transformation. This component was shown to be a heat shock protein, which associates with the receptor to obscure the region understanding transformation came with the discovery that the native receptors for several classes of steroid hormones consist of a steroid-binding subunit responsible for binding to DNA. As shown in Figure 3, interaction with the steroid displaces the heat shock protein making the DNA-binding domain available for interaction with target genes. Native receptors also contain low-molecular-weight components that appear to be required for the association with heat shock protein. Their removal by dialysis or gel filtration eliminates the need for hormones in effecting transformation.

The concept of dissociation from heat shock protein, coupled with the removal of low-molecular-weight factors that participate in this aggregation, serves to explain many of the heretofore puzzling observations regarding receptor transformation. Still to be elucidated is how the steroid hormone effects disruption of the macromolecular complex under physiological conditions and what role, if any, receptor phosphorylation and dephosphorylation play in transformation and nuclear binding (7,15).

Reaction with Target Genes

The biochemical mechanism by which transformed steroid-receptor complexes enhance gene expression is currently an active area of research. Although understanding is still far from complete, many facts have been ascertained concerning the general nature of this process (4-7). It has been established by many investigators that stimulation by transformed steroid-receptor complexes does not involve interaction at the site of transcription, but rather with a "hormone-response element" (HRE), an enhancer located in the promoter area in the 5'-flanking region of the target gene. Palindromic sequences of 13-15 base pairs make up the binding site for the dimeric receptor. The hormone-response elements for progestins and glucocorticoids are similar in composition and interact in some degree with both receptors.

Recognition of the response element appears to reside in the DNA-binding domain of the receptor, since a chimeric protein, formed by replacing this region in the estrogen receptor with the corresponding sequence of the glucocorticoid receptor, activates the expression of a corticoid-inducible but not of an estrogen-inducible gene in the presence of estrogen. As with many protein-DNA interactions, the association of receptor with the response element appears to be mediated by a pair of "zinc fingers," peptide loops involving chelated metal that are located in the highly conserved (C) region in steroid receptors.

Glucocorticoid and mineralocorticoid receptors show close homology in their DNA-binding regions and appear to react with the same gene networks.

Just how the binding of the transformed steroid-receptor complex to hormone-response elements enhances RNA synthesis is not completely elucidated. There is evidence that it involves the participation of other transcription factors. In a cell-free system, stimulation of transcription by activated progestin receptor appears to result from its enhancement of a stable preinitiation complex at the gene promoter. Once it has induced transformation of the receptor, a further role for the steroid in transcription enhancement also is not entirely clear. It has been reported that the presence of hormone is necessary for the binding of transformed glucocorticoid receptor to enhancer elements in intact cells and for progesterone receptor in a cell-free system. However, after activation by heat, salt treatment, or purification, steroid-free receptors for progestins and gluco-corticoids not only bind to their response elements, but the salt-activated progestin receptor stimulates transcription in an *in vitro* system in the absence of steroids. Moreover, certain mutant receptors for glucocorticoids and estrogens, which lack the steroid-binding domain, show a constitutive ability to interact with DNA in the absence of hormone and to stimulate transcription *in vitro*. It appears that the steroid-binding region of the receptor somehow prevents the domains for DNA binding and transcription activation from functioning and that the presence of hormone relieves this inhibition (9).

Summary

Steroid hormone receptors comprise a family of regulatory proteins with many similarities in their structures and modes of action. These receptors are present within target cells in the nucleus and in some, and probably all, cases in the cytoplasm as well. Before exposure to hormone, these receptors exist in combination with heat shock proteins and other entities that prevent their interaction with DNA. Association with the steroid causes disruption of this complex and exposure of the DNA-binding site.

This "transformed" hormone-receptor complex, in dimeric form, then reacts with a hormone-response element in the promoter region of target genes to enhance transcription. Thus, the biological action of steroid hormones is said to involve a two-step mechanism: conversion of the native receptor to a functional transcription factor and reaction of this transformed receptor with responsive genes.

References

1. O'Malley BW, Means AR (1974) Female steroid hormones and target cell nuclei. Science 183:610-620.
2. Yamamoto KR, Alberts, BM (1976) Steroid receptors: elements for modulation of eukaryotic transcription. Annu Rev Biochem 45:721-746.

3. Jensen EV, DeSombre ER (1973) Estrogen-receptor interaction. Estrogenic hormones effect transformation of specific receptor proteins to a biochemically functional form. Science 182:126-134.
4. Evans RM (1989) Molecular characterization of the glucocorticoid receptor. Recent Prog Horm Res 45:1-27.
5. Carson-Jurica MA, Schrader WT, O'Malley BW (1990) Steroid receptor family: structure and functions. Endocrine Rev 11:201-220.
6. Parker MG (ed) (1991) Nuclear hormone receptors. Academic Press, London.
7. Jensen EV (1991) Steroid hormone receptors. In: Seifert G (ed) Current Topics in Pathology, vol 83, Cell receptors. Springer-Verlag, Heidelberg, pp. 365-431.
8. Green S, Chambon P (1986) A superfamily of potentially oncogenic hormone receptors. Nature 324:615-617.
9. Evans RM (1988) The steroid and thyroid hormone receptor superfamily. Science 240:889-895.
10. Walters MR(1985) Steroid hormone receptors and the nucleus. Endocrine Rev 6:512-543.
11. Pratt WB (1987) Transformation of glucocorticoid and progesterone receptors to the DNA-binding state. J Cell Biochem 35:51-68.
12. Gustafsson J-Å, Carlstedt-Duke J, Poellinger L, Okret S, Wikström A-C Brönnegård M, Gillner M, Dong Y, Fuxe K, Cintra A, Härfstrand A, Agnati L (1987) Biochemistry, molecular biology, and physiology of the glucocorticoid receptor. Endocrine Rev 8:185-234.
13. Baulieu E-E, Binart N, Cadepond F, Catelli MG, Chambraud B, Garnier J, Gasc JM, Groyer-Schweizer G, Oblin ME, Radanyi C, Redeuilh G, Renoir JM Sabbah M (1989) Do receptor-associated nuclear proteins explain earliest steps of steroid hormone function? In: Carlstedt-Duke J, Eriksson H, Gustaffson J-Å (eds) The steroid/thyroid hormone receptor family and gene regulation. Birkhäuser Verlag, Basel, pp. 301-318.
14. Pratt WB, Sanchez ER, Bresnick EH, Meshinchi S, Scherrer LC, Dalman FC, Welsh MJ (1989) Interaction of the glucocorticoid receptor with the M_r90,000 heat shock protein: an evolving model of ligand-mediated receptor transformation and translocation. Cancer Res 49:2222s-2229s.
15. Auricchio F (1989) Phosphorylation of steroid receptors. J Steroid Biochem 32:613-622.

4

Control of Uterine Epithelial Growth and Differentiation: Implications for Estrogen-Associated Neoplasia

John A. McLachlan, Retha R. Newbold, Karen G. Nelson, and Kenneth S. Korach

Introduction

Estrogens have been associated with neoplasia in various target organs for many years. Since a consequence of estrogen administration is usually epithelial proliferation in these same target organs, the assumption underlying estrogen-associated neoplasia is that cell proliferation per se is the trigger for this condition. We have tested this assumption in nontarget cells in culture (Syrian hamster embryo cells, SHE cells) and have shown that various estrogens, both natural and synthetic, are capable of neoplastically transforming SHE cells *in vitro* in the absence of any enhanced cell proliferation (1). In fact, additional studies show that these cells lack most classical estrogen-growth responses and are relatively poor in ER (Tsutui et al., in preparation). Thus, at least in this *in vitro* system, cell transformation, the presence of classical ER, and enhanced growth response seem to be separable; however, congruence of ER and cell differentiation could not be determined since no differentiation-specific genes for estrogen action are yet known in this nontarget cell system. We decided, therefore, to study the role of cell proliferation and differentiation in a target tissue which, while relatively deficient in ER, provided marker genes for estrogen-associated cell differentiation. The tissue that met this criterion was the newborn mouse uterine epithelium.

Uterine Pathobiology in Developmentally Estrogenized Mice

It has been known for many years that treatment of newborn mice with estrogen results in abnormal differentiation of the cervicovaginal epithelium with subsequent long-term lesions in the treated adults (2-4). The Bern and Forsberg labs have continued to report findings on the estrogen-imprinted cervicovaginal epithelium and formulate new models for studying hormonal carcinogenesis (see, for example, 5,6).

Previous studies with neonatally estrogenized mice have not demonstrated high yields of malignant epithelial neoplasms in the reproductive tract. Recently, our lab has reported that uterine adenocarcinoma is demonstrable in 90% of mice receiving DES for 5 days neonatally; the induction of these uterine epithelial lesions was age- and dose-related (7). Furthermore, the tumors were estrogen-dependent in that ovariectomy of adult mice with tumors resulted in partial regression, and uterine tumors implanted in nude mice required estrogen for their continued growth and transplacentability. However, cell lines established from these estrogen-dependent uterine epithelial neoplasms lose their ER and estrogen dependency (Hebert et al., unpublished).

Estrogen seems to play two roles in murine uterine tumor induction. First, an induction role where exposure to an exogenous estrogen in the first week of life is apparently necessary for inducing the molecular defect that leads to subsequent tumor formation; indeed, administration of 17β-estradiol, DES, or other DES-related synthetic estrogens results in uterine cancer (7). Secondly, an expression role where ovarian steroids, presumably endogenous estrogens at puberty, are required for the progression of the neonatally induced uterine lesions; animals treated with DES do not express tumors if they are ovariectomized before puberty and the onset of ovarian function (7). Thus, in this model, estrogen is apparently involved in the induction as well as the expression of the growth and differentiation defects that give rise to murine uterine cancer. Similarly, the neonatal hamster uterus appears very sensitive to neoplastic transformation, since following similar DES treatment in the newborn hamster, virtually all the adults express hormone-dependent uterine carcinoma (8).

The induction phase in the mouse is relatively short, requiring only 5 days of treatment occurring at a critical stage of development during the neonatal period. On the other hand, similar short-term treatment of the adult mouse does not induce uterine adenocarcinoma (Newbold and McLachlan, unpublished). Indeed, uterine epithelial neoplasms are rare in mice (9). Even following lifetime feeding of adult mice with DES, the incidence of uterine adenocarcinoma only reaches 1.7% (10); clearly, the adult uterus is responsive to and stimulated by this estrogen, since 95% of the mice demonstrate cystic endometrial hyperplasia. Spontaneous uterine adenocarcinoma in rats is also rare and only reaches 0.5% at two years of age; estrogen treatment in adults induces a variety of nonneoplastic proliferative lesions but rarely cancer (11). Thus, although the mature differentiated rodent uterine epithelium responds to high doses of estrogen with sustained proliferation, it seldom undergoes complete neoplastic transformation.

Ontogeny of Estrogen Response in the Uterus

What, then, are the unique features of the newborn murine uterine epithelium that may contribute to the apparently enhanced transformation response? One of the most obvious is the relative lack of epithelial ER. In the first week of life epithelial ERs are undetectable (12); by day 11 postnatally, about one-half the uterine epithelial cells contain detectable ER; and by day 14 and on, ER can be found in all the epithelial cells. Uterine stromal cells, however, contained ER at all ages examined.

When newborn mice are treated with estrogen in the first week of life, a proliferative response is seen in the ER-deficient epithelium. In fact, estrogen-induced DNA synthesis, as determined by tritiated thymidine labeling, is seen in ER-positive cells as well as cells that do not contain detectable ER (13). On the other hand, the production of an estrogen-inducible protein, lactoferrin, is invariably colocalized with ER. In this immature *in vivo* system, therefore, a secretory pathway associated with mature epithelium segregates with the ER while epithelial proliferation does not necessarily.

In the case of the newborn mouse uterus, there are several hypotheses to explain how ER-deficient epithelial cells can respond to estrogen. One is that the ER is below the limits of detection of our techniques.

Another hypothesis considers that the estrogen signal reaches the epithelium via the ER-rich stroma. Certainly, results in mice have suggested that morphogenesis of the reproductive tract depends on stromal cues (14,15). However, no convincing evidence exists that epithelial proliferation is determined by the stroma alone.

Uterine-Derived Growth Factors and Estrogen Action

An additional pathway for estrogen action in ER-poor cells involves autocrine or paracrine actions of growth factors. The mouse uterus contains numerous growth factors and their cognate receptors, including epidermal growth factor (EGF), transforming growth factor α (TGFα), transforming growth factor βs (TGFβ), insulin-like growth factors (IGF), and colony-stimulating factor (CSF) (16).

EGF may play a role in the ontogeny of hormone response in the mouse uterus, since the EGF receptor is detected in the anlage of the uterine epithelium at very early developmental stages (17). In fact, the appearance of the epithelial EGF receptor precedes the estrogen receptor by almost two weeks (a very long time in early mouse development). Moreover, estrogen apparently regulates the uterine EGF receptor at both the protein and message levels (18,19).

Uterine epithelial cells in serum-free culture derived from either mouse (20) or rabbit (21) respond mitogenically to EGF. In fact, EGF was the most potent mitogen in cultured murine cells that contained, on average, 52,000 EGF binding sites per cell.

That EGF may, in part, mediate an estrogen signal in the mouse uterus was further supported by work from our laboratory demonstrating an estrogen-like state in the uterus and vagina of immature ovariectomized mice treated with slow-release pellets of EGF (22). A wide spectrum of responses associated with estrogen was seen following EGF treatment: epithelial proliferation in the vagina and uterus, vaginal epithelial differentiation including cornification, and uterine epithelial differentiation including morphological changes and estrogen-associated gene expression.

A site for estrogen action could be at the level of formation of the EGF ligand, since studies from our lab (23) and others (24,25) have shown increases in proprio-EGF messenger RNA as well as free ligand. The actual mechanism for activation of EGF-like peptides in the mammalian reproductive tract remains to be established. Indeed, other members of this closely related family may also be involved in uterine response to estrogen, since we have recently found increases in TGFα peptide and message following estrogen treatment in mice (26).

Estrogen Receptor as Protective Against Estrogen-Induced Uterine Cancer: An Hypothesis

Thus, a picture is developing in which the estrogen signal for uterine cell division and differentiation can be transduced through several complementary pathways, which may involve both the ER and growth factors. The relatively undifferentiated, ER-poor, uterine epithelium in the neonatal mouse can divide in response to estrogens, possibly mediated by autocrine or paracrine mechanisms, while the induction of classically estrogen-regulated proteins, such as lactoferrin, requires a functional epithelial ER. This raises the possibility that estrogen-stimulated cell proliferation, in the absence of classical ER pathways associated with control of specific genes that are normally regulated in the adult reproductive tract, may create an environment conductive to the induction of permanent carcinogenic lesions by estrogens. This may, in turn, partially provide an explanation for the relative sensitivity of newborn mouse uterine epithelium to neoplastic transformation. Thus, in this model, the ER may function to protect the mature epithelium by mediating a specific pathway of growth and differentiation. In the immature uterus, cells unable to appropriately differentiate but still able to experience growth stimulation may be the most at risk for neoplastic cell transformation.

Although the presence of a cellular steroid receptor is currently considered as a first step to steroid hormone-associated disease, the association is not yet a complete one (27). For example, it has recently been shown that the early postmenstrual epithelium of the subhuman primate endometrium heterogeneously stains for ER (28) much like the neonatal mouse uterine epithelium (13). Moreover, when treated with estrogen during this luteal-follicular transition phase, ER-negative epithelial cells in the rhesus monkey incorporate tritiated thymidine in their nuclei much like the neonatal mouse does. Finally, the distribution of EGF receptor in the human uterine epithelium (29-31) is also similar to that of the mouse (17).

Thus, the possibility arises that each month the primate endometrium presents relatively undifferentiated cells that are similar to the neonatal mouse epithelium in sensitivity to estrogen-associated cell transformation. In fact, the relationship of ER content to endometrial cancer seems currently confounded; and, in some cases, ER content is associated with increased survival time in ER-positive tumors compared with ER-negative ones (32). Given the remarkably active stem-progenitor cell population in the primate endometrium described by Padykula and her colleagues (33), a strategy to induce ER early in stem cell life may be protective in human endometrial cancer. This strategy is being tested in the newborn mouse uterus.

Conclusions

Administration of estrogen to the newborn mouse is associated with long-term changes in the reproductive tract; one such change is the induction of uterine epithelial neoplasia. Disturbances of uterine growth and differentiation by estrogen is apparently limited to critical developmental stages, particularly the neonatal period, in rodents. A unique feature of the murine uterine epithelium in the first week of life is the relative absence of ERs, a common biochemical marker of the mature, differentiated epithelium. However, these ER-deficient cells are still quite mitogenically responsive to estrogen. Possible mechanisms for the transduction of the estrogen signal in the newborn uterus may involve cues from the ER-rich stroma or autocrine/paracrine growth factors associated with the epithelium. In fact, EGF and its cognate receptor may be important factors in estrogen action in the uterus. Thus, the newborn uterus contains the capacity to respond to estrogen with cell division but, in the relative absence of ER, may adopt an aberrant differentiation program that contributes to neoplastic progression. In this sense, the presence of ER, as a key first step in the differentiation process, may be protective against estrogen-associated cell transformation and uterine cancer.

References

1. McLachlan JA, Wong A, Degen GH, Barrett JC (1982) Morphologic and neoplastic transformation of Syrian hamster embryo fibroblasts by diethylstilbestrol and its analogs. Cancer Research 42: 3040-3045.
2. Takasugi N, Bern HA, DeOme KB (1962) Persistent vaginal cornification in mice. Science 138: 438-439.
3. Dunn TB, Green AW (1963) Cysts of the epididymis, cancer of the cervix, granular cell myoblastoma, and other lesions after estrogen injections in newborn mice. J Natl Cancer Inst 31: 425-455.
4. Forsberg J-G (1966) The effects of estradiol 17β on the epithelium in the mouse vaginal analage. Acta Anat (Basal) 63: 71-88.
5. Bern HA, Edery M, Mills KT, Kohrman AF, Mori T, Larson L (1987) Long-term alterations in histology and steroid receptor levels of the genital tract and mammary gland following neonatal exposure of female BALB/cCrgl mice to various doses of diethylstilbestrol. Cancer Research 47: 4165-4172.

6. Andersson C, Forsberg J-G (1988) Induction of estrogen receptor, peroxidase activity, and epithelial abnormalities in the mouse uterovaginal epithelium after neonatal treatment with diethylstilbestrol. Teratogenesis, Carcinogenesis, Mutagenesis 8: 347-361.

7. Newbold RR, Bullock BC, McLachlan JA (1991) Uterine adenocarcinoma in mice following developmental treatment with estrogens: a model for hormonal carcinogenesis. Cancer Research 50: 7677-7681.

8. Leavitt WW, Evans RW, Hendry WJ III (1982) Etiology of DES-induced uterine tumors in Syrian hamsters. In: WW Leavitt (ed) Hormones and Cancer, Plenum Publishing Corp., New York, pp. 63-69.

9. Johnson LD (1987) Lesions of the female genital system caused by diethylstilbestrol. In TC Jones, U Mohr, RD Hunt (eds) Genital System, Springer-Verlag, New York, pp. 84-109.

10. Highman B, Norvell MJ, Shellenberger T (1977) Pathological changes in female C3H mice continuously fed diets containing diethylstilbestrol or estradiol 17β. J Environ Pathol Toxicol 1: 1-30.

11. Goodman DG, Hildebrandt PK (1987) Adenocarcinoma, endometrium, rat. In: TC Jones, U Mohr, RD Hunt (eds) Genital System, Springer-Verlag, New York, pp. 80-82.

12. Yamashita S, Newbold RR, McLachlan JA, Korach KS (1989) Developmental pattern of estrogen receptor expression in female mouse genital tracts. Endocrinology 125: 2888-2896.

13. Yamashita S, Newbold RR, McLachlan JA, Korach KS (1990) The role of the estrogen receptor in uterine epithelial proliferation and cytodifferentiation in neonatal mice. Endocrinology 127: 2456-2463.

14. Bigsby RM, Cunha GR (1986) Estrogen stimulation of deoxyribonucleic acid synthesis in uterine epithelial cells which lack estrogen receptors. Endocrinology 119: 390-395.

15. Taguchi O, Bigsby RM, Cunha GR (1988) Estrogen responsiveness and the estrogen receptor during development of the murine female reproductive tract. Develop Growth Differ 30: 301-303.

16. McLachlan JA, Nelson KG, Takahashi T, Bossert NL, Newbold RR, and Korach KS (1991) Estrogens and growth factors in the development, growth, and function of the female reproductive tract. In: DW Schomberg (ed) Growth Factors in Reproduction, Springer-Verlag, New York, pp. 197-203.

17. Bossert NL, Nelson KG, Ross KA, Takahashi T, McLachlan JA (1990) Epidermal growth factor binding and receptor distribution in the mouse reproductive tract during development. Dev Biol 142: 75-85.

18. Mukku VR, Stancel GM (1985) Regulation of epidermal growth factors by estrogens. J Biol Chem 260: 9820-9824.

19. Lingham RB, Stancel GM, Loose-Mitchell DS (1988) Estrogen regulation of epidermal growth factor receptor messenger ribonucleic acid. Mol Endo 2: 230-235.

20. Tomooka Y, DiAugustine RP, McLachlan JA (1986) Proliferation of mouse uterine epithelial cells *in vitro*. Endocrinology 118: 1011-1018.
21. Gerschenson LE, Conner EA, Yang J, Anderson M (1979) Hormonal regulation of proliferation in two populations of rabbit endometrial cells in culture. Life Sci 24: 1337-1343.
22. Nelson, KG, Takahashi T, Bossert NL, Walmer DK, McLachlan JA (1991) Epidermal growth factor replaces estrogen in the stimulation of female genital-tract growth and differentiation. Proc Natl Acad Sci USA 88: 21-25.
23. DiAugustine RP, Petrusz P, Bell GI, Brown CF, Korach KS, McLachlan JA, Teng CT (1988) Influence of estrogens on mouse uterine epidermal growth factor precursor protein and messenger ribonucleic acid. Endocrinology 122: 2355-2363.
24. Gonzales F, Lakshmanan J, Hoath S, Fisher DA (1984) Effect of estradiol-17β on uterine epidermal growth factor concentrations in immature mice. Acta Endoc Copenh 105: 425-428.
25. Huet-Hudson YM, Chakraborty C, De SK, Suzuki Y, Andrews GK, Dey SK (1990) Estrogen regulates synthesis of EGF in mouse uterine epithelial cells. Mol Endo 4: 510-523.
26. Nelson KG, Takahashi T, Lee DC, Luetteke, NC, Bossert NL, Eitzman BE, McLachlan JA (1991) TGFα is a potential mediator of estrogen action in the mouse uterus. Endocrinology (In press, 1992).
27. Sheridan PJ, Blum K, Trachtenberg MC (eds) (1988) Steroid Receptors and Disease, Marcel Dekker, New York.
28. Brenner RM, West NB, McClellan MC (1990) Estrogen and progesterone receptors in the reproductive tract of male and female primates. Biol Reprod 42: 11-19.
29. Hofmann GE, Rao CV, Barrows GH, Schultz GS, Sanfilippo JS (1984) Binding sites for epidermal growth factor in human uterine tissues and leiomyomas. J Clin Endocr 58: 880-887.
30. Chegina N, Rao CV, Wakim N, Sanfilippo J (1986) Binding of ^{125}I-epidermal growth factor in human uterus. Cell Tissue Res 246: 543-548.
31. Damjanov I, Mildner B, Knowles BB (1986) Immunohistochemical localization of the epidermal growth factor receptor in normal human tissues. Lab Invest 55: 588-592.
32. Segretti EM, McCarty KS Sr, McCarty KS Jr (1988) Sex steroid receptors in human neoplasia. In: PJ Sheridan, K Blum, MC Trachtenberg (eds), Marcel Dekker, New York, pp. 493-524.
33. Padykula HA, Coles LG, Okulicz, WC, Rapaport SI, McCracken JA, King NA Jr, Longcope C, Kaiserman-Abramof IR (1989) The basalis of the primate endometrium: a bifunctional germinal compartment. Biol Reprod 40: 681-690.)

5

A Novel Protein Kinase Activity Identified from Human Breast Cancer Cell Lines

Alberto Baldi, Denis M. Boyle, Nestor V. Annibali, and James L. Wittliff

Introduction

Protein kinases (PKs) represent a diverse number of enzymes that exert a critical role in posttranslational changes on polypeptide structure and function (1,2). They catalyze the covalent transfer of phosphate from two common donors, ATP or GTP, to serine, threonine, and tyrosine residues located on its own molecule, endogenous cellular or exogenous protein acceptors, or synthetic aminoacidic sequences. Regarding their function it is well established that PKs regulate diverse physiological processes such as metabolic pathways, gene expression, membrane transport of ions and metabolites, cell cycle, nervous transmission, and cell transformation and differentiation (3). At the same time, they are dependent for their regulation on a number of activators or inhibitors with the exception of oncogenic transforming PK (4). The former group, the regulated one, in basal stage exhibited a low level of activity due to interaction of an "autoinhibitory" domain located within the enzyme at the catalytic site in a way that blocked the binding with the substrates (5). The enzyme is activated by an allosteric activator that induces a conformational change in the autoinhibitory domain allowing the enzyme to release its catalytic capability.

The number of regulated or autonomous PKs that have been described has recently risen exponentially considered in the order of 100. The tremendous diversity of the protein kinase family lies on the limited divergence of its catalytic domain, phylogenetic mapping, and the aminoacidic sequences lying outside the catalytic domain where residues involved in enzyme regulation need special consideration.

In this report we described a novel PK candidate isolated from human breast cancer cells that exhibits three different autophosphorylable subunits, all of them containing ATP binding sites.

Protein Kinase Assay from Breast Cancer Cells

When cytosol from two human breast cancer cell lines, MCF-7 and T47D, was associated to a solid polystyrene matrix (as a final step of purification) and incubated in the presence of [Y-^{32}P]ATP, the labeled phosphate was transferred to three major polypeptides whose mobilities in NaDodSO$_4$- polyacrylamide gel electrophoresis corresponded to molecular weights of 57, 47, and 43 kDa (Figure 1).

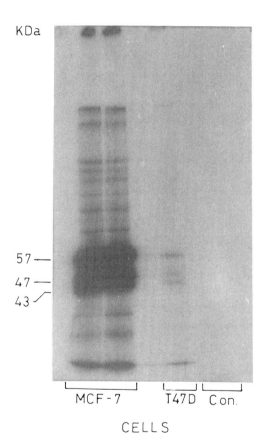

Fig. 1. Left. Autophosphorylation activity of PK from human breast cancer cell lines, MCF-7 (lane 1-2) and T47D (lane 3). Lane 4: Reaction in the absence of MCF-7 immobilized enzyme. Each reaction was performed in 150 μl of P$_{10}$ buffer containing 10 μCi of [Y-^{32}P]-ATP and 10 mM MgCl$_2$ for 30 min at 30°C (See Ref. 10).

Characterization of Protein Kinase Activity: Effectors and Inhibitors

The phosphorylating associated activity was further characterized with respect to divalent cation and cyclic nucleotide requirements as well as for exogenously added calmodulin and its inhibitors. Mg^{2+} (10 mM) was the preferred divalent cation; Ca^{2+} abolished the incorporation of ^{32}P into polypeptides of partially purified preparations in the absence of Mg^{2+}. Mn^{2+} appeared to partially support protein kinase activity. Neither cyclic AMP nor cyclic GMP was found to be stimulatory. Calmodulin plus Ca^{2+} inhibited the reaction. Similar effects were seen with calmidazolium, chlorpromazine, and trifluoperazine. When the partially purified enzyme was preincubated for 15 min with 5'-p-fluorosulfonylbenzoyl adenosine and the reaction continued in the presence of $[Y-^{32}P]ATP-Mg^{2+}$, phosphorylation did not take place. Neither estradiol nor tamoxifen or its 4-OH derivative added to the reaction changed the rate of autophosphorylation. H7 1-(5-isoquinolinylsulfonyl)-2-methylpiperazine, a protein kinase C inhibitor, did not interfere with the kinase reaction. Using MCF-10 T2 breast cancer cell line (provided by Dr. J. Russo from the Michigan Cancer Foundation, Detroit) exposed in culture to several signaling transduction agents, such as FSH, LH, TPA, E2, or hCG. We demonstrated that only hCG and FSH increase PK autocatalytic activity (Baldi A, Annibali N, unpublished).

Determination of the Amino Acid Specificity of the Kinase Activity

As presented in Figure 2 each of the three polypeptides yielded a major species of ^{32}P-amino acid migrating with phophoserine with only traces of phosphothreonine and phosphotyrosine. Therefore, the kinase activity must be considered a serine kinase.

Protein Kinase Activity Eluted in Components I and II After HPLC Is Distinctly Stimulated by Exogenous Phospholipids

Several methodologies were used to fractionate protein kinase entities according to their physicochemical characteristics. These procedures were based on the technique to separate estrogen-receptor isoforms as depicted in Figure 3A where the PK activity migrate with two receptor components. The kinase reaction was also carried out in the presence of exogenously added phosphatidyl serine and phosphtidyl choline (PS/PC) to test the possibility of a stimulatory effect on kinase activity as has been shown for the C kinases (6). As is shown in Figure 3B and autoradiogram in 3C, there was a slightly stimulatory effect of PS/PC on the total ^{32}P-polypeptides formed as measured by TCA-precipitable radioactivity. However, fractions containing components I and II showed different responses with the addition of phosphatidyl choline/phosphatidyl serine (PS/PC) regarding phosphorylation of the 57, 47, and 43 kDa proteins.

The Protein Kinase Exhibited ATP Binding Site

The protein kinase reaction was performed with the ATP analog fluorosulfonylbenzoyl adenosine, 5'-*p*-[adenine-8-14C] (FSBA), (NEN-DUPONT) 40-60 mCi/mmol with no other modification using as a source of enzyme MCF-7 cells. Analysis of the fluorographed polyacrylamide gel electrophoresis shown in Figure 4 reveals identical subunits compared to those obtained when 32P-ATP was used as phosphate donor.

Concluding Remarks

In this report, a new putative protein kinase was identified from human breast cancer cells. Several criteria differentiate this activity from other kinases described in the literature. Thus, divalent cation requirements for Mg^{2+}, but not Ca^{2+} or Mn^{2+}, were demonstrated. When Mg^{2+} and $[Y-^{32}P]ATP$ were present in a reaction mixture containing immobilized PK, three major ^{32}P-labeled phosphopeptides of M_r 57,000, 47,000, and 43,000 were detected on NaDodSO$_4$-polyacrylamide gel electrophoresis. Phosphorylation occurred on serine residues. The activity was cyclic nucleotide and calmodulin-independent; cAMP at high concentrations (1 mM) inhibited autophosphorylation but 0.5 μM did not. The autophosphorylating reaction was slightly inhibited in the presence of calmidazolium and calmodulin kinase inhibitors such as trifluoperazine and

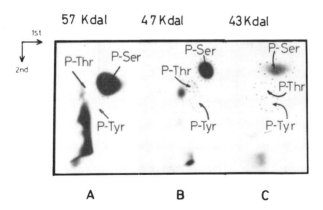

Fig. 2. Right. Phosphoamino acid analysis of autophosphorylated PK subunits from MCF-7 cells. Purified PK was phosphorylated as before and the phosphopeptides resolved by NaDodSO^4-polyacrylamide gel electrophoresis. The three major ^{32}P-peptides were excised individually from the gel and subjected to partial acid hydrolysis as described by Hunter and Sefton (11).

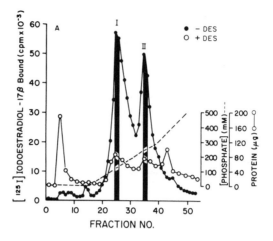

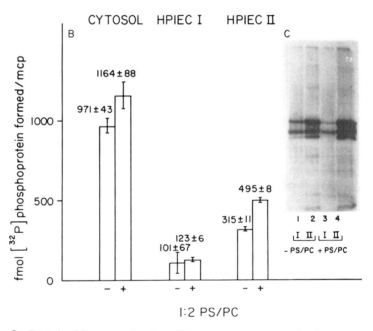

Fig. 3. Protein kinases migrate with estrogen-receptor isoforms on high-performance ion-exchange chromatography (See Ref. 9). Peak fractions used for PK activity are shown as solid bars. These fractions were used after adsorption of PK to solid polystyrene matrix. Panel A: Ion-exchange chromatography analysis of cytosol labeled with ^{125}I-iodoestradiol. Panel B: Quantitation of phosphorylating activity from PK migrating with estrogen isoforms. Panel C: Autoradiogram. Experiments were performed in duplicate. Negative (-) or positive (+) marks indicate the absence or presence of phopholipids in the kinase reaction.

chlorpromazine. When the immobilized kinase was subjected to the disorganizationism phosphorylating assay, but preincubated with 5'-*p*-fluorosulfonylbenzoyl adenosine (an ATP analog that inhibits most PK), kinase activity was abolished. Demonstration of an ATP-binding site is necessary to establish a protein as a kinase. Accordingly, the presence of ATP binding sites on the three kinase subunits (57, 47, and 43 kDa) by labeling with fluorosulfonylbenzoyl-adenosine, 5'-*p*-[adenine-8^{14}C], via perhaps through the covalent modification of lysine residue located at the conserved catalytic core of the enzyme, supports our conclusion that the autophosphorylation associated activity is intrinsic to immobilized PK. We have shown that an agonist ligand (estradiol) or two nonsteroidal antagonists (tamoxifen and 4-OH-tamoxifen) did not change the rate of phosphorylation of the PK in the assay. The importance of these compounds is obvious, since both cell lines used are dependent on estradiol for its growth and for many biochemical events and undergo cell proliferation restriction under antiestrogens (7).

Other characteristics of this enzyme include: the PK was expressed in the "complete" (three subunits) form in breast cancer cells only.   Several fractionation procedures used to partially purify PK indicated that identical methodology is incompatible with other kinase purification. (Results to be published elsewhere). Data from one of such procedures were reported here where the [^{125}I]-labeled estrogen receptor from MCF-7 cells fractionated into two components (I and II) by HPIEC (Fig 3).   Both components showed autophosphorylation associated activity and estrogen binding capacity (8). In addition, component II was stimulated by PS/PC whereas PK isoform I was not. This is especially remarkable since other kinases, recently described as a C-kinase by Nishizuka and co-workers, are stimulated by phospholipids (6). However, a distinct characteristic emerged from this study: Ca^{2+} abolished the

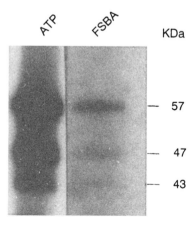

Fig. 4. ATP binding sites lie on the same autophosphorylable PK subunits.

PK described here in the absence of Mg^{2+} ions. C-kinase activity is Ca^{2+}-dependent, indicating that we have not copurified a C-kinase-like enzyme but instead, a new kinase entity. This is also incompatible with the activity of Ca^{2+}-calmodulin-dependent serine kinases (9).

In summary, we have shown a new kinase from human breast cancer cells associated with serine-kinase activity that may be intrinsic to breast cancer cells. The biological significance of the autophosphorylation-associated activity exhibited by this kinase is under extensive study in our laboratory.

References

1. Blackshear PJ, Nairn AC, Kuo JF (1988) Protein Kinases 1988: A current perspective. FASEB J 2:2957-2969.
2. Edelman AM, Krebs EG (1987) Protein serine/threonine kinases. Annu Rev Biochem 56:567-613.
3. Taylor SS (1989) cAMP-dependent protein kinase. J Biol Chem 264:8443-8446.
4. Taylor SS, Buechler JA, Yonemoto W (1990) cAMP-Dependent protein kinase: Framework for a diverse family of regulatory enzymes. Annu Rev Biochem 59:971-1005.
5. Soderling TR (1990) Protein kinases. J Biol Chem 265:1823-1826.
6. Kikkawa U, Kishimoto A, Nishizuka Y (1989) The protein kinase C family: Heterogeneity and its implications. Annu Rev Biochem 58:31-44.
7. Jensen EV, Suzuki T, Kawashima WE, Stumpf WE, Jungblut PW, DeSombre ER (1968) A two-step mechanism for the interaction or estradiol with rat uterus. Proc Natl Acad Sci USA 59:632-638.
8. Boyle DM, Wiehle RD, Shahabi N, Wittliff JL (1985) Rapid high resolution procedure for assessment of estrogen receptor heterogeneity in clinical samples. J Chromatogr 327:369-376.
9. Nairn AC, Hemmings HC, Greengard P (1985) Protein kinases in the brain. Annu Rev Biochem 54:931.
10. Baldi A, Boyle DM, Wittliff JL (1986) Estrogen receptor is associated with protein and phospholipid kinase activities. Biochem Biophys Res Commun 135:597-606.
11. Hunter T, Sefton BM (1980) Transforming gene product of Rous sarcoma virus phosphorylates tyrosine. Proc Natl Acad Sci USA 77:1311-1315.

6

Estrous Cycle Modification of Rat Mammary Carcinoma Induction

Craig W. Beattie and Conwell H. Anderson

Introduction

Mitogenesis, or an increase in cell replication, has been proposed as a major rate-limiting factor in carcinogenesis (1). With respect to breast cancer, excess estrogen has been proposed to lead to increased proliferation of mammary epithelium (2). We have asked the question of whether a hormonally induced alteration(s) in cell proliferation is an integral feature of the multiple rate-limiting events (3) that underlie the chemically induced transformation of normal mammary epithelial cells to their malignant counterparts. Recent observations suggest that the hormonal environment at the time of administration of the direct acting carcinogen methylnitrosourea (MNU) significantly alters the early development and subsequent biology of mammary tumors in the rat without significantly altering the hormonal environment itself (4,5).

Estrous Cycle Dependence of Preneoplastic Lesions

Initial reports suggesting that the rapidity of cellular turnover in relatively undifferentiated rat mammary epithelial structures, such as the terminal end bud or TEB (6), provided additional evidence for the importance of this site in tumor initiation and a logical starting point for investigating the potential impact of a hormonal contribution to mammary cell transformation. The epithelial and myoepithelial cells that comprise the mammary network are clearly able to respond to estrogen(s) relatively early during development. Significant differences exist in mammary epithelial nuclear estrogen-receptor content during the rat estrous or reproductive cycle in 50-55-day-old virgin rats (Table 1). Total nuclear estrogen-receptor content is significantly higher immediately following a preovulatory increase in circulating estradiol during the morning of proestrus and remains elevated over diestrus levels on estrus. Administration of MNU to

65

Table 1. ERN in virgin rat mammary epithelial cells throughout the estrous cycle.

Day of cycle	N	Receptor status	Affinity K_d (10^{-10})	Content fmol/mg DNA
Metestrus	5	Unoccupied	1.9 ± 0.7	45.0 ± 5.1
Diestrus	3	Total	4.2 ± 1.4	41.1 ± 7.5
Proestrus	4	Unoccupied	1.9 ± 0.2	76.5 ± 15.6
	4	Total	1.8 ± 0.2	106.0 ± 10.5[a]
Estrus	5	Unoccupied	2.3 ± 0.1	44.7 ± 3.5
	3	Total	4.1 ± 0.2	64.1 ± 7.5

[a] $p < 0.01$ vs. diestrus.

Table 2. Incidence of MNU-induced abnormalities in rat mammary gland post-MNU injection on proestrus, estrus, and diestrus.

	Hyperplastic Alveolar Abnormalities Nodules (HAN) Cycle day				Ductal and Ductal-Alveolar Hyperplasia Cycle day				TEB Abnormalities Cycle day				Tumors Cycle day				Mean No. per Rat[d]
Week	E	PE	DE	C[a]	E	PE	DE	C	E	PE	DE	C	E	PE	DE	C	E + PE+ DE
1[b]	1	1	0	0	0	0	2	6	3	1	0	0	0	0	0	0	13/6 = 2.2
2	0	1	0	0	0	1	0	0	6	4	1	0	0	0	0	0	13/6 = 2.2
3	3	3	0	0	2	2	1	8	5	1	6	0	0	0	0	0	28/6 = 4.7
4	4	1	0	0	3	3	2	0	1	4	2	1	0	0	0	0	20/6 = 3.3
5	2	0	3	0	9	3	8	2	3	2	1	0	1	0	0	0	33/6 = 5.5
6	8	2	1	2	9	8	5	0	2	0	2	0	0	1	0	0	39/6 = 6.5
Σ[f]	17	8	5	2	23	18	17	3	22	21	10	8	1	1	0	0	
10[c]	1	2	4	0	6	25	14	0	1	4	2	0	1	15	8	0	59/12 = 4.9 24/12[e]= 2.0 Total 6.9
12	4	1	1	0	15	9	15	1	1	0	1	0	8	17	6	0	47/12 =3.9 31/12[e]= 2.6 Total 6.5

[a] Control - saline injected killed randomly
[b] Two animals per week per cycle stage
[c] Four animals per week per cycle stage
[d] Sum of abnormalities in MNU-treated excluding tumors/total no. rats per week per cycle stage.
[e] No. tumor/no. rats.
[f] Summation 1 through 6 weeks.

regularly cycling, 50-55-day-old, virgin, Sprague-Dawley rats results in a significant number of TEB abnormalities in the mammary glands of rats within one week following injection on proestrus and estrus when compared with injection on diestrus, with significantly more carcinomas arising in rats injected on proestrus. (Figure 1 and Table 2). Ductal and ductal-alveolar hyperplasias and hyperplastic alveolar nodules appeared during the third week post-MNU, with the latter most numerous in glands from rats injected on estrus. Adenocarcinomas arose randomly from both the proximal and distal ductal network, not solely as the result of proliferation of individual peripherally located TEBs, by 10-12 weeks post-MNU with significantly more tumors found in rats injected on proestrus than diestrus or estrus. The increased incidence of mammary carcinomas arising from potentially preneoplastic histologic abnormalities on proestrus and estrus suggests the estrous cycle not only influences the site, but the incidence and latency of preneoplastic changes (Figure 2 and Table 2).

Cell Cycle Alterations in Response to Carcinogen

However, it would appear that significant differences in the proliferation rate of cells comprising the TEBs do not underlie the estrous cycle dependent development of preneoplastic hyperplasias, tumor latency, and number (4,5; Table 3). Computer analysis (7) of the time course of [^{3}H]-thymidine incorporation into the mitoses of cells comprising TEB during proestrus, estrus, and diestrus suggests that there was no significant difference in G_1 or S phase, the stages of the cell cycle most susceptible to DNA adduct formation (8) (Table 3). If a physiologic hormonal stimulus modifies the proliferative rate of cells within the structures most likely to be affected by a direct carcinogenic insult, it is not apparent from these observations.

The recovery of cell proliferation within TEBs following carcinogen presentation on proestrus, estrus, or diestrus may be more complex, however (Figure 3). The initial peak of the labeled mitosis wave (LMW) in TEB is significantly extended following MNU irrespective of the time of administration (Figure 3). The extension while no doubt due to a combination of the direct cytotoxic and mutagenic effects of the carcinogen appears significantly longer in rats injected on proestrus relative to diestrus. The second peak of the LMW is also delayed. Full recovery of the LMW takes approximately 48-56 hr and is not dependent on the stage of the estrous cycle on which MNU is administered (Anderson CH, Beattie CW, unpublished). This apparent increase in [^{3}H]-thymidine incorporation into TEB (mitoses) 8-16 hr post-MNU on proestrus relative to diestrus appears associated with a similar and selective quantitative increase in O^6-methylguanine DNA adduct formation 8-25 hr-post-MNU administration on proestrus and estrus relative to diestrus (9). Whether this brief alteration in TEB cell cycle dynamics, as well as those that may be present in terminal ducts and ductal-alveoli, is sufficient to produce the observed differences in tumor development remains to be determined. Although DNA

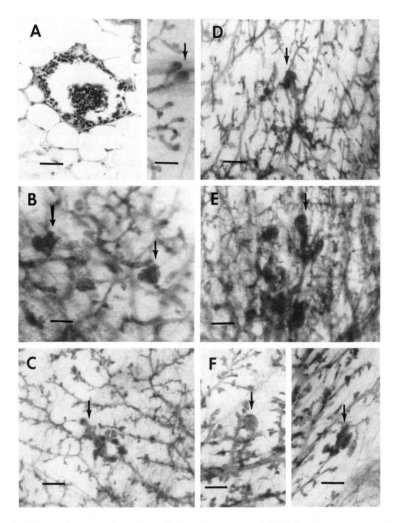

Fig. 1. Photomicrographs of small dysplasias seen in thick wholemount of rat mammary glands after MNU. These are recognized as denser and/or larger structures than surrounding normal tissue. A. Two large TEB in wholemount (arrow right) and a histological section of a TEB (left; scale bar, 40 μm) with intraductal hyperplasia. B, C, and D. Ductal alveolar hyperplasias have both ducts and alveoli out of proportion to normal tissue. E. Ductal hyperplasias show large ducts and dense bulbous endings. F. Two HAN at arrows. Scale bars, 500 μm.

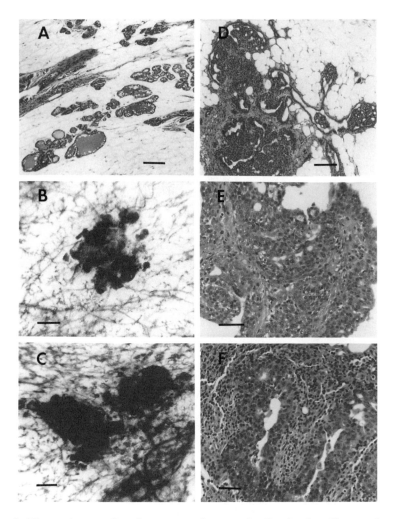

Fig. 2. Photomicrographs of tumors and cysts. A. Cystic alveoli are enlarged and fluid filled, but do not have enhanced cellularity (scale bar, 100 μm). B and C. Two small tumors in wholemounts which are not obviously encapsulated (scale bar, 500 μm), and D. the histology typical of these microtumors (scale bar, 100 μm). E and F. Histological sections of tumors show adenocarcinomas with pleomorphic, multilayered epithelial cells. Lymphocytic invasion is prominent in F (scale bar, 40 μm).

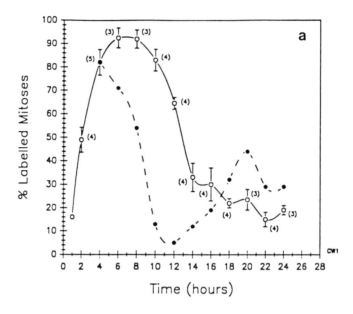

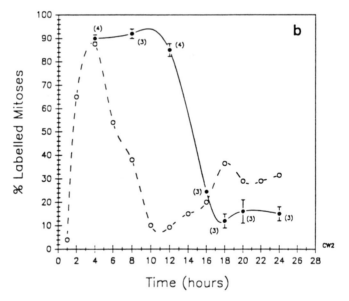

Fig. 3. A. MNU-induced delay in LMW in TEB isolated from rats injected on diestrus. [³H] Thd was injected 1 hr prior to MNU (50 mg/kg iv) and rats killed at the times (post[³H] Thd) shown. Dashed line is the normal LMW on diestrus. B. MNU-induced delay in LMW in TEB isolated from rats on proestrus. Dashed line is the normal LMW on proestrus.

Table 3. Cell cycle parameters of rat mammary gland TEB.

| | Cycle Stage | | |
	Metestrus/ Diestrus	Proestrus	Estrus
Cycle	18.8	19.9	15.4
G_1	10.5	12.1	7.8
S	4.9	4.9	4.3
G_2	1.9	1.5	2.3

replication is essential to the initiation of carcinogenesis and subsequent tumorigenesis (10,11), our observations clearly suggest that any mutagenic effects induced by a carcinogenic (and cytotoxic) dose of MNU that may lead to a higher tumor yield are not likely to be accompanied by a direct, immediate MNU-induced increase in TEB cellular proliferation or tumor promoter-like effects (1). However, it is apparent that, in the rat, physiologic increases in potentially mitogenic hormones may alter the way a direct-acting carcinogen affects cell cycle at those sites that give rise to the preneoplastic lesions and eventual adenocarcinomas of the mammary gland.

If mammary epithelial sensitivity to chemical carcinogenesis, and by inference, the expression of molecules that repair potentially mutagenic lesions in DNA, is directly and solely dependent on a mitogenic stimulus, any increase in repair might be associated with or result from an increase in target cell proliferation. Since each phase of the cell cycle in TEBs appears similar this is probably not the case. However, DNA adducts such as the mutagenic O^6-methylguanine do appear to be increased in rats injected on proestrus (9). Whether this is the result of a quantitative decrease in repair protein(s) in mammary epithelial cells awaits the quantitation of these proteins in mammary epithelial cells at different stages of the estrous cycle prior to carcinogen exposure.

Conclusions

In summary, rats injected with MNU on proestrus and estrus develop abnormal TEB sooner and in greater number than rats injected on diestrus. These results, while supporting the theory that the hormonal environment at the time of MNU administration significantly alters early development of mammary tumors in the rat, also clearly suggest that a significant estrous cycle induced in the increased proliferation rate of cells comprising TEBs is not responsible for those developmental differences.

Acknowledgments

Supported by NCI 5 R01 CA45355-03. The authors thank A. Shilkaitis for preparing the micrographs and D. Gardner for manuscript preparation.

References

1. Ames BN, LS Gold (1990) Too many rodent carcinogens: Mitogenesis increases mutagenesis. Science 249:970-971.
2. Henderson BE, Ross R, Bernstein L (1988) Estrogens as a cause of human cancer. Cancer Res 48:246-253.
3. Weinstein IB (1988) The origins of human cancer: molecular mechanisms of carcinogenesis and their implication for cancer prevention and treatment. Cancer Res 48:4135-4143.
4. Braun RJ, Pezzuto JM, Anderson CH, et al (1989) Estrous cycle status alters N-methyl-N-nitrosourea (NMU) induced rat mammary tumor growth and regression. Cancer Lett 48:205-211.
5. Anderson CH, Hussain RA, Han HC, et al (1991) Estrous cycle dependence of nitrosomethylurea (NMU)-induced preneoplastic lesions in rat mammary gland. Cancer Lett 56:77-84.
6. Russo J, Russo IH (1980) Influence of differentiation and cell kinetics on the susceptibility of the rat mammary gland to carcinogenesis. Cancer Res 40:2677-2687.
7. Steel GG (1977) In Growth kinetics of tumors. Clarendon Press, Oxford, pp. 120-146.
8. Kaufmann WK, Kaufman DG, Rice JM, et al (1981) Reversible inhibition of rat hepatocyte to proliferation by hydrocortisone and its effect on cell cycle-dependent hepatocarcinogenesis by N-methyl-N-nitrosourea. Cancer Res 41:4653-4660.
9. Ratko TA, Braun RJ, Pezzuto JM et al (1988) Estrous cycle modification of rat mammary gland DNA alkylation by N-methyl-N-nitrosourea. Cancer Res 48:3090-3093.
10. Warwick GP (1971) Effect of the cell cycle on carcinogenesis. Fed Proc 30:1760-1765.
11. Bertram JS, Heidelberger C (1974) Cell cycle dependence of oncogenic transformation induced by N-methyl-N'-nitro-N-nitrosoguanidine in culture. Cancer Res 34:526-537.

7

Hormones, Cell Proliferation, and Mammary Carcinogenesis

Satyabrata Nandi, Raphael C. Guzman, and Shigeki Miyamoto

Introduction

Cell proliferation in tissues and organs is essential to carcinogenesis (1). The classical hormones from ovary, adrenal cortex, and anterior pituitary have been shown to be essential for cell proliferation in the mammary glands, as well as for the carcinogenesis induced in mammary epithelial cells (MEC) by viruses, radiation, and chemical carcinogens. However, this does not explain the origin of the various precancerous and cancerous lesions observed in the mammary glands of rodents and of humans, nor does it explain the mechanisms by which the observed hormonal actions occur.

One of the chief interests of our laboratory has been the analysis of the role of mitogenic factors, including hormones, in the normal to neoplastic transformation. We have also concerned ourselves with the genesis of the various lesions observed in the mammary glands of mice, rats, and humans exposed to endogenous and exogenous carcinogens. Such studies are inherently difficult to accomplish in the complex *in vivo* environment, where many variables are difficult to control. Thus, during the last 12 years, we have been developing an *in vitro* collagen matrix culture system which allows 3-dimensional growth of MEC under serum-free, defined conditions.

Our studies thus far indicate that MEC, proliferating in 3-dimensional patterns under these culture conditions, maintain many of their *in vivo*-like characteristics even after prolonged growth *in vitro*. These characteristics include cellular polarity, the ability to respond to mammogenic hormones, and the ability to synthesize casein, both in culture and after transplantation, back into a host animal.

Utilizing this system, we have begun to analyze the role of hormonal and nonhormonal agents on MEC proliferation and on the chemical carcinogen-induced transformation of virgin adult mouse MECs. In the following discussion, we summarize current findings that have allowed us to form a working hypothesis concerning the role of the classical hormones on mammary gland proliferation, as well as the genesis of various lesions in this gland. For

73

the sake of brevity, this report is confined largely to the work of our own laboratory.

Cell Proliferation

During the last 60 years, mammary cell proliferation has been studied with a variety of *in vivo* and *in vitro* methods in rodents (2,3), clearly establishing multihormonal requirements as well as dependencies upon the stromal components of the fat pad for MEC proliferation *in vivo* during different physiological states. Recent studies have implicated growth factors and extracellular matrix components as well (2,4-6).

Using our collagen matrix culture system, we have studied agents causing proliferation of MEC from adult virgin BALB/c female mice. The following summarizes our findings to date: (1) Insulin or IGF-1 must be present for any mitogen to result in proliferation *in vitro*. (2) Hormones (e.g. progesterone, corticosterone, prolactin) that are mammogenic *in vivo* are also mitogenic *in vitro*. (3) Estrogen is neither mitogenic nor shows any additive or synergistic effects with other mitogens, but estrogen can induce progesterone receptors *in vitro*. (4) A variety of growth factors and nonhormonal agents stimulate MEC proliferation *in vitro*. (5) All mitogens (including the classical hormones) can be classified into three groups according to mode of action. Group 1 consists of factors (including prolactin, progesterone, corticosterone, aldosterone, EGF, Basic FGF, and TGFα) that require specific receptors for their action. Group 2 consists of various diffusible agents (c-AMP, lithium ion [Li$^+$], 12-*O*-tetradecanoylphorbol-13-acetate [TPA], dilinoleoyl phosphatidic acid [18:2 PA] and dilinoleoyl phosphatidic serine). Group 3 contains agents (such as linoleic acid and its metabolites) called "comitogens," causing proliferation of MECs only when combined with factors from Groups 1 or 2.

All the agents mentioned above, except for TPA, allow the proliferation of luminal epithelial cells that are capable of producing casein in the presence of insulin, cortisol, and prolactin. The response of MECs to diffusible agents that are neither hormones nor peptide growth factors suggests the existence of intracellular signal transduction pathways separate from the receptor-mediated pathways. At present, we believe that multiple growth-regulating pathways are probably operative in different physiological states and/or different parts of the mammary tree.

Cell Transformation

Our goal was to develop an *in vitro* transformation system of high efficiency that would parallel events in mice subjected to chemical carcinogens *in vivo*. *In vivo* studies (7,8) show the development of ductal hyperplasias (DHs) in virgin mice subjected to chemical carcinogens. On transplantation into cleared fat pads of syngeneic hosts, these DHs develop into tumors. In contrast, pituitary-isografted mice given the same carcinogens develop hyperplastic alveolar nodules (HANs) predominately, as well as direct tumors that are not preceded by identifiable preneoplastic states. Like DHs, HANs give rise to tumors following transplantation.

Using our collagen matrix culture system, we have reported (9-11) successful tranformations of MECs from adult virgin BALB/c mice when these cells were exposed *in vitro* to *N*-nitroso-*N*-methyl urea (MNU) in the presence of a variety of mitogens. These results, along with some of our recent unpublished work, are summarized here.

(1) *In vivo*-like DHs, HANs, and direct tumors were observed following exposure of MECs *in vitro* to MNU. (2) DHs were the predominant lesions observed in the presence of the mitogens EGF and FGF. (3) HANs and direct tumors were the predominant lesions in MECs exposed to MNU in media containing progesterone + prolactin or lithium. (4) Most HANs and tumors induced by MNU in the presence of progesterone + prolactin contained an activated K-*ras* with G to A transitional mutation in the 12th codon. This oncogene activtion has not been detected in lesions induced in the presence of other mitogens. (5) The highest incidence of lesions occurred in MECs exposed to MNU in the presence of the mitogens progesterone + prolactin or lithium. The proliferative potential of mitogens were as follows: Li^+ ~ bFGF > EGF > progesterone + prolactin.

Finally, in a recent *in vivo* experiment, we observed that pituitary-isografted BALB/c mice treated with a single dose of MNU developed a high incidence of HANs and direct tumors. Most of these lesions contained activated K-*ras* mutations similar to those observed in the lesions induced *in vitro* with MNU in the presence of progesterone + prolactin. These results suggest: (1) MEC can be transformed *in vitro* to preneoplastic and neoplastic states similar to those found *in vivo*. (2) Mitogen-induced cell proliferation is essential for tranformation, but there is not a direct correlation between the degree of cell proliferation and the incidence of transformation. (3) The mitogenic environment around the time of carcinogen exposure probably determines the incidence, phenotype, and the nature of oncogene activation in the induced lesions.

The notion that the type of mitogen determines the frequency and phenotype of tranformants could be derived only through our use of primary MEC in serum-free defined media. This exciting possibility may have far-reaching influence on our thinking about the regulation of proliferation in MECs from different parts of the mammary tree, as well as the origins of different types of mammary lesions.

Working Hypothesis

A major question is why there are so many different types of lesions in the mammary glands of animals and humans. We now think that different parts of the mammary tree respond to different mitogens. At the same time, it is the mitogenic environment, the nature of the carcinogen, and the time of exposure of the MECs to carcinogens that determines the phenotype of the mammary lesions. This correlates well with current findings from several laboratories which show that different parts of the mammary tree respond to different hormones and mitogens and also show differences in the nature of growth factors produced (3,5,12-14).

The roles of classical hormones (estrogen, progesterone, prolactin, etc.) in MEC proliferation and in the determination of the frequency and pheontype of lesions appear to be quite complex. We now think that hormones are the upstream regulators of MEC proliferation, and that they also stimulate different parts of the mammary tree and of the stromal components to produce different growth factors. These factors in turn act locally either as autocrine or paracrine factors, singly or in conjunction with the classical hormones, to stimulate proliferation of MEC at different parts of the mammary tree and at different physiological states.

Conclusions

Although we are still far from a complete understanding of the mechanisms involved, we have made much progress in determining the role of hormones in the proliferation and transformations of mouse MEC. Without the development of our *in vitro* collagen matrix culture system and the serum-free media for studies of epithelial cells *in vitro*, much of this progress would not have been possible. Exciting work can now be undertaken, using these *in vitro* techniques, to analyze and elucidate the cellular alterations associated with the genesis of various mammary lesions, as well as of the genetic events associated with these changes.

Acknowledgments

This work was supported by Grants CA-05388, CA-40160, and CA-09041 awarded by the National Institutes of Health, Department of Health and Human Services.

References

1. Preston-Martin S, Pike MG, Ross RK, Jones PA, Henderson BE (1990) Increased cell division as a cause of human cancer. Cancer Res 50:7415-7421.
2. Imagawa W, Bandyopadhyay GK, Nandi S (1991) Regulation of mammary epithelial cell growth in mice and rats. Endo Rev 11:494-523.
3. Daniel CW, Silberstein GB (1987) Postnatal development of the rodent mammary gland. In: Neville, M. C., Daniel, C. W. (eds) The Mammary Gland: Development, Regulation and Function. Plenum Publishing Corp., New York, pp. 3-36.

4. Levay-Young BK, Imagawa W, Yang J, Richards JE, Guzman RC, Nandi S (1987) Primary culture system for mammary biology studies. In: Medina D, Kidwell W, Heppner G, Anderson E. (eds) Cellular and Molecular Biology of Mammary Cancer. Plenum Publishing Corp., New York. pp. 181-203.

5. Yang J, Nandi S (1983) Growth of cultured cells using collagen as substrate. Int Rev Cytol 81:249-286.

6. Snedeker SM, Brown CF, DiAugustine RP (1991) Expression and functional properties of transforming growth factor α and epidermal growth factor during mouse mammary gland ductal morphogenesis. Proc Nat Acad Sci USA 88:276-280.

7. Medina D (1974) Mammary tumorigenesis in carcinogen-treated mice. II. Dependence on hormone stimulation for tumorigenesis. J Nat Cancer Inst 53:223-226.

8. Medina D, Warner MR (1978) Mammary tumorigenesis in chemical carcinogen-treated mice. IV. Induction of mammary ductal hyperplasia. J Nat Cancer Inst 47:331-337.

9. Guzman RC, Osborn RC, Bartley JC, Imagawa W, Asch BB, Nandi S (1987) *In vitro* transformation of mouse mammary epithelial cells grown serum-free inside collagen gels. Cancer Res 47:275-280.

10. Miyamoto S, Guzman RC, Osborn RC, Nandi S. (1988) Neoplastic transformation of mouse mammary epithelial cells by *in vitro* exposure to N-methyl-N-nitrosourea. Proc Nat Acad Sci USA 85:447-481.

11. Miyamoto S, Sukumar S, Guzman RC, Osborn RC, Nandi S (1990) Transforming C-K-*ras* mutation is an early event in mouse mammary carcinogenesis induced *in vitro* by *N*-methyl-*N*-nitrosourea. Mol Cell Biol 10:1593-1599.

12. Bresciani F (1968) Topography of DNA synthesis in the mammary gland of the C3H mouse and its control by ovarian hormones: an autoradiographic study. Cell and Tissue Kinet 1:51-63.

13. Du Bois M, Elias JJ (1984) Subpopulations of cells in immature mouse mammary gland as detected by proliferative responses to hormones in organ culture. Dev Biol 106:70-75.

14. Liscia DS, Merlo G, Ciardiello F, Kim N, Smith GH, Callahan R, Solomon DS (1990) Transforming growth factor—α messenger RNA localization in the developing adult rat and human mammary gland by *in situ* hybridization. Dev Biol 140:123-131.

PART 3. ESTROGEN METABOLISM AND CARCINOGENICITY

INTRODUCTION

Factors Influencing the Metabolism and Action of Estradiol

Allan H. Conney, Lisa A. Suchar, Shuzo Okumura, and Richard L. Chang

The mechanism(s) of carcinogenesis by estradiol and other estrogens is unknown. A direct stimulatory effect of estradiol on proliferation and growth of target tissues as well as the metabolism of estrogens to chemically reactive intermediates that covalently bind to critical cellular targets are possible early steps in the carcinogenic process.

Inhibition of Metabolism-Mediated Covalent Binding of Estradiol to Protein

Incubation of estradiol with hepatic enzymes results in the formation of water-soluble metabolites and protein-bound adducts (1,2). Although estradiol and estrone are metabolized extensively to protein-bound products, either small amounts or no DNA bound adducts are formed (3,4). The available evidence suggests that catechol estrogens and the corresponding o-quinone-semiquinones are metabolic intermediates in the formation of protein-bound adducts (2,5). In addition, recent studies have shown that 16α-hydroxyestrone can covalently bind to cellular proteins including the estrogen receptor (6).

The castrated male hamster is susceptible to estrogen-induced kidney and liver tumorigenesis (7). In accord with an inhibitory effect of ascorbic acid on the liver microsomal metabolism of estradiol to protein-bound products (5), high-dietary ascorbic acid has been reported to inhibit estrogen-induced tumorigenesis in the hamster (8). These results suggest that metabolism-mediated covalent binding of estradiol may play a role in estradiol-induced carcinogenesis. We recently found that ascorbyl palmitate (lipophilic derivative of ascorbic acid) and tannic acid (polyphenolic plant substance) are more potent than ascorbic acid as inhibitors of metabolism-mediated covalent binding of estradiol to protein (Figure 1). We also found that a mixture of polyphenolic compounds in green tea has a strong inhibitory effect on the metabolism-mediated covalent binding

81

of estradiol to protein (unpublished). It would be of interest to determine whether these substances and other naturally occurring polyphenolic antioxidants commonly ingested in our diet have an inhibitory effect on estrogen-induced tumorigenesis.

Complex Metabolism of Estradiol by Liver Microsomes

We recently developed an HPLC system for separating a large number of potential metabolites of estradiol (9), and we have used this HPLC system for studying the NADPH-dependent metabolism of estradiol by liver microsomes from castrated male hamsters. Although metabolites with the chromatographic mobility of estrone, 2-hydroxyestradiol, 4-hydroxyestradiol, and 16α-hydroxyestradiol (most frequently observed microsomal metabolites of estradiol) were found, more than ten additional metabolites were also observed. The results of our studies indicate that the metabolism of estradiol by liver microsomes from the castrated male hamster is very complex. Although considerable attention has focused on the possible role of 16α-hydroxyestradiol (possesses estrogenic activity), 16α-hydroxyestrone (possesses estrogenic activity and forms protein adducts) and the estrogen catechols (nonestrogenic intermediates that form protein adducts) in the carcinogenic process, more research is needed on the biological activities of these and the many other metabolites of estradiol.

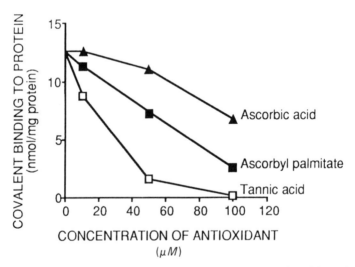

Fig. 1. Effect of ascorbic acid, ascorbyl palmitate, and tannic acid on the liver microsomal metabolism of estradiol to protein-bound adducts.   Liver microsomes (1 mg protein) from castrated male hamsters were incubated for 30 min at 37°C in the presence of [4-^{14}C] estradiol (50 μM), NADPH (1 mM), Tris-HCl buffer (pH 7.4; 150 mM) and inhibitor (10-100 μM) in a final volume of 5 ml.

Factors Influencing the 2- and 16α-Hydroxylation of Estradiol

The levels of microsomal cytochrome P-450 enzymes that metabolize xenobiotics, endogenous estrogens, and other steroid hormones are influenced by life-style, treatment with drugs, environmental chemicals, and by dietary changes (10). The induction by phenobarbital of increased levels of hepatic monooxygenases, which metabolize estradiol and estrone in rats, is associated with enhanced *in vivo* estrogen metabolism and with a decreased uterotropic action of estradiol and estrone (10). Cigarette smoking, treatment with indole-3-carbinol (present in cruciferous vegetables), as well as increasing the ratio of protein to carbohydrate in the diet increases the 2-hydroxylation of estradiol in humans, whereas obesity, high-fat diets, hypothyroidism, and cimetidine therapy are associated with decreased 2-hydroxylation (11,12).

Recent studies suggest that an increased ratio of 2- to 16α-hydroxylation of estradiol may be associated with a decreased risk for breast cancer in mice and with a decreased risk of endometrial and breast cancer in women. Treatment of female C3H/OuJ mice with indole-3-carbinol stimulates the hepatic 2-hydroxylation of estradiol and decreases the development of spontaneous breast tumors (13). Women with breast or endometrial cancer have been reported to have enhanced 16α-hydroxylase activity (14). High rates of hepatic 16α-hydroxylation are associated with an increased incidence of breast tumors in several mouse strains (15). In addition, cigarette smoking stimulates the 2-hydroxylation of estradiol in women (11), and cigarette smokers have a decreased risk for endometrial cancer and an increased risk for osteomalacia (16,17). These are changes in disease patterns that are associated with decreased estrogen action. Treatment of rodents with dioxin enhances the 2-hydroxylation of estradiol (18) and reduces the incidence of tumors in estrogen-responsive tissues, such as the pituitary, uterus, breast, and adrenal gland (19). Preliminary studies suggest that women exposed to dioxin from the chemical plant explosion at Seveso, Italy, may have a decreased risk for breast cancer (20). The results of these studies suggest a need for further research to fully explore the relationship between estrogen-induced cancers and the pathways of estrogen metabolism and to determine whether increasing the ratio of 2- to 16α-hydroxylation of estradiol will decrease the risk for endometrial and breast cancer in women with a high risk for developing these tumors.

Acknowledgments

We thank the Schering-Plough Corporation and Kyowa Hakko Kogyo Co., Ltd. for their help in the support of these studies. Partial support for these studies also came from NIH Grant CA-49756. We thank Deborah Bachorik and Diana Lim for their help in the preparation of this manuscript.

References

1. Riegel IL, Mueller GC (1954) Formation of a protein-bound metabolite of estradiol-16-C^{14} by rat liver homogenates. J Biol Chem 210:249-257.
2. Marks F, Hecker E (1969) Metabolism and mechanism of action of oestrogens. XII. Structure and mechanism of formation of water-soluble and protein-bound metabolites of oestrone in rat-liver microsomes *in vitro* and *in vivo*. Biochim Biophys Acta 187:250-265.
3. Caviezel M, Lutz WK, Minini U, et al (1984) Interaction of estrone and estradiol with DNA and protein of liver and kidney in rat and hamster *in vivo* and *in vitro*. Arch Toxicol 55:97-103.
4. Brueggemeier RW, Kimball JG, Kraft F (1984) Estrogen metabolism in rat liver microsomal and isolated hepatocyte preparations-I. Metabolite formation and irreversible binding to cellular macromolecules. Biochem Pharmacol 33:3853-3859.
5. Haaf H, Li SA, Li JJ (1987) Covalent binding of estrogen metabolites to hamster liver microsomal proteins: inhibition by ascorbic acid and catechol-O-methyl transferase. Carcinogenesis 8:209-215.
6. Swaneck GE, Fishman J (1988) Covalent binding of the endogenous estrogen 16α-hydroxyestrone to estradiol receptor in human breast cancer cells: characterization and intracellular localization. Proc Natl Acad Sci USA 85:7831-7835.
7. Li JJ, Li SA (1987) Estrogen carcinogenesis in Syrian hamster tissues: role of metabolism. Fed Proc 46:1858-1863.
8. Liehr JG, Roy D, Gladek A (1989) Mechanism of inhibition of estrogen-induced renal carcinogenesis in male Syrian hamsters with vitamin C. Carcinogenesis 10:1983-1988.
9. Suchar LA, Chang RL, Conney AH (1991) HPLC method for the separation of estradiol metabolites formed by rat liver microsomes. First International Symposium on Hormonal Carcinogenesis, Cancun, Mexico.
10. Conney AH (1982) Induction of microsomal enzymes by foreign chemicals and carcinogenesis by polycyclic aromatic hydrocarbons: GHA Clowes Memorial Lecture. Cancer Res 42:4875-4917.
11. Michnovicz JJ, Fishman J (1990) Increased oxidative metabolism of oestrogens in male and female smokers. In: Wald N, Baron J. Smoking and Hormone Related Disorders. Oxford University Press 197-207.
12. Michnovicz JJ, Bradlow L (1990) Dietary and pharmacological control of estradiol metabolism in humans. Ann NY Acad Sci 595:291-299.
13. Bradlow HL, Michnovicz JJ, Telang NT, et al. Effects of dietary indole-3-carbinol on estradiol metabolism and spontaneous mammary tumors in mice. Submitted for publication.
14. Fishman J, Schneider J, Hershcopf RJ, et al (1984) Increased estrogen 16α-hydroxylase activity in women with breast and endometrial cancer. J Steroid Biochem 20:1077-1081.

15. Bradlow HL, Hershcopf RJ, Martucci CP, et al (1985) Estradiol 16α-hydroxylation in the mouse correlates with mammary tumor incidence and presence of murine mammary tumor virus: A possible model for the hormonal etiology of breast cancer in humans. Proc Natl Acad Sci USA 82:6295-6299.

16. Lesko SM, Rosenberg L, Kaufman DW, et al (1985) Cigarette smoking and the risk of endometrial cancer. N Engl J Med 313:593-596.

17. Baron JA, LaVecchia C, Levi F (1990) The antiestrogenic effect of cigarette smoking in women. Am J Obstet Gynecol 162:502-514.

18. Graham MJ, Lucier GW, Linko P (1988) Increases in cytochrome P-450 mediated 17β-estradiol 2-hydroxylase activity in rat liver microsomes after both acute administration and subchronic administration of 2,3,7,8-tetrachlorodibenzo-p-dioxin in a two-stage hepatocarcinogenesis model. Carcinogenesis 9:1935-1941.

19. Kociba RJ, Keyes DG, Beyer JE, et al (1978) Results of a two-year chronic toxicity and oncogenicity study of 2,3,7,8-tetrachlorodibenzo-p-dioxin in rats. Toxicol Appl Pharmacol 46:279-303.

20. Bertazzi PA, Zocchetti C, Pesatori AC, et al (1989) Ten-year mortality study of the population involved in the Seveso incident in 1976. Am J Epidemiol 129:1187-1200.

8

Interactions of Carcinogenic Estrogens with Microtubular Proteins

Manfred Metzler, Erika Pfeiffer, Werner Köhl, and Robert Schnitzler

Introduction

Although the carcinogenic effects of certain estrogens, including the endogenous steroid estradiol-17ß (E_2) and the synthetic stilbene estrogen diethylstilbestrol (DES), have been amply demonstrated in various animal species (1), the mechanisms of estrogen carcinogenicity remain elusive. It is generally accepted that estrogens stimulate cell proliferation in target tissues and may thereby act as tumor promoters. However, the question of whether carcinogenic estrogens are able to cause genetic damage and act as initiators of neoplasia is still a matter of debate.

Recent studies with a series of steroidal and stilbene estrogens in the male Syrian golden hamster have shown that high hormonal activity is a prerequisite but does not suffice for the induction of renal tumors, as some strong estrogens proved to be weakly carcinogenic or even noncarcinogenic in this animal model (2,3). Both steroidal and stilbene estrogens have been shown to undergo oxidative biotransformation involving reactive electrophilic intermediates (4). Therefore, it has been proposed that metabolic activation may play an important role in the mechanism of estrogen-mediated carcinogenesis (3-5)

Part of the reluctance to consider estrogens as tumor initiators may be due to the fact that these compounds do not readily form DNA adducts and fail to induce DNA damage and gene mutations in bacterial or mammalian cells (6). However, recent studies in Syrian hamster embryo (SHE) cells *in vitro* have shown that carcinogenic estrogens act as chromosomal mutagens, leading to near-diploid aneuploidy (7,8). The induction of numerical chromosomal aberrations has been proposed as a genetic event underlying the estrogen-mediated neoplastic transformation of SHE cells.

This hypothesis has stimulated our interest in the biochemical mechanisms of aneuploidy induction by estrogens. The present paper reports on the covalent and noncovalent binding of estrogens of diverse structures to microtubular proteins (MTPs), the role of metabolic activation in this binding, and the effect of estrogen/MTP interaction on microtubule (MT) assembly. Data on the induction of micronuclei by various steroidal and stilbene estrogens in SHE and other cells *in vitro* are also provided.

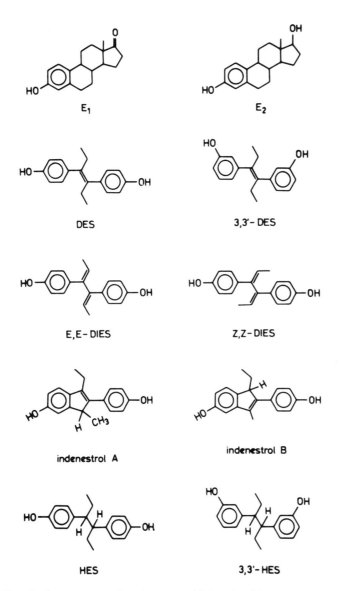

Fig. 1. Chemical structures of various steroidal and stilbene estrogens.

Estrogens, Cell Transformation, and Peroxidative Metabolism

When the steroidal estrogens estrone (E_1), E_2, and estriol (E_3) were tested together with their 2- and 4-hydroxy derivatives (chemical structures, see Fig. 1), the catechol compounds, although weaker estrogens, were more potent transforming agents than the parent molecules (9). Similarly, in a series of structurally related stilbene estrogens, there was no correlation between estrogenicity and potency for cell transformation (10). For example, the powerful estrogens E,E-dienestrol (E,E-DIES) and erythro-hexestrol (erythro-HES, chemical structures, see Fig. 1) were poor transformants. Rather than estrogenicity, a structure allowing peroxidative metabolism to a quinoid intermediate appeared to be important for cell transformation. Such structural features included the catechol group in steroidal estrogens and the stilbene double bond and two free hydroxy groups located in para-position at the aromatic rings in stilbene estrogens (Fig. 2).

Peroxidative metabolism of DES to Z,Z-dienestrol (Z,Z-DIES) through DES-4',4"-quinone has been demonstrated in SHE cells and is most likely mediated by prostaglandin-H-synthase (11).

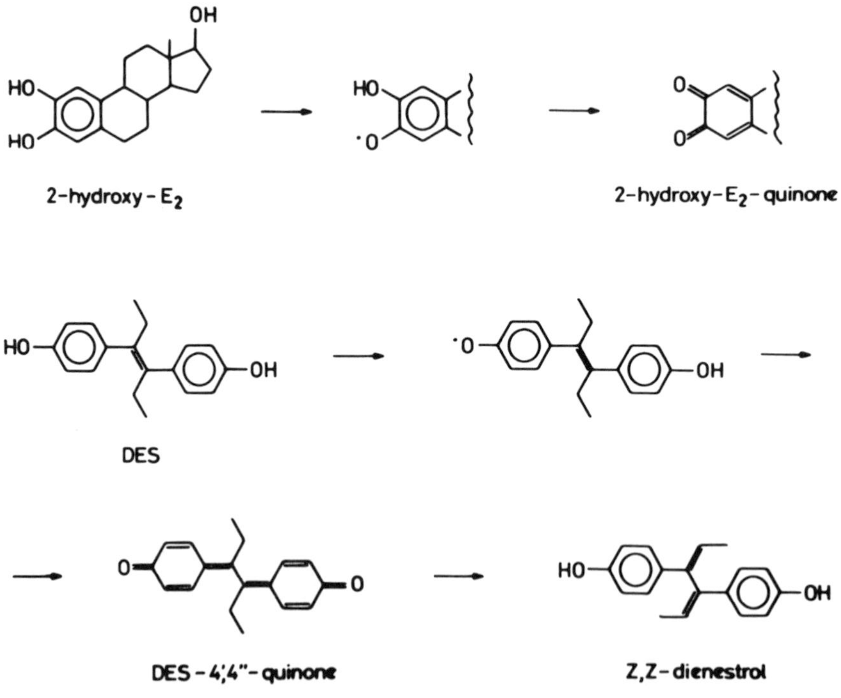

Fig. 2. Peroxidase-mediated quinone formation of steroidal catechol estrogens and stilbene estrogens.

The importance of the quinone pathway is supported by the observation (12) that 3,3'-DES and indenestrol B (see Fig. 1), both of which cannot form quinones, are devoid of SHE cell transforming activity, in contrast to indenestrol A, which is readily oxidized to the respective quinone.

Inhibition of MT Assembly Under Cell-Free Conditions

Following the observation of several investigators (13) that DES can interfere with the polymerization of microtubular proteins (MTP) to microtubules (MT) in a cell-free system, we have previously reported that the quinones of DES and indenestrol A are powerful inhibitors of MT assembly (13,14).

We have now tested a series of steroidal and stilbene estrogens both without and with peroxidase-mediated activation for inhibition of MT polymerization *in vitro* (see Pfeiffer and Metzler, this volume). In the absence of peroxidative oxidation, neither E_1 and E_2 nor their 2- and 4-hydroxy metabolites caused any inhibition of MT assembly. However, all catechol estrogens, but not the parent steroids E_1 and E_2, proved to be strong inhibitors after oxidation to quinone metabolites. For stilbene estrogens, the results were less straightforward. Even without metabolic activation, an inhibitory effect on MT polymerization was observed with all the stilbenes studied, although to a varying degree. Some stilbene estrogens prone to quinone formation, e.g., indenestrol A and 3'-, 5'-, 3"-, 5"-tetrafluoro-DES, were poor inhibitors without peroxidative oxidation

Table 1. Decrease in free sulfhydryl groups of MTP and inhibition of MT assembly. Compounds marked with * were oxidized to quinones prior to incubation with MTP. Sulfhydryl groups were determined with Ellman's reagent.

Compound	Concentration	Sulfhydryl groups lost per tubulin dimer	Inhibition
2-Hydroxy-E_2*	40 μM	1.3	48%
	80 μM	2.0	100%
E-DES*	40 μM	0.0	39%
	80 μM	0.0	100%
p-Benzoquinone	20 μM	1.0	46%
N-Ethylmaleimide	10 μM	0.35	16%

but became powerful inhibitors after oxidation. Thus, our results with steroidal and stilbene estrogens support the notion that peroxidase-mediated quinone formation is important for the inhibition of MT polymerization and possibly also for aneuploidy induction.

Covalent Binding of Quinone Metabolites to MTP

Previous investigations with radioactively labeled compounds have shown that DES, indenestrol A, 2-hydroxy-E_2, and 2-hydroxy-EE_2, but not HES, E_2, and EE_2, bind covalently to MTP after peroxidase-mediated activation (14,15). Covalent binding to MTP occurred more avidly than to bovine serum albumin, suggesting functional groups in MTP with a high reactivity toward the quinone intermediates. According to polyacrylamide electrophoresis followed by autoradiography, ß-tubulin was the component of MTP with the preferential binding.

In our recent study (Pfeiffer and Metzler, this volume), covalent binding of the 2- and 4-hydroxy derivatives of E_1 and E_2 after peroxidative activation was detected by UV spectroscopy. Both the quinone intermediates of the catechol estrogens and their MTP adducts gave rise to characteristic UV absorbances.

The binding to MTP of the quinones derived from 2-hydroxy-E_2 and from DES was studied in more detail. MTP was incubated with oxidized 2-hydroxy-E_2 and DES at various concentrations, and the sulfhydryl groups of MTP were determined by titration with Ellman's reagent (16) (5,5'-dithiobis[2-nitrobenzoic acid]) before and after reaction with the quinones (Table 1). In addition, the inhibition of MT assembly caused by the quinones was determined. p-Benzoquinone and N-ethylmaleimide were included in this study for comparison (Table 1). At concentrations leading to 50% inhibition of MT polymerization, 2-hydroxy-E_2 and p-benzoquinone, but not DES, led to a decrease in the number of free sulfhydryl groups in MTP by one per tubulin dimer. This suggests that the quinone of 2-hydroxy-E_2 but not of DES, binds covalently to a cysteine moiety in MTP.

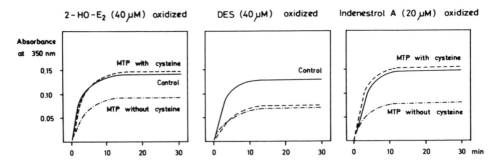

Fig. 3. Effect of cysteine on the inhibition of MT assembly by quinones of different steroidal and stilbene estrogens.

The notion that sulfhydryl groups are implicated in the MTP binding of 2-hydroxy-E_2 quinone is supported by the finding that addition of cysteine to the quinone prior to incubation with MTP completely prevented the inhibition of MT assembly (Fig. 3, left panel). With DES quinone, cysteine had no such effect (Fig. 3, center panel), whereas the quinone of indenestrol A could obviously be trapped with cysteine, according to the result of the MT assembly study (Fig. 3, right panel).

Binding to Tubulin vs. Microtubule-Associated Proteins

MTP consists of dimers of α- and ß-tubulin (about 85%) and of several microtubule-associated proteins (MAPs, 15%). It can be separated into fractions containing tubulin dimers and the predominating MAPs (MAP-1 and MAP-2) by chromatography on phosphocellulose. As both tubulin and MAPs contain sulfhydryl groups, it is conceivable that both MTP components react with quinones. The question then arises which of these quinone adducts is relevant for the inhibition of MT assembly.

When purified tubulin and MAPs were separately incubated with the peroxidation products of 2-hydroxy-E_2, it was indeed observed by UV spectroscopy that the quinone reacted with both protein fractions. After adding cysteine to trap any excess of the quinone, the quinone adduct of tubulin (tubulin-Q) was reconstituted with untreated MAPs, and the quinone adduct of the MAPs (MAP-Q) was combined with untreated tubulin at a ratio corresponding to that of MTP. When the polymerization of these reconstituted systems was measured (Table 2), it turned out that tubulin-Q but not MAP-Q had an inhibitory effect on MT assembly. The extent of inhibition in the reconstituted

Table 2. Effect of quinone adduct formation with tubulin and MAPs on MT polymerization. 2-Hydroxy-E_2 (40 μM) was oxidized with horseradish peroxidase/H_2O_2 to its quinone Q. Aliquots were then incubated with tubulin and MAPs at 37°C for 20 min. The concentration of the quinone corresponded to 40 μM 2-hydroxy-E_2. Cysteine (200 μM) was added to trap unreacted Q, and the adduct solutions were reconstituted with untreated material to obtain a mixture of 85% tubulin and 15% MAPs. Assembly of MT was compared to control consisting of untreated tubulin and MAPs.

System	MT Polymerization (%)
Tubulin + MAPs	100
Tubulin-Q + MAPs	67
Tubulin + MAPs-Q	102

system was about the same as in intact MTPs at this concentration of 2-hydroxy-E_2.

Induction of Micronuclei in Cultured Cells

Binding to MTP and inhibition of MT assembly under cell-free conditions indicate the potential of a compound to act as an aneuploidogen. In intact cells, however, this potential may or may not be expressed. For example, it is conceivable that cells lack the enzymatic capability for metabolic activation or lead to a rapid inactivation of the compound. Therefore it is crucial to study the aneuploidogenic effects in cells *in vitro*. So far, this has been done for only a few stilbene and steroidal estrogens, mostly in SHE cells (6-8).

Although SHE cells are capable of peroxidative metabolism, this enzymatic activity appears to be rather low (11). Therefore, our laboratory and others are employing sheep seminal vesicle (SSV) cells for the study of estrogen-mediated genetic toxicity, because these cells are known to have a high level of prostaglandin-H-synthase. Instead of karyotyping cells, which is tedious, our laboratory has chosen the approach of determining micronuclei (see Schnitzler and Metzler, this volume). In order to distinguish between micronuclei (MN) containing an entire chromosome (indicative for aneuploidogens) from those containing only a chromosome fragment (indicative for clastogens), we are scoring MN for the presence of chromatids by CREST antikinetochore immunofluorescence staining.

As described in more detail in the chapter by Schnitzler and Metzler (this volume), several steroidal estrogens including E_2, 2-hydroxy-E_2 and 4-hydroxy-E_2, as well as the stilbene estrogens DES, 3,3'-DES, indenestrol A and indenestrol B were tested for MN induction in SHE and SSV cells. MN were found in all cases, but only DES gave rise to a high frequency of kinetochore-positive MN. This emphasizes the marked aneuploidogenic effect of DES and suggests that the other estrogens, in addition to acting as aneuploidogens, may have additional effects at the chromosomal level.

Conclusion

The dissociation of estrogenicity from neoplastic transformation both *in vivo* in the male Syrian hamster kidney and *in vitro* in Syrian hamster embryo cells, together with the identification of reactive estrogen metabolites, makes a case for an important role of metabolic activation in the mechanism of estrogen-mediated carcinogenesis. The present study on the interaction of estrogens and their peroxidative metabolites with microtubular proteins (MTP) under cell-free conditions supports this notion. Based on the hypothesis that binding of estrogen metabolites to MTP can disturb microtubule (MT) formation and thereby lead to the induction of aneuploidy, which has been proposed as an early genetic event in cell transformation, we have shown that steroidal estrogens need metabolic activation, presumably to quinones, and covalent binding in order to inhibit MT assembly. With most stilbene estrogens, inhibition was observed already prior to metabolic activation, but was in some cases markedly enhanced by peroxidative metabolism. Thus, not all estrogens need metabolic activation in order to interfere with MT formation. In intact cells in culture, induction of kinetochore-positive micronuclei also implied an interaction of both steroidal and stilbene estrogens with the mitotic spindle, although the relatively high percentage of kinetochore-negative micronuclei observed with some estrogens suggests that other mechanisms may also be involved.

Acknowledgments

This study was supported by the Deutsche Forschungsgemeinschaft (Sonderforschungsbereich 172). We thank Mrs. Anita Strohauer for typing the manuscript.

References

1. IARC Monographs on the Evaluation of the Carcinogenic Risk of Chemicals to Humans, Vol. 21: Sex Hormones (II), International Agency for Research on Cancer, Lyon (France) 1979.
2. Li JJ, Li SA, Klicka JK, Parsons JA, Lam LKT (1983) Relative carcinogenic activity of various synthetic and natural estrogens in the Syrian hamster kidney. Cancer Res 43:5200-5204.
3. Liehr JG (1983) 2-Fluoroestradiol. Separation of estrogenicity from carcinogenicity. Molec Pharmacol 23:278-281.
4. Metzler M (1984) Metabolism of stilbene estrogens and steroidal estrogens in relation to carcinogenicity. Arch Toxicol 55:104-109.
5. Li JJ, Li SA (1987) Estrogen carcinogenesis in Syrian hamster tissues: role of metabolism. Fed Proc 46:1858-1863.
6. Degen GH, Metzler M (1987) Sex hormones and neoplasia: genotoxic effects in short term assays. Arch Toxicol Suppl 10:264-278.
7. Tsutsui T, Maizumi H, McLachlan JA, Barrett JC (1983) Aneuploidy induction and cell transformation by diethylstilbestrol: a possible chromosomal mechanism in carcinogenesis. Cancer Res 43:3814-3821.
8. Tsutsui T, Suzuki N, Fukuda S, Sato M, Maizumi H, McLachlan JA, Barrett JC (1987) 17ß-Estradiol-induced cell transformation and aneuploidy of Syrian hamster embryo cells in culture. Carcinogenesis 8:1715-1719.
9. Wong A, Degen GH, Bryan PC, Barrett JC, McLachlan JA (1983) Transformation of Syrian hamster embryo cells by steroidal estrogens and their catechol derivatives. Proc Am Assoc Cancer Res 24:182.

10. McLachlan JA, Wong A, Degen GH, Barrett JC (1982) Morphological and neoplastic transformation of Syrian hamster embryo fibroblasts by diethylstilbestrol and analogs. Cancer Res 42:3040-3045.

11. Degen GH, Wong A, Eling TE, Barrett JC, McLachlan JA (1983) Involvement of prostaglandin synthetase in the peroxidative metabolism of diethylstilbestrol in Syrian hamster embryo fibroblast cell cultures. Cancer Res 43:992-996.

12. Pechan R, Seibel K, Metzler M (1992) Cell transformation in vitro by tamoxifen and structurally related compounds. Anticancer Res, in press.

13. Epe B, Harttig UH, Schiffmann D, Metzler M (1989) Microtubular proteins as cellular targets for carcinogenic estrogens and other carcinogens. In: Mechanisms of Chromosome Distribution and Aneuploidy (Resnick MA, Vig BK, Eds) Allan R Liss Inc, New York 1989, pp 345-351.

14. Epe B, Harttig U, Stopper H, Metzler M (1990) Covalent binding of reactive estrogen metabolites to microtubular protein as a possible mechanism of aneuploidy induction and neoplastic cell transformation. Environ Health Perspect 88:123-127.

15. Epe B, Hegler J, Metzler M (1987) Site-specific covalent binding of stilbene-type and steroidal estrogens to tubulin following metabolic activation in vitro. Carcinogenesis 8:1271-1275.

16. Ellman GL (1959) Tissue sulfhydryl groups. Arch Biochem Biophys 82:70-77.

9

Differential Interactions of Estradiol Metabolites with the Estrogen Receptor: Genomic Consequences and Tumorigenesis

Jack Fishman and George Swaneck

The incidence of breast cancer in the human has been rising and is now such that one out of nine women will develop the disease in her lifetime and one out of 18 will die from it. Ample epidemiological evidence indicates that the incidence is not a random process, but that both exogenous and endogenous factors enhance the risk for breast cancer (1). A prime candidate among the endogenous factors influencing the risk for the disease is the female sex hormone estradiol and its metabolites. While animal evidence is unequivocal that estrogens play an essential role in the etiology of breast tumors (2), in humans the evidence of estrogen participation in breast cancer incidence is indirect but nevertheless convincing (3). Numerous studies have, therefore, been directed to unearth a difference in the estrogen secretion and metabolism in breast cancer patients relative to unaffected controls, but these efforts have been frustrated by the technical difficulties of measuring the very low levels of these hormones which also undergo complex patterns of excretion and conjugation in body fluids. A second, and possibly more important factor why no consistent differences have become apparent is the likelihood that the initiation of the breast tumor, or carcinogenesis, precedes its clinical diagnosis by a period of 20 or more years. Hence analysis of the estrogen milieu at the time of diagnosis may reveal little about its features at the time of carcinogenesis. This time lag issue has been addressed in a prospective as well as retrospective manner. In the former, cohorts identified as at risk for genetic or environmental reasons have been compared to those without these enhanced risk characteristics (4-6). Some differences were observed, but these have so far not been confirmed in other studies (7,8). In the retrospective approach we sought to identify components of the estrogenic profile that do not change with age or reproductive status of the woman, and hence, can be considered at the time of measurement to be representative of the situation at the time of tumor initiation.

We studied the *in vivo* metabolism of estradiol in peri- and postmenopausal women with and without cancer by a radiometric procedure and showed that of the three main pathways of the oxidative metabolism of estradiol (Figure 1), only 16α-hydroxylation was increased in the women with breast cancer (9,10). This observation was supported by studies in the mouse mammary tumor model where 16α-hydroxylation correlated with mammary tumor incidence in different mouse strains (11,12) and where this enzyme activity was shown to be enhanced by the presence of the mouse mammary tumor virus. Furthermore, numerous epidemiological factors in humans associated with greater breast cancer risk, such as body weight or composition (13), diet (14,15), and family history (16), correlated exceptionally well with the presence of excess of 16α-hydroxylated metabolites of the female hormone relative to the 2-hydroxylated forms. These observations led us to study the biological properties of the 16α-hydroxylated metabolites, estriol, and 16α-hydroxyestrone. Our attention focused on 16α-hydroxyestrone whose biology has been explored relatively little compared to that of estriol which is the dominant estrogen of pregnancy and was considered at one time as an antiestrogen or an impeded estrogen (17). We found that 16α-hydroxyestrone, while a relatively poor ligand for the estrogen receptor, was very much a potent estrogen (18,19). To assign a carcinogenic role in the breast tissue, specificity implies the participation of the estrogen receptor, a protein whose nature and role as a transcription factor has been in the forefront of molecular biology research (20-22). An important issue in defining the biological end points of the hormone and hormone-receptor complex is the role of the nature of the binding of the former to the latter. The present conventional perception is that all estrogens, natural or synthetic, react with the steroid binding elements of the estrogen receptor in a similar reversible fashion with the

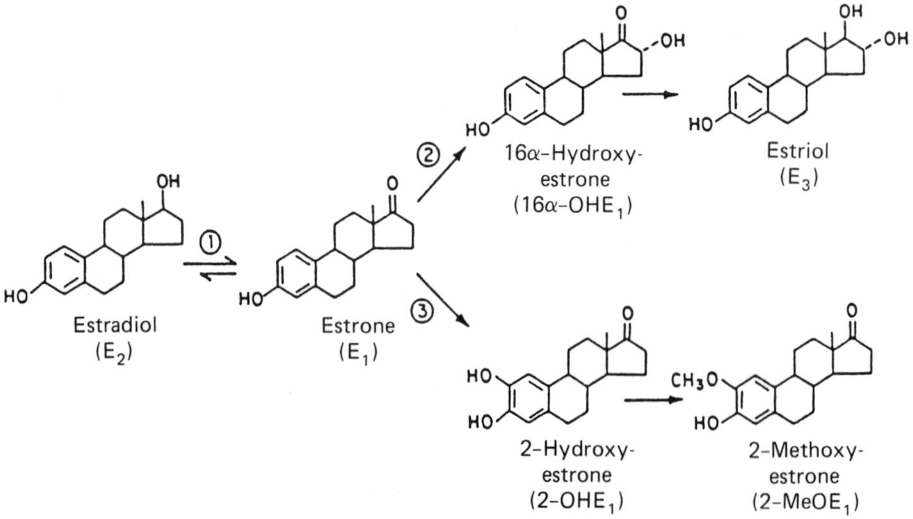

Fig. 1. Oxidative metabolism of 17β-estradiol.

sole difference residing in the affinity of the binding. While such conventional binding of 16α-hydroxyestrone to the receptor was found to be reversible and to be of much lower affinity than estradiol, this metabolite was shown to uniquely form an irreversible covalent linkage with the estrogen receptor (23). This bonding occurs via a stabilized Schiff base formation with primary amino groups, presumably on lysine residues, followed by a Heyns rearrangement resulting in the formation of a covalent secondary amine bond (Figure 2). This bond formation was chemical in nature, was time- and temperature-dependent, and required no enzyme participation. It was demonstrated in the MCF-7 cell cultures and was remarkably specific for the estrogen receptor relative to similar interaction with nonspecific proteins (24).

The association of excess 16α-hydroxyestrone formation with increased breast cancer risk and the identification of the nonclassical irreversible interaction of this metabolite with the estrogen receptor suggested a possible mechanism for the link between this estradiol metabolite and carcinogenesis in the breast. Such a linkage, however, required that the irreversible binding of 16α-hydroxyestrone with the estrogen receptor influenced the transcriptive functions of the receptor and resulted in altered gene expression. Because the covalent binding was time-dependent, in contrast to the classical reversible interaction, it was possible to distinguish the biological consequence of the two types of bindings by observing the changes induced with time of exposure of the target tissue to 16α-hydroxyestrone. The studies were carried out in MCF-7 cell cultures where the time element could be emphasized, since only when a significant portion of the

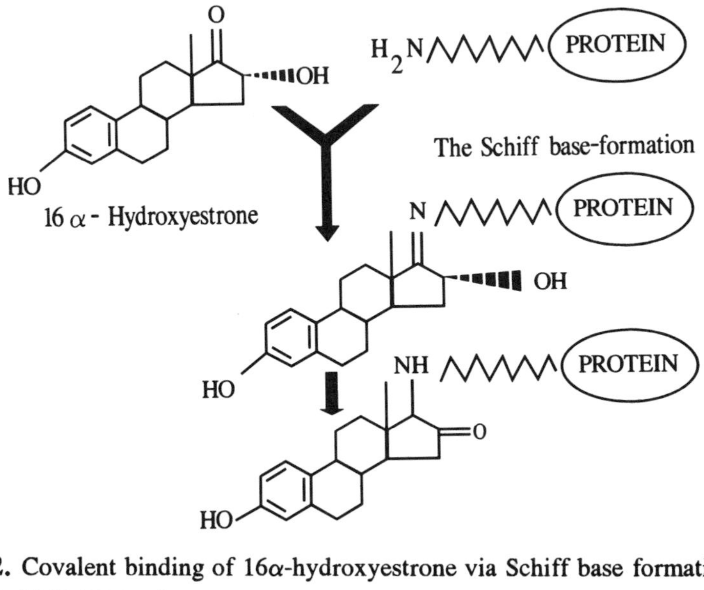

Fig. 2. Covalent binding of 16α-hydroxyestrone via Schiff base formation and Heyns rearrangement.

cells contained the irreversibly bound receptor would the biological changes occasioned by this binding be detectable above the background levels of the classically reversibly bound receptor containing cells. *A priori* we already had evidence of a possible genomic effect of the irreversible binding of 16α-hydroxyestrone to the receptor—the great increase in the half-life or turnover of the receptor. Several experiments employing different methodologies have demonstrated that the estrogen receptor has a half-life of only several hours (25). To allow the accumulation of irreversibly bound receptor containing cells over a period of days or weeks, clearly this characteristic of the receptor had to be altered, and the life of irreversibly bound receptor had to be greatly prolonged relative to the classical hormone-receptor complex.

MCF-7 human breast cancer cells obtained from the Michigan Cancer Foundation (Detroit, MI) were grown in plastic T-150 flasks in Dulbecco's modified Eagle's medium (DMEM) in the absence of any estrogenic stimulation by culture in phenol red-free medium containing 7.5 % fetal calf serum treated twice with dextran-coated charcoal (DCC) to remove endogenous steroids and in the presence of 1 ng/ml insulin. To determine the effects of estradiol and 16α-OHE1 on estrogen-receptor and PR levels, MCF-7 cells were harvested and seeded into T-75 flasks at a density of 1.5 x 10^6 cells/T-75 flask. Cells were exposed to 1 x $10^{-8}M$ estradiol or 1 x $10^{-8}M$ 16α-OHE1 and control cells received the same volume of vehicle per flask (0.1 % ethanol). Treatment of cells was extended over a period of 6 to 8 weeks. When cells reached confluence, they were harvested and replated at a density of 1:3. During treatment, culture medium was changed every 2 days.

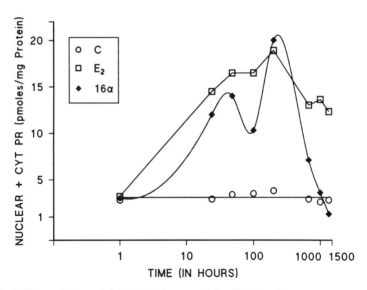

Fig. 3. Effects of E_2 and 16α OH E_1 on cellular PR levels.

Receptor Binding Activity Measurements: Before binding assays, estradiol-treated cells were washed 3 times during a 2 hour period and refed with fresh medium in the absence of estradiol to remove free steroid. This treatment was shown to deplete the cells of unbound estradiol prior to the exchange assay and PR assays were done using radiolabeled R5020. Nuclear exchange assays were performed at 30°C for 30 min in the presence of 2 x 10^8M [^{3}H]-estradiol. In order to measure nonspecific binding, parallel assays were done in the presence of 100-fold excess nonradiolabeled estradiol. Assays were completed after 30 min when tubes were placed at 4°C and bound radioactive estradiol was measured after precipitation with 5% protamine sulfate. Progesterone binding activities were determined in combined nuclear and cytosol fractions using 2 x 10^8M [^{3}H]-R5020 at 4°C for 4 hours. Nonspecific binding was assessed in parallel assays in the presence of 100-fold excess nonradiolabeled R5020. Samples were precipitated in the presence of 5% protamine sulfate. Specific binding was calculated as the difference between total and nonspecific binding per mg of DNA.

Studies on Cell Proliferation: MCF-7 cells that had been grown for more than one year in DMEM in the absence of estrogenic stimulation, e.g., 7.5% fetal calf serum treated twice with DCC and in phenol red-free conditions were exposed to 10^8M estradiol or 10^8 16α-OHE1 for 1 and 4 weeks. Control cells received only the vehicle at a final concentration of 0.1% ethanol. One day after seeding at a density of 7 x 10^5 cells/25 cm^2 flask in DMEM (day 0), attached cells were harvested from 3 x T-25 flasks from each group. Their viability was assessed by exclusion of Trypan blue solution and their number was determined in duplicate samples from each flask using a Coulter cell counter. Viability was 95-97% of total cell number in the three experimental groups.

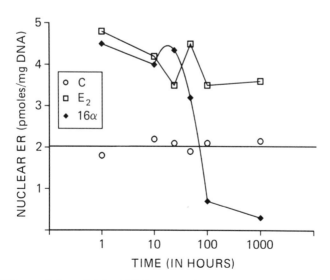

Fig. 4. Effects of E$_2$ and 16α OH E$_1$ on nuclear ER levels.

Studies of MCF-7 cells cultured in the presence of either 16α-hydroxyestrone or estradiol over a period of 6 weeks showed clearly that estradiol caused an increase in the progesterone receptor, considered a classical product of estrogen-dependent gene activation (26-28). The hormone induced the expected short-term rise in the progesterone receptor, which was maintained over the six-week period of the study. In contrast, the cultures exposed to 16α-hydroxyestrone exhibited an initial rise in progesterone receptor commensurate with the classical reversible binding of the metabolite, but upon prolonged exposure and irreversible complex formation, the levels of progesterone receptor decreased to below control values (Figure 3). Although the effect of estrogen on the induction of the estrogen receptor in MCF-7 cells was less well defined and exhibited a more complex temporal pattern (29-31), a distinction was found between the short-term 16α-hydroxyestrone exposure cultures, which showed an increase in the nuclear estrogen receptor, while upon long-term exposure to 16α-hydroxyestrone the estrogen-receptor presence was virtually eliminated (Figure 4). In contrast, the cells exposed to estradiol failed to show this differentiation and maintained a consistent presence of estrogen receptor after induction (Figure 4). These results could be interpreted as providing evidence that the irreversibly bound 16α-hydroxyestrone estrogen-receptor complex was transcriptionally inactive, a finding of lesser interest than if that binding resulted in differential gene expression. We therefore examined yet another biological response of the exposure of MCF-7 cells to estrogens, cell proliferation (Figure 5) (32). That response of the cells to 16α-hydroxyestrone did not differ significantly from that achieved with estradiol irrespective of time indicating that the genomic actions induced by estrogens involved in cell proliferation were not affected by the irreversible binding of the estrogen receptor with 16α-hydroxyestrone. While clearly, alternative explanations are possible, such as an excessive proliferative response of the unaffected cells, the most plausible rationalization is that the

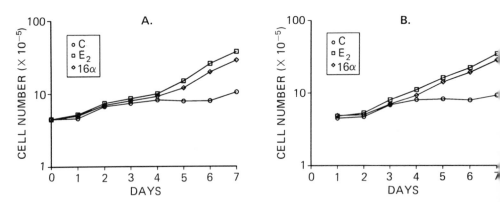

Fig. 5.1. Cell proliferation effects of E_2 and 16α OH E_1 (A) after 1 week and (B) after 4 weeks.

irreversible binding of 16α-hydroxyestrone to the estrogen receptor results in differential genomic expression in which receptor recycling and progesterone-receptor and estrogen receptor synthesis are diminished or abolished, while cellular proliferation is unaffected. These findings could provide the framework of a biochemical mechanism relating 16α-hydroxyestrone excess to target-site carcinogenesis. The enhanced possibility of the 16α-hydroxyestrone-estrogen receptor irreversible interaction, which is linked to an increased 16α-hydroxyestrone/estradiol ratio, and receptor availability could lead to genomic changes leading eventually to cell transformation. Whether this concept has merit requires further investigation, and a series of studies are presently underway to either provide further supportive evidence for this hypothesis or to diminish its relevance.

References

1. Willett W (1989) The search for the causes of breast and colon cancer. Nature 338:389-394.
2. Jensen EV, DeSombre ER (1972) Epidemiology of breast cancer. Annual Review of Biochem 41:203-230.
3. Lippman M (1988) Diagnosis and management of breast cancer. Epidemiology of Breast Cancer, W.B. Saunders and Co., pp. 1-9.
4. Bulbrook RD, Moore JW, Clark GMG et al (1978) Plasma oestradiol and progesterone levels in women with varying degrees of risk of breast cancer. Eur J Cancer 14:1369-1371.
5. Pike MC, Cassagrande JT, Brown JB et al (1977) Composition of urinary and plasma hormone levels in daughters of breast cancer patients and controls. J Natl Cancer Inst 59:1351-1354.
6. Morgan RW, Vakil DV, Brown JB et al (1978) Estrogen profiles in young women: effect of maternal history of breast cancer. J Natl Cancer Inst 60:965-968.
7. Fishman J, Fukushima DK, O'Connor J, Rosenfeld RS, Lynch HT, Lynch JF, Guirgis H, Maloney K (1978) Plasma hormone profiles of young women at risk for familial breast cancer. Cancer Res 38:4006-4011.
8. Fishman J, Fukushima DK, O'Connor J, Lynch H (1979) Low urinary estrogen glucuronides in women at risk for familial breast cancer. Science 204:1089-1091.
9. Fishman J, Bradlow HL, Schneider J, Anderson KE, Kappas A (1980) Radiometric analysis of biological oxidation in man: sex differences in estradiol metabolism. Proc Natl Acad Sci USA 77:4957-4960.
10. Schneider J, Kinne D, Fracchia A, Pierce V, Anderson KE, Bradlow HL, Fishman J (1982) Abnormal oxidative metabolism of estradiol in women with breast cancer. Proc. Natl. Acad. Sci. USA 79:3047-3051.
11. Bradlow HL, Hershcopf RJ, Martucci CP Fishman J (1985) Estradiol 16α-hydroxylation in the mouse correlates with mammary tumor incidence and presence of murine mammary tumor virus: a possible

model for the hormonal etiology of breast cancer in humans. Proc Natl Acad Sci USA 82: 6295- 6299.

12.   Bradlow HL, Hershcopf R, Martucci C Fishman J (1986) 16α-Hydroxylation of estradiol: a possible risk marker for breast cancer. Annals NY Acad Sci 464: 138-151.

13.   Schneider J. Bradlow HL, Strain G, Levin J, Anderson K, Fishman J (1983) Effects of obesity on estradiol metabolism: decreased formation of nonuterotropic metabolites. J Clin Endocrinol Metab 56:973-978.

14.   Anderson KE, Kappas A, Conney AH, Bradlow HL, Fishman J (1984) The influence of dietary protein and carbohydrate on the principal oxidative biotransformations of estradiol in normal subjects. J Clin Endocrinol Metab 59:103-107.

15.   Miller AB (1977) Role of nutrition in the etiology of breast cancer. Cancer Res 39:2704-2706.

16.   Osborne MP, Rosen PP, Lesser ML, Schwartz MK, Menendez-Botet CJ, Fishman J, Kinne DW, Beattie EJ, Jr (1983) The relationship between family history, exposure to exogenous hormones and estrogen receptor protein in breast cancer. Cancer 51:2134-2138.

17.   Lemon HM (1969) Endocrine influences on human mammary cancer formation. Cancer 23:781-784.

18.   Martucci C, Fishman J (1977) Direction of estradiol metabolism as a control of its hormonal action - uterotrophic activity of estradiol metabolite. Endocrinology 101: 1709-1715.

19.   Fishman J, Martucci C (1980) Biological properties of 16α-hydroxyestrone: implications in estrogen physiology and pathophysiology. J Clin Endocrinol Metab 51: 611-615.

20.   Beato M (1989) Gene regulation by steroid hormones. Cell 56:335-344.

21.   Picard D, Salser SJ, Yamamoto KR (1988) A movable and regulable inactivation function within the steroid binding domain of the glucocorticoid receptor. Cell 54:1073-1080.

22.   Picard D, Kumar V, Chambon P, Yamamoto KR (1990) Signal transduction by steroid hormones: nuclear localization is differentially regulated in estrogen and glucocorticoid receptors. Cell Regulation 1:291-299.

23.   Swaneck GE, Fishman J (1980) Covalent binding of the endogenous estrogen 16α-hydroxyestrone to estradiol receptor in human breast cancer cells: Characterization and intranuclear localization. Proc Natl Acad Sci USA 85: 7831-7835.

24.   Yu S, Fishman J (1985) Interaction of histones with estrogens - covalent adduct formation with 16α- hydroxyestrone. Biochemistry 24: 8017-8021.

25.   Katzenellenbogen JA, Katzenellenbogen BS (1984) Affinity labeling of receptors for steroid and thyroid hormones. Vit Horm 41:213-274.

26. Horwitz KB, Tava DT, Thilagar AK, Hensen EM, McGuire, WL (1978) Steroid receptor analyses of nine human breast cancer cell lines. Cancer Res 38:2434-2437.

27. Horwitz KB, McGuire WL (1978) Estrogen control of progesterone receptor in human breast cancer. Correlation with nuclear processing of estrogen receptor. J Biol Chem 253:2223-2228.

28. Westley B, Rochefort H (1980) A secreted glycoprotein induced by estrogen in human breast cancer cell lines. Cell 20: 353-362.

29. Kassis JA, Sakai D, Walent JH, Gorski J (1984) Primary cultures of estrogen-responsive cells from rat uteri: induction of progesterone receptors and a secreted protein. Endocrinology 114:1558-1566.

30. Piva R, Bianchini E, Kumar VL, Chambon P, del Senno L (1988) Estrogen induced increase of estrogen receptor RNA in human breast cancer cells. Biochem Biophys Res Commun 155:943-949.

31. Piva R, Kumar VL, Hanau S, Rimondi AP, Pansini S, Mollica G, del Senno L (1989) Abnormal methylation of estrogen receptor gene and reduced estrogen receptor RNA levels in human endometrial carcinomas. J Steroid Biochem 32:1-4.

32. Dickson RB, Lippman ME (1987) Estrogenic regulation of growth and polypeptides growth factor secretion in human breast carcinoma. Endocrine Rev 8:29-43.

10

Oxidation of Estrogens and Other Steroids by Cytochrome P-450 Enzymes: Relevance to Tumorigenesis

F. Peter Guengerich

Introduction

There is a considerable body of epidemiological evidence available to support the view that hormone levels influence several kinds of human cancer. Further, there are many experimental models for hormonal carcinogenesis. Estrogens can cause or augment endometrial cancer, probably by their effects on cell proliferation. Similarly, higher estrogen and progesterone levels increase breast cancer risk. However, the use of the artificial steroids in oral contraceptives can reduce endometrial cancer risk (1). The androgen testosterone may be a factor in prostatic cancer.

The association between estrogen levels and cancer is complex. Depletion of estrogen levels through reduced synthesis has been a popular strategy (2), and the increased degradation of 17β-estradiol has been considered as a mechanism for the reduced incidence of tumors in hormonally responsive tissues after exposure to 2,3,7,8-tetrachlorodibenzo-p-dioxin. However, there is also a considerable body of evidence linking the cytochrome P-450 (P-450)-mediated oxidation of steroids with experimental tumors, particularly in the case of estrogens (3). For instance, 16α-hydroxylation in the mouse is correlated with mammary tumor incidence and the presence of a mammary tumor virus. Also, comparison of animal models suggests that catechols derived from estrogen 2- and 4-hydroxylation may be important in the estrogen-induced hamster kidney tumor model. However, in contrast to the situation with some artificial stilbene hormones, where oxidation can lead to defined DNA adducts, no direct link for tumor initiation or promotion has been defined. Estrogen administration has been shown to result in the formation of specific although uncharacterized DNA adducts that seem to arise from reactions with chemicals endogenous to the body.

These complex relationships are outlined in Figure 1. In the course of our work we have been interested in defining which of the many P-450 enzymes are most important in particular reactions involving steroids and nonsteroidal genotoxic carcinogens, particularly in humans. This information should be vital in making interpretations about the role of steroid metabolism in hormone-associated cancer.

Roles of P-450 Enzymes in 17β-Estradiol Hydroxylation

In rat liver, the 2-hydroxylation of 17β-estradiol is modulated by a variety of factors. It has been demonstrated that the P-450s responsible for the hepatic activity are mainly P-450 1A2, P-450 2C11, and a P-450 3A family enzyme (4). The P-450 3A family is now known to consist of several genes and its complexity is not fully understood, however, the inducibility of catalytic activity by phenobarbital and pregnenolone-16α-carbonitrile would argue that P-450 3A1 is involved in this reaction, but this conclusion must be considered tentative. The pattern of 4-hydroxylation appears to resemble that of 2-hydroxylation with regard to the enzymes involved, the rates are considerably lower (4). Although the amounts of these three P-450s are modulated by a variety of factors, including induction, hormonal influences, and the degree to which a single P-450 is responsible for this catalytic activity as a function of the animal experiment. P-450 3A enzymes are expressed in extrahepatic tissues, but apparently P-450 1A2 and 2C11 are not.

In human liver, the bulk of 17β-estradiol 2- and 4-hydroxylation appears to be due to P-450 3A4 (5), and the verification of this activity has been demonstrated in a recombinant enzyme assay. Recently Ball et al. (6) have proposed different assignments of both rat and human enzyme activities, however, these findings must be questioned in light of the very low specific activities reported.

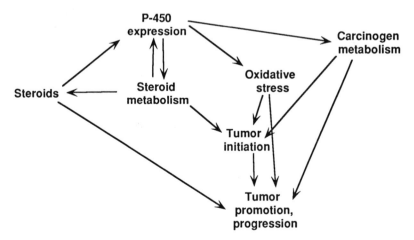

Fig. 1. Events related to hormonal and other chemical-induced carcinogenesis.

It would appear that P-450 1A1, which is essentially an extrahepatic enzyme in humans, is capable of catalyzing 17β-estradiol 2-hydroxylation, as shown by inducibility by 2,3,7,8-tetrachlorodibenzo-p-dioxin in cultured MCF-7 breast tumor cells. The significance of such a response is presently unclear.

Roles of P-450 Enzymes in 17α-Ethinylestradiol Hydroxylation

The metabolism of 17α-ethinylestradiol is of interest in consideration of its extensive use as an (estrogenic) oral contraceptive. Little is actually known regarding the catalytic specificity of the rat enzymes involved in 2-hydroxylation, the major oxidative reaction involved in its biotransformation. The results of Ball et al.'s (6) studies in rats and humans are questionable because of the low activities reported. In humans, P-450 3A4 appears to have the major role in the 2-hydroxylation reaction (7). This conclusion is consonant with the known induction of the enzyme by rifampicin and the history of that agent in enhancing the elimination of 17α-ethinylestradiol with the resulting lack of clinical effectiveness.

At least four different P-450 3A family genes have been reported, but P-450 3A4 appears to be dominant in human liver. A minor P-450, P-450 3A5, is ~ 88% identical to P-450 3A4 in its primary sequence, it has a somewhat less 17β-estradiol 2-hydroxylation activity than P-450 3A4, but much less 17α-ethinylestradiol 2-hydroxylation activity.

P-450 Enzymes Involved in the Oxidation of Other Steroids

The aromatase, P-450 19A, is involved in the formation of estrogens and is a target in the treatment of cancers of the breast and other tissues (2). In steroidogenic tissues, a number of steroids are processed by enzymes in the P-450 11, 17, and 21 families. In human liver, a number of reactions, particularly several 6β-hydroxylations, are attributed largely to P-450 3A4 (Table 1). The 6β-hydroxylation of cortisol is of particular interest because the measurement of the ratio of 6-hydroxycortisol to cortisol in the liver may provide a useful noninvasive measure of P-450 3A4 levels. It should be emphasized that the P-450s involved in many steroid oxidations remain to be elucidated. In some cases, the similarity of the primary sequences of the human enzymes to closely related forms in experimental animals is not a particularly good guide to their function. For instance, we have recently purified P-450 2A3 from human liver, although the primary sequence is highly identical to that of rat P-450 2A1, an enzyme whose most distinguishing catalytic activity is testosterone 7α-hydroxylation, the human enzyme is unable to hydroxylate testosterone at all.

Table 1. Steroid hydroxylation reactions catalyzed by human cytochrome P-450 3A4.

17β-Estradiol 2-hydroxylation
17β-Estradiol 4-hydroxylation
17α-Ethynylestradiol 2-hydroxylation
17α-Ethynylestradiol ácetylene oxidation (enzyme inactivation)
Gestodene acetylene oxidation (enzyme inactivation)
Testosterone 6b-hydroxylation
Androstendione 6b-hydroxylation
Cortisol 6b-hydroxylation
Progesterone 6b-hydroxylation
Dehydroepiandrosterone 3-sulfate 16a-hydroxylation

Moduation of Levels of Human P-450s

The regulation of P-450 gene expression is a complex matter. Considerable work has been done in experimental animal and cellular models, and advances have been made in understanding some of the events involved in the regulation of certain P-450s. Considerable effort will be required to understand how all of the P-450s are regulated in humans.

Some of the factors that modulate human P-450 3A4 activity are cited in Table 2. Rodents are notorious for dramatizing gender differences in metabolism (4). However, such an effect does not appear to be operative for human P-450 3A4. A somewhat higher extent of excretion of 17β-estradiol is seen in males than in females, but this observation can be explained in terms of gender-specific sulfation, and there does not appear to be a difference among the sexes in P-450 3A4 levels.

However, considerable inter-individual human variation exists in metabolism of estrogens, and this is well-documented in the case of 17α-ethinylestradiol. In addition, in many instances there is considerable variation within an individual over a period of time. Rifampicin and barbiturates are known to enhance *in vivo* rates of 2-hydroxylation and to induce P-450 3A4. Dexamethasone may also induce human P-450 3A4, although this suggestion is based upon the animal ortholog and a careful study with this drug alone has not been carried out. Kappas et al. (8) have shown that 17β-estradiol 2-hydroxylation is enhanced by feeding a high-protein diet, which may result in P-450 3A4 induction, as a high-protein diet is known to induce the oxidations of some other drugs.

As well as induction of steroid hydroxylation, enzyme inhibition can be important. Macrolide antibiotics such as rifampicin and, to a lesser extent, erythromycin can be oxidized to nitroso derivatives that complex the ferrous P-450 iron. The acetylenic steroids can act as mechanism-based inactivators. To some extent this occurs with 17α-ethinylestradiol (7), but the progestogenic

Table 2. Factors known or suspected to modulate human P-450 3A4 activity.

        Increased activity
                Rifampicin
                Barbiturates
                Dexamethasone
                High-protein diet (?)
                Certain flavones (?)

        Decreased activity
                Certain macrolide antibiotics
                Gestodene
                Naringenin and other flavones

---

oral contraceptive component, gestodene, seems to be considerably more potent *in vitro* (9) and *in vivo* studies. Other P-450 3A4 reactions are also inhibited *in vitro* (9). Finally, some food components can also show substantial effects. Recently, the consumption of moderate amounts of grapefruit juice has been shown to have a dramatic effect in inhibiting the P-450 3A4-dependent oxidation of dihydropyridine drugs. In addition, grapefruit juice also inhibits *in vivo* 6β-hydroxycortisol excretion, as would be expected (J.D. Groopman, unpublished). The effect is postulated to be due to naringenin, a principal flavonoid in the fruit. Indeed, naringenin can inhibit P-450 3A4-dependent nifedipine oxidation and activation of aflatoxin B_1 *in vitro*. Therefore, the contribution of other natural products cannot be ruled out. Moreover, each substrate needs to be considered individually, since it has been shown that 7,8-benzoflavone stimulates aflatoxin B_1 8,9-oxidation, but inhibits the 3-hydroxylation that leads the formation of aflatoxin Q_1.

Conclusions

P-450s are important because they are the principal enzymes involved in the biotransformation of steroids, and alterations in their catalytic activities can lead to changes in the levels of the parent compounds or their metabolites. Major roles for individual rat and human P-450s have been implicated in a number of key steroid hydroxylations. Many of the experimental rodent models are complex and there are considerable hormonal effects in the regulation of P-450 enzymes involved in steroid hydroxylation. The available information points to a major role of human P-450 3A4 in the 2-hydroxylation of estrogens and the 6β-hydroxylation of a number of other steroids. Factors that influence the level of this enzyme and steroid hydroxylation may influence hormone-induced carcinogenesis depending upon the roles of the steroids and their biotransformation products such as quinones.

Acknowledgments

This research was supported in part by U.S. Public Health Service grants CA 44353, ES 00267, and ES 01590.

References

1. Preston-Martin S, Pike MC, Ross RK, Jones PA, Henderson BE (1990) Increased cell division as a cause of human cancer. Cancer Res 50:7415-7421.
2. Brodie AMH (1985) Aromatase inhibition and its pharmacologic implications. Biochem Pharmacol 34:3213-3219.
3. Li JJ, Li SA (1987) Estrogen carcinogenesis in Syrian hamster tissues: role of metabolism. Fed Proc 46:1858-1863.
4. Dannan GA, Porubek DJ, Nelson SD, Waxman DJ, Guengerich FP (1986) 17β-Estradiol 2- and 4-hydroxylation catalyzed by rat hepatic cytochrome P-450: roles of individual forms, inductive effects, developmental patterns, and alterations by gonadectomy and hormone replacement. Endocrinology 118:1952-1960.
5. Guengerich FP, Martin MV, Beaune PH, Kremers P, Wolff T, Waxman DJ (1986) Characterization of rat and human liver microsomal cytochrome P-450 forms involved in nifedipine oxidation, a prototype for genetic polymorphism in oxidative drug metabolism. J Biol Chem 261:5051-5060.
6. Ball SE, Forrester LM, Wolf CR, Back DJ (1990) Differences in the cytochrome P-450 isoenzymes involved in the 2-hydroxylation of oestradiol and 17α-ethinyloestradiol. Biochem J 267:221-226.
7. Guengerich FP (1988) Oxidation of 17α-ethynylestradiol by human liver cytochrome P-450. Mol Pharmacol 33:500-508.
8. Kappas A, Anderson KE, Conney AH, Pantuck EJ, Fishman J, Bradlow HL (1983) Nutrition-endocrine interactions: induction of reciprocal changes in the D^4-5a-reduction of testosterone and the cytochrome P-450-dependent oxidation of estradiol by dietary macronutrients in man. Proc Natl Acad Sci USA 80:7646-7649.
9. Guengerich FP (1990) Mechanism-based inactivation of human liver cytochrome P-450 IIIA4 by gestodene. Chem Res Toxicol 3:363-371.

11

Metabolism of Moxestrol in the Hamster Kidney: Significance for Estrogen Carcinogenesis

Sara Antonia Li and Jonathan J. Li

Introduction

Moxestrol [11β-methoxy-17-ethinyl-1,3,5(10)-estratriene-3,17β-diol or R 2858] is a potent estrogen in both animals and humans (1,2) and is used in Europe as a postmenopausal agent. Its estrogenic potency, depending on the biologic or biochemical parameters used, is approximately 10 to 100 times higher than 17β-estradiol (E_2) (1) and about 5 times more potent than ethynylestradiol (EE_2) (2). Its hormonal effectiveness has been attributed to the stability of the complex it forms with the estrogen receptor (3), its lower affinity for serum plasma proteins (1), and also the degree to which it is metabolized (4). In the hamster estrogen-induced-renal adenocarcinoma model, Moxestrol and EE_2 exhibited similar estrogenic activities. Moxestrol, however, displayed potent tumorigenic activity at this organ site, eliciting 100% tumor incidence (5,6). In contrast, its parent compound EE_2 exhibits only modest 10% renal tumor incidence when similarly administered. Since metabolism has been postulated by us (7) and others (8-10) to play a significant if not crucial role in neoplastic transformation of the hamster kidney, it becomes evidently pertinent to investigate the metabolism of Moxestrol in the kidney and liver of this species.

Estrogenic Activity

Raynaud et al. have made extensive studies of Moxestrol in humans (11) and in a number of mammalian species (4). Using rat uterus, these workers compared the estrogenic activity of E_2, EE_2, and methoxy derivatives of both of these two estrogens. Since Moxestrol did not bind appreciably to plasma proteins, this property was considered significant in contributing to the very strong uterotropic activity of Moxestrol despite its somewhat lower affinity for the uterine estrogen receptor relative to E_2 or EE_2. It was concluded that the properties of high-uterine uptake and lack of plasma protein binding of this substituted synthetic steroidal estrogen were important factors leading to its potent estrogenic activity

(4). Our studies of competitive binding to estrogen receptor in hamster renal tumor cytosol, inducibility of progesterone receptor in the nontransformed hamster kidney, and the levels of serum prolactin in estrogenized animals treated with Moxestrol for four months, indicate that Moxestrol is as estrogenic as E_2, or diethylstilbestrol (DES) in the hamster kidney model (Table 1). Moreover, Moxestrol and EE_2 were nearly equally capable of inducing cell proliferation of primary hamster proximal tubular epithelium in culture under serum-free chemically defined conditions at physiological concentrations (12). Recently, however, we have shown that EE_2 elicited hyperplasias in different cortical cells in the hamster kidney than either Moxestrol, E_2, or DES *in vivo*, and that EE_2 only rarely gave rise to preneoplastic interstitial foci (13); thus providing a rationale for its weak tumorigenic activity.

Carcinogenic Activity of Steroidal Estrogens in the Hamster Kidney

Purdy et al. (14) have reported that DES, E_2, and EE_2 cause morphologic transformation of Balb/c 3T3 cells *in vitro*. These transformed cells grow as multicellular tumor spheroids and cause tumor formation when injected into NIH nude mice. In contrast, Moxestrol did not lead to any detectable morphologic transformation of Balb/c 3T3 cells, and this was attributed to its lack of ability to be appreciably metabolized to catechol products. However, using the hamster kidney model, Liehr (15) reported an 80% tumor incidence using Moxestrol. Our laboratory (6) found that Moxestrol is as effective as E_2 and DES in producing 100% renal tumor incidence after nine months of treatment with a similar number of combined tumor foci in each animal as the other potent carcinogenic estrogens (Table 2). It is clear from these studies that Moxestrol is highly tumorigenic in the hamster kidney and compares favorably with other potent carcinogenic estrogens. In marked contrast, EE_2 induces only one or two very small tumor foci in only 10% of animals similarly treated (16).

Moxestrol Metabolism in Various Species

In the last decade, a pertinent etiologic role for the metabolism of estrogens in neoplastic transformation has been postulated (17). While there is considerable evidence that estrogens are capable of undergoing oxidative metabolism to form catechols and then ortho-semiquinone and -quinone intermediates via a number of enzymatic pathways, including horseradish peroxidase, mushroom tyrosinase, medullary prostaglandin H-synthetase, and phenobarbital-induced cytochrome P-450 oxidase, evidence is still lacking on whether these reactions are relevant to tumor formation in an estrogen-induced site. While estrogen hydroxylase activity has been shown in the hamster liver and kidney (18), confounding evidence indicates that these activities are markedly reduced by chronic estrogen treatment (19). This finding has also been confirmed in present studies.

Table 1. Hormonal Parameters of Natural and Synthetic Steroidal Estrogens[a]

Estrogen[b]	Competitive Binding % Inhibition[c]	Induction Prog Receptor fmol/mg P	Serum Prolactin ng/ml[d]
17β-Estradiol	92 $\pm$ 1	49 $\pm$ 6	390 $\pm$ 76
Estrone	85 $\pm$ 1	47 $\pm$ 1	378 $\pm$ 58
Ethinylestradiol	91 $\pm$ 1	56 $\pm$ 3	210 $\pm$ 55
Moxestrol	85 $\pm$ 2	60 $\pm$ 2	330 $\pm$ 65

[a] Results are expressed as the mean $\pm$ SEM.
[b] Duration of treatment was 3.5 months for the induction of progesterone receptor and serum prolactin levels, and 9-10 months for the competitive binding of the estrogen receptor.
[c] Competitive binding of radioinert estrogens for estrogen receptor was carried out on cytosols obtained from hamster estrogen-induced renal carcinomas, with 5 nM [^{3}H]-estradiol alone or in combination with competitive nonradioactive compounds at 100-fold excess.
[d] Serum prolactin levels were assayed by the Nb_2 node rat lymphoma cell bioassay.

Table 2. Tumorigenic Parameters of Natural and Synthetic Steroidal Estrogens

Estrogen[a]	No. Animals with Tumors/n	% Tumor Incidence	Combined No. Tumor Nod.[b]
17β-Estradiol	20/20	100	18 $\pm$ 4
Estrone	20/20	100	14 $\pm$ 5
Ethinylestradiol	2/20	10	2 $\pm$ 1
Moxestrol	20/20	100	18 $\pm$ 3

[a] Duration of treatment was 9.0-10.0 months. After the initial pellet implantation, additional estrogenic compound pellets were implanted every 2.5 months.
[b] Values represent the mean number of tumor foci per animal in each group $\pm$ SEM.

In regard to Moxestrol metabolism, it has been shown that humans and rats metabolize this synthetic estrogen to appreciable quantities of 16β-hydroxy Moxestrol and only low amounts of 2- and 4-hydroxy catechols (4,11). On the other hand, the major metabolic route in baboons was 2- and 4-hydroxylation, with complete absence of 16-hydroxylation. In the dog, however, the metabolism of Moxestrol is essentially absent. Therefore, it is clear from these data that the species and tissue are important considerations in Moxestrol metabolism. The authors concluded that the low concentration of catechol estrogens formed with Moxestrol, in most cases, is a result of the 11β-methoxy group effectively impeding hydroxylation at C-2 and C-4 owing to steric hindrance. In an attempt to compare estrogen carcinogenicity and catechol formation, Liehr et al. (15) reported that Moxestrol had the lowest rate of catechol formation when compared to E_2 and other potent estrogen carcinogens of the hamster kidney. In the same study, using microsomes from BALB/c 3T3 cells, these authors reported that Moxestrol was also a very poor substrate for 2- and or 4-hydroxylase activity, which was consistent with its lack of ability to transform these cells *in vitro*.

Estrone Metabolism in the Hamster Kidney

The oxidative metabolism of radiolabeled estrone and Moxestrol was carried out by a modified method described previously by us (20). We have previously reported that following incubation with [^{14}C]-estrone with hamster liver microsomes derived from castrated hamsters, six major and five minor metabolites were observed in addition to a large nonpolar fraction and a small amount of conversion of estrone to 17β-estradiol (20). In contrast, five major and two minor estrone metabolites were found after HPLC separation employing hamster kidney microsomes. Interestingly, there was a substantial conversion of estrone to 17β-estradiol, but the nonpolar peak was distinctly smaller compared to hamster liver microsomal incubations (Fig. 1). Only 61% of the parent compound remained. The hydroxy metabolites 7α, 6α, 6β, 2-, and 4-hydroxyestrone, as well as the 6-ketoestrone and 17β-estradiol were conclusively identified from known standards, on the basis of their mass spectra and retention time. Hamster kidney microsomes converted estrone largely to 2-hydroxyestrone and 17β-estradiol and smaller quantities of the 6α- and 6β-hydroxyestrone. Hamster kidney homogenates yielded mainly 2-hydroxyestrone, a monohydroxy estradiol metabolite, and 17β-estradiol. Except for homogenates, catechol intermediates represented 14% of the metabolized estrone.

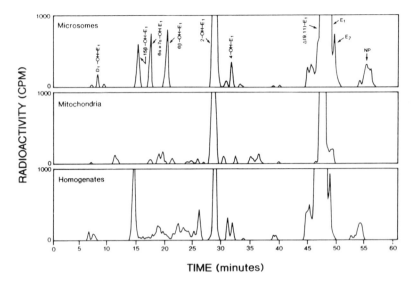

Figure 1. Representative HPLC profiles of [14C]-estrone metabolites in hamster kidney microsomes, mitochondria and homogenates. Incubations consisted of 7-8 mg kidney microsomal protein, 50 μM [14C]-estrone, 1 mM ascorbate and 2 mM NADPH. HPLC separation was carried out using a linear gradient of 52-72% methanol in water in 42 min, followed by 10 min elution with 100% methanol.

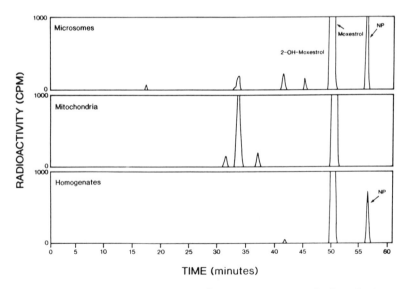

Figure 2. Typical HPLC profiles of [3H]-Moxestrol metabolites in hamster kidney microsomes, mitochondria, and homogenates. Details of the incubations are described under figure 1.

Moxestrol Metabolism in the Hamster Kidney

In marked contrast, incubations of hamster kidney microsomes with [³H]-Moxestrol (Fig. 2) yielded variable trace amounts of 2-hydroxy Moxestrol with the nonpolar material representing the largest peak (3%). Typically, 94-97% of the Moxestrol remained unmetabolized. Mitochondrial incubations of the hamster kidney yielded two minor metabolites and a substantial amount of an unknown metabolite; evidently not a catechol intermediate. It is highly significant that both whole kidney homogenates and isolated fresh proximal tubules incubated with radioactive Moxestrol resulted in negligible amounts of catechol Moxestrol intermediates (< 0.1%) (Fig. 3).

Conclusions

The quantity of 2-/4-hydroxyestrone found in kidney microsomes of the hamster represented over 14% of the total metabolites formed, whereas similar microsomal incubations with Moxestrol yielded no or negligible amounts of catechol intermediates. Since 94-97% of Moxestrol remained unmetabolized compared to 64% of estrone, these findings strongly weaken the belief that catechol estrogens and their subsequent semiquinone, quinone products, and redox recycling play a significant role in the tumorigenicity of Moxestrol. Based on these findings, we believe that this conclusion is valid for other potent tumorigenic estrogens as well that are capable of effecting tumor formation in the hamster kidney, particularly, when we and others have shown that the metabolism of estrogens is sharply and rapidly reduced in renal microsomes when derived from estrogenized castrated male hamsters.

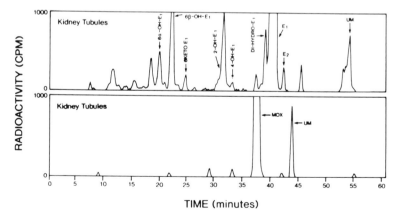

Figure 3. Representative HPLC profiles of [¹⁴C]-estrone and [³H]-Moxestrol. Kidney tubules were prepared as described previously by us (12), and the incubations were performed as indicated under Figure 1.

References

1. Raynaud JP (1973) Influence of rat estradiol binding plasma protein (EBP) on uterotrophic activity. Steroids 21:249-258.
2. Robyn C, M Vekemans, M Rozencweig, D Chigot and JP Raynaud (1978) Double-blind crossover clinical pharmacology study comparing Moxestrol (R-2858) and ethinyl estradiol in postmenopausal women. J Clin Pharmcol 18:29-34.
3. Bouton MM and JP Raynaud (1979) The relevance of interaction kinetics in determining biological response to estrogens. Endocrinology 105:509-515.
4. Salmon J, D Coussediere, C Cousty and JP Raynaud (1983) Pharmacokinetics and metabolism of Moxestrol in animals, rat, dog and monkey. J. Steroid Biochem 19:1223-1234.
5. Li JJ and SA Li (1990) Estrogen carcinogenesis in hamster tissues: A critical review. Endocrine Rev 11:524-531.
6. Li JJ, SA Li, TD Oberley, M Metzler and JA Parsons (1993) Further comparisons of carcinogenic activities of various natural and synthetic estrogens in the hamster kidney: Relation to proximal tubular cell proliferation in-vitro. Cancer Res, In press.
7. Li JJ and SA Li (1987) Estrogen carcinogenesis in Syrian hamster tissues: role of metabolism. Federation Proc 46:1858-1863.
8. Gotteschlich R and M Metzler (1980) Metabolic fate of diethylstilbestrol in Syrian golden hamster, a susceptible species for diethylstilbestrol carcinogenicity. Xenobiotica 10:317-327.
9. Liehr JG (1984) Modulation of estrogen-induced carcinogenesis by chemical modifications. Arch Toxicol 55: 119-122.
10. Tsibris JCM and PM McGuire (1977) Microsomal activation of estrogens and binding to nucleic acids and proteins. Biochem Biophys Res Commun 78:411-417.
11. Salmon J, D Coussediere, C Cousty and JP Raynaud (1983) Pharmacokinetics and metabolism of moxestrol in humans. J Steroid Biochem 18:565-573.
12. Oberley TD, Lauchner LJ, Pugh TD, Gonzalez A, Boldfarb S, Li SA, Li JJ (1989) Specific estrogen-induced cell proliferation of cultured syrian hamster renal proximal tubular cells in serum-free chemically defined media. Proc Natl Acad Sci USA 86:2107-2111.
13. Oberley TD, A Gonzalez, LJ Lauchner, LW Oberley and JJ Li (1991) Characterization of early kidney lesions in estrogen-induced tumors in the Syrian hamster. Cancer Res. 51;1922-1929.
14. Purdy RH, JW Goldzieher, PW Le Quesne, S Abdel-Baky, CK Durocher, PH Moore and JS Rhim (1982) Active intermediates in carcinogenesis. In Merriam GR & Lipsett MB (eds): Catechol Estrogens, New York: Raven Press, Chapt 13.

15. Liehr JG, RH Purdy, JS Baran, EF Nutting, F Colton, E Randerath and K Randerath (1987) Correlation of aromatic hydroxylation of 11β-substituted estrogens with morphological transformation *in vitro* but not with *in vivo* tumor induction by these hormones. Cancer Res 47: 2583-2588.
16. Li JJ, SA Li, JK Klicka, JA Parsons and LKT Lam (1983) Relative carcinogenic activity of various synthetic and natural estrogens in the hamster kidney. Cancer Res 43:5200-5204.
17. Li JJ and S Nandi (1990) Hormones and carcinogenesis: laboratory studies. In: Becker KL (ed) Principles and practice of endocrinology and metabolism. J.B. Lippincott Co. Philadelphia, Chap. 225.
18. Li SA, JK Klicka and JJ Li (1985) Estrogen 2-/4-hydroxylase activity, catechol estrogen formation and implications for estrogen carcinogenesis. Cancer Res 45:181-185.
19. Liehr JG (1990) Genotoxic effects of estrogens. Mutat Res 238:269-276.
20. Haaf H, M Metzler and JJ Li (1992) Metabolism of [^{14}C]-estrone in hamster and rat hepatic and renal microsomes: Species-, sex- and age-specific differences. J Steroid Biochem. In Press.

PART 4. HORMONES AND TUMOR PROMOTION

INTRODUCTION

Inhibition of Tumor Promotion by Antihormonal Agents

Leonard J. Lerner

Hormones are regulatory substances. They stimulate, inhibit, or modulate physiological processes throughout the body. Growth and development and normal bodily functions would be impossible without these products of the endocrine system.

Excessive amounts of hormones can be detrimental, but excess activity by these substances is usually self-limiting through feedback mechanisms that reduce secretion or release of that hormone. Other mechanisms for controlling hormonal activity involve receptor desensitization through reduction in the numbers or binding potency of these proteins; increased metabolism and/or excretion of the hormone; secretions of counteracting hormones; or by other means.

Administration of natural synthetic hormonal compounds having estrogenic activity for a prolonged period of time or in large dosages has been associated with an increased incidence of cancers. There is a lack of evidence to demonstrate that estrogens in the absence of other factors are causative of these cancers.

Factors involved in estrogen-associated neoplasms include genetics, since different strains and species of animals exhibit different susceptibilities, and there are family-associated increased risks in humans. Additional factors include viruses, radiation, and chemical carcinogens.

The cooperative nature of a hormone and a chemical carcinogen is demonstrated in the DMBA (dimethylbenzanthracene) mammary tumors in the rat. Tumor induction by DMBA administration depends on the presence of endogenous or exogenous estrogen. Removal of estrogen by ovariectomy or by treating the animal with an antiestrogen blocks tumor growth (1,2). Inhibition of the tumor with an estrogen antagonist continues for as long as treatment is continued, but growth resumes soon after cessation of such treatment (3). Similarly, administration of an estrogen to a rat whose DMBA-induced mammary tumor was suppressed by ovariectomy allows for a resumption of growth of that tumor.

The experience gained through three decades of antiestrogen use in women with breast cancer demonstrates that progression of the tumor can be inhibited and that complete disease-free status is attainable in many women. Even more exciting are the findings that adjuvant tamoxifen therapy may have prevented the development of primary tumors in the counterlateral breasts of the treated women (4,5).

Studies in animals and humans with the relatively nontoxic antiestrogens in breast tumors favored by an estrogenic environment are encouraging the investigation of long-term antihormonal therapy in women apparently free of disease but having familial history of breast cancers and other risk factors.

The availability of receptor antagonists for all classes of steroid hormones (2,6-9) as well as inhibitors of the biosynthesis of such hormones should allow for better investigation of the involvement of steroid hormones in growth phenomena and carcinogenesis. Similarly the identification of various growth factors apparently induced by hormones should stimulate the search for, or the synthesis of, specific inhibitors of those growth factors. All of these inhibitors should have clinical utility as well as help elucidate the sequential events involved in hormonal carcinogenesis.

References

1. Jordan VC, Dix CJ, Allen KE (1979) The effectiveness of a long-term treatment in a laboratory model for adjuvant hormone therapy of breast cancer. In: Salmon SE, Jones SE (eds) Adjuvant therapy for cancer, II. Grune and Stratten, New York, pp 19-26.
2. Lerner LJ, Jordan VC (1990) Development of antiestrogens and their use in breast cancer: Eight Cain Memorial Award Lecture. Cancer Res 50:4177-4189.
3. Robinson SP, Maul DA, Jordan VC (1988) Antitumor actions of toremifene in the 7,12-dimethylbenzanthracene (DMBA)-induced rat mammary tumor model. Eur J Cancer Clin Oncol 24:1817-1821.
4. Cuzik J, Baum M (1985) Tamoxifen and contralateral breast cancer. Lancet 2:282.
5. Forander T, Rutquist LE, Cedermark B, Glas U, Mattson A, Siljversward JD, Skoog L, Somell A, Theve T, Wilking N, Askergren J, Hjolmar ML (1989) Adjuvant tamoxifen in early breast cancer: occurrence of new primary cancers. Lancet 1:117-120.
6. Lerner LJ, Holthaus FJ, Jr, Thompson CR (1958) A non-steroidal estrogen antagonist 1-(p-2-diethylaminoethoxy-phenyl)-1-phenyl-2-p-methoxyphenyl ethanol. Endocrinology 63:295-318.
7. Lerner LJ, Bianchi A, Borman A (1960) A-norprogesterone, an androgen antagonist. Proc Soc Exp Biol Med 103:172-175.
8. Lerner LJ (1964) Hormone antagonists: Inhibitors of specific activities of estrogen and androgen. Recent Progress in Hormone Res 20:435-490.

9. Herrman W, Wyss R, Riondel A, Philbert D, Teutsch G, Sakiz E, Baulieu EE (1982) Effect d'un steriode anti-progesterone chez la femme: interruption du cycle menstruel et de las grossesse au debut. C R Acad Sci Serie III 294:933-938.

12

Sexual Dimorphism of Hepatic Steroid Metabolism and Its Significance for Chemical Hepatocarcinogenesis

Christopher Liddle, Catherine Legraverend, Agneta Blanck, Inger Porsch-Hällström, Agneta Mode, and Jan-Åke Gustafsson

Introduction

Hepatic cytochrome P-450 (P-450) is a family of enzyme forms predominantly located in the smooth endoplasmic reticulum of hepatocytes. These enzymes are active in the metabolism of an extensive range of endogenous and xenobiotic compounds. P-450s can be classified as being constitutive or inducible. By definition, constitutive forms of P-450 are found in normal untreated animals, while inducible P-450s increase in concentration, often from undetectable levels, following exposure to certain xenobiotic compounds.

Constitutive P-450s appear to be subject to complex hormonal regulation. In rats and some other rodents there is a pronounced sexual dimorphism of hepatic oxidative metabolism due to different expression of P-450 enzyme forms between the sexes. The rat 2C11 and 2C13 genes encode two male-specific P-450s: a testosterone 16α-hydroxylase and a testosterone 6β-hydroxylase, respectively. The 2C12 gene product is a female-specific steroid sulfate 15β-hydroxylase. Previous studies in rats, predominantly performed *in vivo*, have indicated that the pattern of growth hormone (GH) release from the pituitary gland is a major determinant of this sex difference (1). The male pattern of GH-secretion is characterized by regular bursts every 3-4 h with low, often undetectable, levels in between, whereas the female pattern of secretion is irregular with higher basal levels (2). "Feminization" of a number of male liver functions has been achieved by elevating the basal serum level of GH, e.g., by continuous GH infusion (3, 4). Other hormones, such as glucocorticoids and iodothyronines (1), have also been implicated in the regulation of constitutive P-450s.

Experimental hepatocarcinogenesis in the rat has been shown to be sex-specific in a number of different models (5-7). Following treatment according to the resistant hepatocyte model (RH-model) (8) foci of enzyme-altered cells grow faster in the male than in the female rat liver, and males develop hepatocellular carcinomas earlier than female rats (7). This sex difference occurs during promotion/selection of diethylnitrosamine (DEN)-initiated cells with dietary 2-acetylaminofluorene (2-AAF) and a 2/3 partial hepatectomy (PH). GH has tentatively been identified as the hormone responsible for the observed sexual dimorphism in focal growth (2,9). An understanding of the hormonal regulation of constitutive P-450 enzyme forms is likely to help clarify the role of GH and other hormones in hepatic carcinogenesis.

Hormonal Regulation of Male Sexually Differentiated P-450s in Primary Cultured Rat Hepatocytes

Introduction

A major limitation of *in vivo* models to study hormonal regulation of P-450 is determining whether the actions of hormones on individual hepatic P-450 enzymes are direct or mediated by secondary hormonal changes. Difficulty in constitutively expressing mRNA or protein for male-specific forms of P-450 using *in vitro* models, such as primary cell cultures, has impeded efforts to examine the direct actions of hormones on these enzyme forms. Some male-specific P-450s, such as forms 2C11 and 2C13, are not subject to any known xenobiotic induction and cannot be studied using this approach. It has been previously demonstrated that when primary hepatocytes are cultured on a laminin-rich basement membrane matrix (Matrigel), the cells maintain the ability to express specialized hepatic proteins, including albumin, and following the addition of GH to culture medium, the constitutive female-specific P-450, form 2C12 (10).

Our purpose was to determine if primary cultures of hepatocytes, such as those previously used for the expression of P-450 2C12, could be used for the study of some male-specific rat P-450 enzyme forms (2C11 and 2C13) as measured by steady-state mRNA concentrations and to investigate the direct regulatory actions of GH, glucocorticoids, and iodothyronines on these enzyme forms.

Results and Discussion

Hepatocyte mRNA concentrations for both male-specific P-450s decayed rapidly during the first 24 h in culture in modified Waymouth medium. However, by day 3 the constitutive expression of 2C13 mRNA had begun to increase and by day 7 the level was 86% of that observed in livers from normal male rats. Expression of 2C11 mRNA remained low until day 3, but increased by day 5 when the level was 43% of normal. No further increase in 2C11 mRNA occurred after day 5.

The presence of bovine GH (100 ng/ml) in the culture medium almost completely suppressed the expression of 2C11 mRNA in hepatocytes when measured on days 3, 5 and 7. In contrast, GH only reduced 2C13 message to approximately 50% of that found in untreated control cells. However, when cells were cultured in the presence of (10^{-8} M) dexamethasone (DEX), 2C13 levels were reduced. This resulted in 2C13 mRNA being 20%, 30%, and 22% of control on days 3, 5 and 7 respectively. Interestingly, the negative regulatory effect of DEX on 2C13 was more profound than that of GH. DEX treatment caused a moderate increase in 2C11 expression, being 350% of control on day 3, 127% on day 5 and 225% on day 7. Treatment of cells with (10^9 M) L-triiodothyronine (T3) had no consistent effects on the expression of mRNA for 2C13 in either culture medium, though it did appear to cause some repression of 2C11. When cells were treated with combinations of hormones, in either medium, the following patterns emerged. GH exerted the dominant regulatory effect on 2C11 expression resulting in marked down-regulation of message for this form even in the presence of DEX. In contrast, the combined action of GH and DEX on 2C13 expression appeared to be additive, resulting in marked suppression of this form. Again T3 was found to have no effect on 2C13. Effects on 2C11 were minor and variable.

In summary, these findings demonstrate that primary cultured rat hepatocytes are a suitable model to examine the regulation of at least some constitutive male-specific P-450s. GH acts directly on rat hepatocytes at a pretranslation level to down-regulate the expression of these forms. Glucocorticoids also exert direct pretranslational action on these forms, specifically to increase the expression of mRNA for P-450 2C11 and to decrease that for 2C13.

Transcriptional Regulation of Rat P-450 IIC Gene Subfamily Members by the Sexually Dimorphic Pattern of GH Secretion

Introduction

We have examined the issue of whether the direct and divergent effects of GH on the hepatic expression of the 2C11, 2C12, and 2C13 mRNAs are exerted at the transcriptional level both *in vivo* and in primary cultures of rat hepatocytes. Our previous attempts to investigate the exact level of pretranslational regulation by GH of 2C11 and 2C12 have been hampered by the high degree of nucleic acid homology (71-88%) characteristic of the rat class 2C P450 gene subfamily. To this end, we developed a specific and sensitive run-on assay that clearly discriminates between members of the P-450 2C gene subfamily.

Results and Discussion

Equal amounts of nascent [^{32}P]UTP-labeled RNA were hybridized, under conditions where the signal is proportional to the amount of input RNA, to an excess of full-length cDNA coding for the 2C11, 2C12, or 2C13 gene. cDNAs for β-actin and tyrosine aminotransferase (TAT) were included as controls: β-actin as a housekeeping gene, TAT as the accumulation of its mRNA was previously reported not to be affected by GH treatment in hepatocyte cultures. The comparison by nuclear run-on analysis of liver nuclei isolated from two adult males and two adult females demonstrates that signals for the male-specific 2C11 and 2C13 transcripts are barely detectable with female nuclei and signals for the female-specific 2C12 transcript are very weak with male nuclei indicating that at least *in vivo*, the sex-specificity is tightly controlled at the transcriptional level.

We also examined the effects of hypophysectomy (Hx) as well as the two GH-substitution treatments for 1, 3 and 6 days on the rates of initiation of transcription in Hx males and females, and two clearly distinct patterns of transcriptional regulation by GH emerged from densitometric analysis of autoradiographs. The first pattern, induced by single daily (male-like) injections of GH into Hx animals of both sexes, resulted in the increased transcription of the 2C11 gene at a level comparable to that of normal males within 3 days, as well as a slight increase in the 2C13 gene transcription above Hx level. The second pattern induced after continuous (female-like) infusion of GH, consisted of a rapid suppression of 2C13 gene transcription (90% at day 1), while the transcription of the 2C12 gene increased above the normal female levels within 6 days. As has been previously reported, Hx females respond better than Hx males to both types of GH treatments. Transcription of the TAT and 2C13 genes remained higher in Hx males than in Hx females indicating that not all sex differences are abolished 2 to 3 weeks after hypophysectomy.

Having established the different patterns of GH administration in the control of transcription of 2C11, 2C12, and 2C13 genes *in vivo*, we went on to investigate if similar events occurred in hepatocytes maintained in a hormonally defined environment. When 3-day-old male hepatocyte cultures on Matrigel were treated with 50 ng bovine GH/ml, the transcription of the female-specific P-450 2C12 gene was increased within 2 hours, with an 11-fold induction after 20 h. The male-specific 2C11 and 2C13 genes were repressed by 70% and 60%, respectively, at 20 h. In agreement with the previously reported lack of GH effect on the TAT mRNA accumulation in culture, we found the transcription of the TAT gene to be unaffected by GH.

These findings clearly demonstrate that the constitutive members of the P-450 2C subfamily are directly regulated by GH at the level of transcription.

Aberrant Regulation of Two Sex-Specific Forms of P-450 in Liver Nodules from Male and Female Rats

Introduction

Several enzymes that contribute to the resistance of liver nodules to a variety of toxic agents, including P-450 species mediating different pathways in the metabolism of 2-AAF and the sulfotransferase catalyzing N,O-sulfaction of N-hydroxy-2-AAF, have been shown to be sex-specific and regulated by GH. In addition to the suggested involvement of GH in sex-differentiated liver carcinogenesis, we have previously demonstrated an attenuated sex differentiation of a number of P-450 mediated reactions toward steroid and xenobiotic substrates in liver nodules when compared with surrounding tissue. This might indicate that nodular tissue is withdrawn from the normal endocrine regulation of rat liver, an escape of possible significance for the preneoplastic state. Studies of sex-specific P-450 forms may represent a tool towards a better understanding of the regulation of P-450 system in hepatocyte nodules.

The present study was designed to investigate how P-450s 2C11 and 2C12 are regulated at the mRNA and protein levels in preneoplastic lesions from male and female rats treated according to the RH model and to study whether the normal GH-regulation of these genes is affected in nodular tissue.

Results and Discussion

A 3- to 11-fold decrease in the mRNA expression of the male-predominant P-450 2C11 was observed in nodules and hepatomas from male livers at the different time intervals after initiation, when compared with surrounding tissue. The expression of the female-predominant P-450 2C12 was increased two- to eightfold in the same nodules and hepatomas vs. the surrounding liver. Western blot analysis of microsomal preparations confirmed that the alterations in P-450 mRNA expression in nodules vs. surrounding liver from male rats were reflected in similar changes at the protein level. No significant differences in the mRNA expression of these P-450 enzyme forms were observed in female nodules vs. surrounding liver.

When nodule-bearing male rats received bovine GH infusion for one week before sacrifice, 8 months postinitiation, the surrounding liver responded with a ninefold decrease in the expression of P-450 2C11 and a 14-fold increase in the expression of P-450 2C12. The expression of 2C11 in nodules decreased fivefold following GH treatment, whereas no effect was seen with respect to the nodular expression of 2C12. Treatment of nodule-bearing males with human GH, 11 months postinitiation, caused an efficient induction of 2C12 both in nodules (ninefold) and in surrounding tissue (14-fold), with an expression in nodules exceeding that of surrounding liver. P-450 2C11 expression was markedly decreased in nodules and surrounding liver following human GH treatment.

A decreased expression of P-450 2C12 mRNA was observed in response to Hx of nodule-bearing female rats, both in nodules and in surrounding tissue. No differences in DNA content in the total nucleic acid samples were observed between the different tissues of Hx and intact animals. P-450 2C11 expression was below the detection level both in nodular and surrounding liver from intact and Hx nodule-bearing female rats.

In conclusion, our findings strongly support the view that nodules, to some extent, respond in an aberrant way to the endocrine regulation of rat liver. Further studies are needed to elucidate the mechanisms behind the induction of these alterations in response to hormonal manipulation and to evaluate their relevance in terms of sex-differentiated hepatocarcinogenesis.

Acknowledgments

This study was supported by a grant from the Swedish Medical Research Council (No. 03X-06807).

References

1. Mode A, Wiersma-Larsson E, Ström A, Zaphiropoulos PG, Gustafsson J-Å (1989) A dual role of growth hormone as a feminizing and masculinizing factor in the control of sex-specific cytochrome P-450 isozymes in rat liver. J Endocrinol 120:311-317.
2. Edén S (1979) Age and sex related differences in episodic growth hormone secretion in the rat. Endocrinology 105:555-560.
3. Mode A, Norstedt G, Simic B, Eneroth P, Gustafsson J-Å (1981) Continuous infusion of growth hormone feminizes hepatic steroid metabolism in the rat. Endocrinology 108:2103-2108.
4. Blanck A, Åström A, Hansson T, DePierre J, Gustafsson J-Å (1986) Pituitary regulation of cytochrome P-450-mediated metabolism of steroids and xenobiotics in rat liver microsomes. Carcinogenesis 7:575-582.
5. Stasney J, Paschkis KE, Cantarow A, Rothenberg MS (1947) Neoplasms in rats with 2-acetylaminofluorene and sex hormones. Cancer Res 7:356-362.
6. Wogan GN, Newberne PM (1967) Dose-response characteristics of aflatoxin B_1 carcinogenesis in the rat. Cancer Res 27:2370-2376.
7. Blanck A, Hansson T, Gustafsson J-Å, Ericksson LC (1986) Pituitary grafts modify sex differences in liver tumor formation in the rat following initiation with diethylnitrosamine and different promotion regimens. Carcinogenesis 7:981-985.
8. Solt D, Farber E (1976) New principle for the analysis of chemical carcinogenesis. Nature 262:701-703.
9. Blanck A, Hansson T, Eriksson LC, Gustafsson J-Å (1987) Growth hormone modifies the growth rate of enzyme-altered foci in male rats treated according to the resistant hepatocyte model. Carcinogenesis 8:1585-1588.
10. Guzelian PS, Li D, Schuetz EG, Thomas P, Levin W, Mode A, Gustafsson J-Å (1988) Sex change in cytochrome P-450 phenotype by growth hormone treatment of adult rat hepatocytes maintained in a culture system on Matrigel. Proc Natl Acad Sci USA 85:9783-9787.

13

Growth Stimulation and Tumor Promotion in Rat Liver by Ethynyl Estradiol and Other Estrogens

James D. Yager

Introduction

During the mid 1970s, a series of case reports were published that described a strong association in women between prolonged oral contraceptive (OC) use and the appearance of liver neoplasms (1,2). Based on clinical observations, which included a few examples of regression of the liver neoplasms following cessation of OC use, and the experimental demonstrations that synthetic estrogens were not mutagenic, we hypothesized that the synthetic steroidal estrogens would be promoters of hepatocarcinogenesis (3). Subsequently, we (3) and others (2,4) demonstrated that mestranol (17-α ethynyl estradiol 3-methyl ether) and ethynyl estradiol (EE) are promoters of the appearance of preneoplastic foci and hepatocellular carcinomas in several strains of female rats. The strength of the promoting ability of these estrogens compared to several other promoters in the rat model of hepatocarcinogenesis is indicated by calculation of their promotion indices (PI), which are a function of the volume fraction of treated liver occupied by altered hepatic foci (AHF), divided by the volume fraction of control liver occupied by AHF, times the dose of promoting agent administered per week (5). The PI of phenobarbital, a classic liver promoter, was calculated to be 140, whereas the PIs for mestranol, EE, and 2,3,7,8-tetrachlorodibenzo-p-dioxin (TCDD) were calculated to be 54,000, 93,000, and 28,000,000, respectively. Thus, while the synthetic steroidal estrogens are considerably less potent than TCDD, they are approximately 400-700 times more potent than phenobarbital. In addition, both mestranol and EE treatment results in the appearance of AHF in the livers of noninitiated rats. However, studies on these two estrogens conducted in two laboratories failed to demonstrate significant genotoxic effects or ability to initiate hepatocarcinogenesis.

A property shared by most, if not all, tumor promoters is their ability to stimulate cell proliferation. Results from our laboratory (3) and others (6) have also shown this to be true for the synthetic steroidal estrogens. In the remainder of this paper, the DNA synthetic response upon EE treatment and the cellular events associated with it will be reviewed. In addition, new preliminary data on the effects of other estrogenic chemicals are also presented.

Materials and Methods

The details of the methodology used for the experiments being described have been published previously (3,7-9). In addition, brief descriptions of the experimental approaches and methods will be presented along with the results.

Results and Discussion

Effects of EE on Liver DNA Synthesis

Figure 1 shows the time course of liver DNA synthesis following treatment of female rats with EE using time-release tablets; animals fed phenobarbital in their diet are included for comparison (3). Both promoters induced a rapid threefold to fourfold increase in ^{3}H-thymidine incorporation (2 hr exposure) into liver DNA. DNA synthesis remained elevated through at least 7 days, but was at control levels at 14 and 21 days. For EE, the increase measured at 24 hr followed a dose response between 0.1 and 2.5 μg/day (3). Ochs et al. (6) have shown by autoradiography that this predominately represents DNA synthesis in hepatocytes. The level of DNA synthesis 24 hr after a 2/3 surgical partial hepatectomy would be approximately fourfold to fivefold greater than that induced by EE, whereas elevated DNA synthesis persists longer with EE treatment (3). However, if enhanced DNA synthesis is an important aspect of the mechanism of promotion by EE, one would expect that an elevated level of DNA synthesis would persist throughout the period of EE treatment and not return to control levels within 14 to 21 days as seen here. As indicated, these results were obtained using a 2 hr exposure to ^{3}H-thymidine. This method is considerably less sensitive than use of osmotic minipumps to administer ^{3}H-thymidine or bromodeoxyuridine over a 3 to 10 day labeling period (10). Thus, an experiment is currently under way where the latter approach is being used to address the important question of whether a persistent low level elevation of liver DNA synthesis is associated with chronic EE treatment.

Table 1 lists several potential causes of increased liver cell proliferation. Liver growth can occur in response to hepatotoxicity, metabolic stress, and the presence of growth factors or comitogens. Obviously, it is important to determine which of these mechanisms is responsible for liver growth caused by any xenobiotic agent. The most sensitive experimental approach for determining hepatotoxicity is the use of the prelabeled liver technique (3). Liver DNA is

Table 1. Liver growth.

Regenerative/Repair Growth
A. In response to surgical removal of a portion of the liver
B. In response to xenobiotics at hepatotoxic doses
CCl_4
3'Me DAB
Choline deficiency

Additive Growth
A. In response to xenobiotics at nonhepatotoxic doses
Phenobarbital and other barbiturates
Hypolipidemic agents
B. In response to liver growth factors and comitogens
Growth factors
EGF/TGF-a
HepGFs (HPTA, HPTB, HGF)
Comitogens
Norepinephrine
Phenobarbital?

(Adapted from slide in presentation by R. Jirtle at 1990 SOT Meeting)

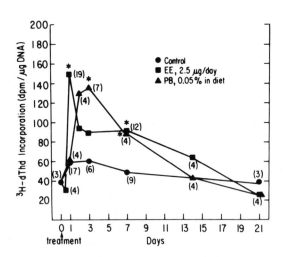

Fig. 1. Time course of liver DNA synthesis following treatment with EE (2.5 μg/day delivered via time release tablet) or phenobarbital (0.05% in the diet). This figure was taken from (3) with permission.

prelabeled using multiple injections of ^{3}H-thymidine following surgical partial hepatectomy. After allowing a 2-week period for recovery, the rats are then exposed to the test agent and at various times thereafter, days to weeks, the amount of label remaining in liver DNA is determined. As liver cells die, their DNA is degraded, which is reflected in a loss of prelabel. This loss is cumulative, and thus, this technique is a very sensitive indicator of hepatotoxicity. When such an experiment was conducted using mestranol and EE, the results were negative, indicating a lack of hepatotoxicity at the low doses (2.5-5.0 μg/day/rat) employed. These results indicated that the synthetic estrogens should be classified as xenobiotics able to stimulate additive growth at nonhepatotoxic doses.

Mechanisms of Liver Growth Stimulation by EE

Serum Factor(s)

Several laboratories have identified and characterized liver cell growth factors from the sera of partially hepatectomized rats [see (9) for references]. In preliminary experiments, we found that sera from EE-treated rats, fractionated on Sephadex G-200, contained elevated levels of a factor(s) stimulatory for hepatocyte DNA synthesis. This activity eluted from the column at a point consistent with a molecular weight of approximately 135 kDa and could be inactivated by heat and trypsin. In addition, the increase in activity stimulatory for hepatocyte DNA synthesis in the Sephadex G-200 fractions was also accompanied by increased competition with ^{125}I-epidermal growth factor (EGF) for specific binding to rat liver membranes. Antibody to EGF did not block the DNA synthesis stimulatory activity of these fractions. These results suggest that EE treatment enhances the level in serum of a factor(s) that appears to be a hepatocyte growth factor. Very preliminary evidence suggests that it may be in the EGF family. If so, this factor would be distinct from hepatocyte growth factor whose receptor was recently shown to be the *met* oncogene (11).

Effects on DNA Synthesis in Cultured Hepatocytes

The rat hepatocyte primary culture system was used to determine whether EE and other estrogens had direct growth stimulatory effects as reflected by stimulation of DNA synthesis (7). Figure 2 shows the effects of EE alone and together with EGF on hepatocyte DNA synthesis. EE alone caused a small, approximately twofold increase in incorporation, whereas with EGF alone the increase was 11-fold over control. However, in cultures treated with both EE and EGF, DNA synthesis was increased 32-fold above control levels.

If the response to EE + EGF were additive, the fold increase would have been 13-fold rather than the 32-fold actually observed. Statistical analysis of this data revealed a significant interaction between EE and EGF. Additional studies

Table 2. Summary of results obtained with EE in cultured hepatocytes.

1. >95% of EE is rapidly metabolized to polar conjugates within 4 hr, thus accounting for the relatively high concentrations required to enhance EGF responsiveness (8).

2. EE treatment causes a > twofold increase in ^{125}I-EGF cell surface specific binding and in total cellular EGF receptor protein (7,9).

3. The mechanism of the increase in EGF receptor involves a twofold increase in receptor protein half-life, not increased transcription or protein synthesis (9).

where hepatocytes were pretreated with EE prior to addition of EGF revealed that EE enhances DNA synthesis in response to EGF (7).

Table 2 presents a summary of the major results obtained in subsequent studies on the metabolism of EE and the mechanism of its stimulatory effects on hepatocyte EGF responsiveness.

Effects of Other Xenobiotics with Estrogenic Activity

More recently, we have begun to investigate whether other chemicals with estrogenic activity, such as diethylstilbestrol (DES), DDT, the zearalenone mycotoxins and selected phytoestrogens, have activities similar to EE on hepatocyte DNA synthesis. The rationale for pursuing this line of investigation

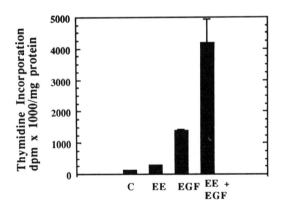

Fig. 2. Hepatocyte cultures were exposed to EE (15 μM) and/or EGF (25 ng/ml) for 0-30 hr and to ^{3}H-thymidine for 30-48 hr. Mean $\pm$ SD of triplicate cultures. Adapted from Table 1 in (7).

is that use of nonsteroidal estrogens would (1) provide information pertaining to structure/activity, estrogen-receptor affinity relationships; and (2) the potential for natural product estrogens to affect liver DNA synthesis and thus perhaps to be promoters of hepatocarcinogenesis. The effects of DES, α-zearalenol (alpha Z), mestranol (Mes), and EE alone (at a concentrations of 3 μM) $\pm$ EGF on hepatocyte DNA synthesis are shown in Figure 3. ^{3}H-thymidine incorporation into control cultures was 610 $\pm$ 50 dpm/culture. EGF alone induced a 13.5-fold increase. In the cultures treated with the estrogens alone, the fold increases, over control, were: DES, 2.2; alpha Z, 1.8; Mes, 3.8; and EE, 3.7. In contrast, when both the estrogens and EGF were present together, the fold increases over control were: DES + EGF, 32.4; alpha Z + EGF, 24.5; Mes + EGF, 55; and EE + EGF, 39. Clearly, the response of the hepatocytes to the combination of estrogen and EGF was more than additive of the response to either alone. In addition, the mycotoxin estrogen alpha zearalenol was the least effective, consistent with its reduced affinity for the estrogen receptor. That mestranol appeared to be most effective might be due to persistence in the cultures due to slower metabolism; however, this requires further investigation. Finally, these results clearly show that the ability of EE to cause enhanced EGF responsiveness is not due to its steroidal structure and further supports the role for the estrogen receptor in this process.

Concluding Remarks

The results of our studies have shown that the synthetic estrogens are strong promoters of hepatocarcinogenesis. In addition, EE stimulates increased liver

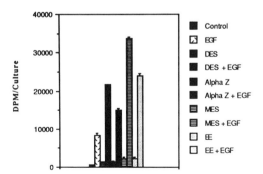

Fig. 3. The effects of diethylstilbesterol (DES), alpha zearalenol (alpha Z), mestranol (Mes) and EE $\pm$ EGF on DNA synthesis (^{3}H-thymidine incorporation into DNA) in cultured rat hepatocytes. The experimental protocol was as described previously (7). The estrogens were present at a concentration of 3 μM and EGF at 20 ng/ml. Each bar represents the mean $\pm$ range of duplicate cultures.

DNA synthesis. However, it is not yet clear whether this is associated in a causal way with its promoting activity, especially since increased DNA synthesis was only transient as determined using 2 hr exposure to ^{3}H-thymidine. This question is presently being reexamined using more sensitive methodology. With regard to the mechanism of effect of EE, our results clearly show that the estrogens are not direct-acting mitogens for liver. Rather, in accord with the causes of liver cell proliferation listed in Table 2, the estrogens should be classified as comitogens for liver. However, since the role of EGF, if any, in liver growth is not clear, it is important to now determine whether EE also enhances the growth stimulatory activity of hepatocyte growth factor which is more likely to be important in mediating liver growth *in vivo*. Finally, our most recent results show that several other estrogens, including the nonsteroidal synthetic estrogen, DES, as well as the mycotoxin estrogen, alpha zearalenol, are also able to enhance hepatocyte responsiveness to EGF. Based on these results, we predict that these estrogens will also stimulate cell proliferation *in vivo* at nonhepatotoxic doses and might also be promoters of hepatocarcinogenesis.

Acknowledgments

This work was supported by PHS NCI grant CA36701. I am also indeted to Dr. Y. Eric Shi who carried out much of the previously published work with the cultured hepatocytes, to Dr. Joanne Zurlo for her constructive, critical comments, and to Ms. Jane Miller for excellent technical assistance.

References

1. Molina, R, Martinez, L, Salas, O, et al (1989) Combined oral contraceptives and liver cancer. Int J Cancer 43:254-259.
2. Porter, LE, Van Thiel, DH Eagon, PK, (1987) Estrogens and progestins as tumor inducers. Semin Liver Dis 7:24-31.
3. Yager, J., Roebuck, BD, Paluszcyk, TL Memoli, VA (1986) Effects of ethinyl estradiol and tamoxifen on liver DNA turnover and new synthesis and appearance of gamma glutamyl transpeptidase-positive foci in female rats. Carcinogenesis 7:2007-2014.
4. Campen, DB, Sloop, TC, Maronpot, RR, Lucier, GW (1987) Continued development of hepatic γ-glutamyltranspeptidase-positive foci upon withdrawal of 17 α-ethinyl estradiol in diethylnitrosamine-initiated rats. Cancer Res 47:2328-2333.
5. Dragan, Y, Xu, Y-D, Pitot, HC (1991) Tumor promotion as a target for estrogen/antiestrogen effects in rat hepatocarcinogenesis. Prev Med 20: 15-26.
6. Ochs, H, Dusterberg, B, Gunzel, P, Schulte-Hermann, R (1986) Effect of tumor promoting contraceptive steroids on growth and drug metabolizing enzymes in rat liver. Cancer Res 46:1224-1232.

7. Shi, YE Yager, JD (1989) Effects of the liver tumor promoter ethinyl estradiol on epidermal growth factor-induced DNA synthesis and epidermal growth factor receptor levels in cultured rat hepatocytes. Cancer Res 49: 3574-3580.

8. Standeven, AM, Shi, YE, Sinclair, JF, Sinclair, PR Yager, JD (1990) Metabolism of the liver tumor promoter ethinyl estradiol by primary cultures of rat hepatocytes. Toxicol Applied Pharmacol 102:486-496.

9. Shi, YE, Yager, JD (1990) Regulation of rat hepatocyte epidermal growth factor receptor by the liver tumor promoter ethinyl estradiol. Carcinogenesis 11:1103-1109.

10. Eldridge, SR, Tilbury, LF, Goldsworthy, TL, Butterworth, BE (1990) Measurement of chemically induced cell proliferation in rodent liver and kidney: a comparison of 5-bromo-2'-deoxyuridine and [^{3}H] thymidine administered by injection or osmotic pump. Carcinogenesis 11:2245-2251.

11. Bottaro, DP, Rubin, JS, Faletto, DL, et al. (1991) Identification of the hepatocyte growth factor receptor as the c-*met* proto-oncogene product. Science 251:802-804.

14

Growth Factors in Murine Mammary Adenocarcinomas Induced by Progestins

Eduardo H. Charreau, Patricia Elizalde, Fabiana Guerra,
Claudia Lanari, Edith Kordon, and
Christiane Dosne Pasqualini

Introduction

Cellular proliferation involves different regulatory molecules that include hormones and growth factors. Interestingly, progestins can stimulate as well as inhibit the growth of tumors depending on the experimental design (1). In mammary cancer, polypeptide growth factors, such as EGF, TGFα, TGFβ, and IGF-I, IGF-II, may play either an autocrine or a paracrine role. The present study investigates the presence of these factors and their receptors in mammary adenocarcinomas induced by medroxyprogesterone acetate (MPA).

Induction of Mammary Adenocarcinomas by MPA

Long-term administration of depot MPA in BALB/c female mice leads to the development of mammary tumors with an actuarial incidence of 79% and an average latency of 52 weeks (2). They are metastatic cystic adenocarcinomas of the Dunn B type and are preceded by ductal preneoplastic lesions (3). *In vivo* syngeneic passages have led to the establishment of hormone-dependent (MPA-

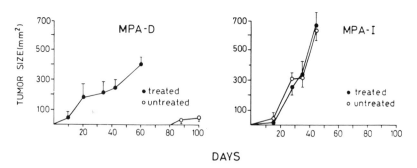

Fig. 1. Examples of MPA-D and MPA-I tumor growth.

Table 1. Concentration of IGF-I & IGF-II in tumor lines.

	IGF-I[a]	IGF-II[a]
MPA-D	58.3 ± 6.6 ($n=14$)	65 ± 6.2 ($n=3$)
MPA-D+MPA	56.5 ± 7.2 ($n=15$)	465 ± 57 ($n=3$)
MPA-I	62.5 ± 7.8 ($n=10$)	531 ± 45 ($n=3$)

[a]Values are expressed in ng/g tissue

D) and hormone-independent (MPA-I) lines (4); we have studied 3 MPA-D and 1 MPA-I lines (Fig. 1).

It is important to note that MPA-D tumors were obtained from mice both treated with 40 mg of MPA depot (MPA-D + MPA) and untreated (MPA-D), in which the tumors grew very slowly.

While all MPA-D lines presented high receptor contents of estradiol (20-254 fmol/mg protein), progesterone (63-710), and prolactin (50-75), the MPA-I lines studied yielded a low content (0-36; 0-13; 15-50, respectively) (5).

IGF-I & IGF-II in MPA-D & MPA-I Tumor Lines

Both IGF-I and II were isolated from tumor samples by acid-ethanol extraction (6) and characterized by molecular sieve chromatography on C18 columns, evaluating IGF-I by a specific radioimmunoassay and IGF-II by a radioreceptor assay. IGF-I expression was studied by Northern blot using a cDNA probe. Tumor concentration of immunoreactive IGF-I was similar for MPA-D+MPA, MPA-D, and MPA-I lines (Table 1).

However, with Northern blot analysis a clear regulation of IGF-I mRNA by MPA was observed in MPA-D tumors (Fig 2). Two IGF-I transcripts of approximately 4.7 and 1.4 Kb were revealed in MPA-I and MPA-D + MPA tumors. Rehybridization of Northern blot with a human GAPD cDNA probe showed equal RNA loading in all lanes. Thus, IGF-I expression appears to be regulated by progestins in MPA-D tumor lines. Although no changes were observed in endogenous IGF-I concentration after MPA treatment, the apparent difference with IGF-I-mRNA expression may be due to the fact that growth factor production has overloaded the reservoir capacity of the tumors so that the amount secreted is not being evaluated. In this sense, mRNA levels of IGF-I may better reflect the real situation of IGF-I synthesis.

On the other hand, definite MPA regulation of IGF-II protein level was detected by measuring tumor concentration (Table 1).

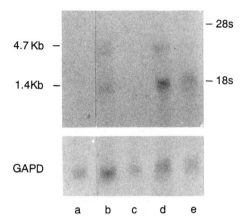

Fig. 2. IGF-I mRNA expression in MPA-D (a,c), MPA-D + MPA (b,d) and MPA-I (e) tumors.

Insulin-Like Growth Factor Receptors

Binding studies of IGF receptors were performed on washed microsomal pellets to avoid interference by the possible presence of IGF serum binding proteins. In all tumors tested we found specific type I & II IGF receptors. Scatchard analysis of the binding data showed the presence of high (K_D = 3.4 x 10^{-12} M, Q = 22.5 fmol/mg protein) and low (K_D = 1.3 x 10^{-10} M, Q = 143 fmol/mg protein) affinity binding sites.

Affinity cross-linking of ^{125}I-IGF-I and further analysis by SDS polyacrylamide gel electrophoresis under reducing conditions showed two labeled bands on autoradiograms. The more intensely labeled band appeared in the Mr 130,000 Da region corresponding to type I IGF receptors.

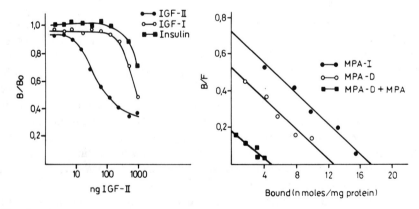

Fig. 3. IGF-II binding studies: (left) specificity (right) Scatchard analysis.

A second less intensive component of an apparent Mr of 260,000 Da could represent type II IGF receptors. No modulation of IGF-I receptors by MPA was observed.

Competitive binding with ^{125}I-IGF II showed that half-maximal displacement was observed with 5nM IGF-II; insulin and IGF-I were tenfold less effective in these competition studies (Fig.3). IGF-II binds only to its own receptor as seen in the affinity labeling studies with ^{125}I-IGF-II. Under reducing conditions, only a 260 KDa band was detected. No cross-linking to 130 KDa type I IGF receptor subunit was detected at nM concentrations of IGF-II. Scatchard analysis of IGF-II binding showed a single class of binding sites with an apparent K_D of 1-5 nM. Moreover, a clear MPA regulation of IGF-II receptors was evident (Fig.3): MPA-D + MPA exhibited much fewer binding sites than MPA-D or MPA-I tumors.

Epidermal and Transforming Growth Factors α and ß

We have previously demonstrated that the presence of EGF receptors is correlated with an autonomous pattern of tumor growth, since they were nondetectable in MPA-D and measurable in MPA-I tumors (3,5). Interestingly, in the acid ethanol extracts of all tumors tested, it was not possible to identify EGF or TGFα, nor could TGFα be detected by Northern blot analysis.

Recently, we have demonstrated the presence of TGFß-like polypeptides (6): in MPA-D and MPA-D + MPA tumors, a high molecular weight (43 KDa) TGFß-like activity was purified by Bio-Gel P-60 chromatography. This TGFß was able to confer the neoplastic phenotype to NRK-49 F cells without the addition of EGF, although its activity could be potentiated by EGF. It did not compete for binding to EGF receptors, had no mitogenic activity on monolayer cultures of NRK fibroblasts and was a potent inhibitor of DNA synthesis induced by EGF and insulin. Another TGFβ with a 13 KDa Mr was isolated from MPA-D and MPA-I tumors, showing the same biological properties as the 43 KDa one, except that in the absence of EGF it did not stimulate soft agar growth of NRK-49F cells. The *in vivo* synthesis of both factors in MPA-D tumors appears to be under MPA control, since their tissue content is much lower in MPA-D + MPA than in MPA-D tumors. In addition, when TGFß$_1$ gene expression was investigated, MPA regulation of its mRNA level was observed. The reported 2.5 Kb mRNA transcript was only detected in MPA-D tumors without MPA treatment. No expression of TGFß$_1$ was detected either in MPA-D + MPA or in MPA-I tumors. Thus, in all tumor lines capable of responding to MPA by increasing their proliferating rate, the hormone inhibits TGFß$_1$ expression. Moreover, TGFß$_1$ receptors were observed in membrane preparations of these tumors. Scatchard analysis revealed the presence of high-affinity (K_D 1-2 x $10^{-9}M$) binding sites. In the affinity labeling studies one labeled species with an apparent Mr of 250-300 K_D was detected.

Conclusions

Recent evidence in favor of progestin stimulation of mammary cancer cells is accumulating (1). In this report, we have demonstrated the presence of IGF-I and II and their corresponding membrane receptors in both hormone-dependent and independent *in vivo* transplants of mammary adenocarcinomas induced by MPA in female BALB/c mice. Although progestin regulation of IGF-I tumor content or a modification in membrane receptors could not be detected, when IGF-I mRNA expression was studied, a modulation of its message by MPA was clearly evident.

We are aware that there are a number of problems in attempting to draw conclusions on how the data on progestin regulation of growth factor gene expression can be related to potential autocrine mechanisms, since our data on IGF-I gene expression and tumor content do not follow the same pattern. There are a number of regulatory steps between mRNA production and the appearance of biologically active growth factor. Therefore, progestins could modulate the level of IGF-I gene transcription without a comparative effect on the biologically active product. It is possible that IGF-I production has overloaded the reservoir capacity of the tumor cells and in consequence the MPA modulation of its synthesis could not be evidenced. Until such data are available, the relationship between progestin control of IGF-I mRNA expression and IGF-I tumor content will remain unclear. Yee *et al.* (7) have demonstrated that IGF-I mRNA was expressed in the stromal but not in the epithelial cells of mammary tumors; they have postulated that IGF-I may be a paracrine growth factor for mammary epithelial cells and an autocrine factor for stromal cells. Considering these findings, stromal cells present in the mammary tumors assayed herein may be a source of IGF-I. Only future *in situ* hybridization studies will address whether IGF-I is synthetized by the epithelial or stromal malignant cells.

What is evident from our limited data is that MPA regulates IGF-II production as well as membrane receptors in the hormone-dependent tumor lines. IGF-II, which is also synthesized and secreted by hormone-dependent and independent mammary tumors (8), increases the growth rate of breast cancer cells. Activation of some biological responses or transducing systems has been attributed to the interaction of IGF-II on its specific type II receptor. However, its mitogenic activity was thought to be mediated mostly by interaction with type I receptors. In our experimental tumor model, the cross-linking experiments as well as competitive binding data suggest that IGF-II binds with high affinity only to type II receptors, and it is possible that the proliferative effect of IGF-II, if any, on these tumor cells is mediated predominantly through the type II receptor. In this sense, the effect of MPA could be accounted for by a progestin down-regulation of IGF-II receptors as the result of an increase in IGF-II production and an autocrine type II receptor-mediated endocitosis.

Other growth factors may be involved in the proliferative effect of progestins. It has been demonstrated that EGF expression in T-47D, ZR-75, and MDA-MB468 cells is regulated by progestins in a steroid-specific, time- and concentration-dependent manner; in these cells, the expression of TGFα is increased while other steroid hormones have no effect (1); in contrast, TGFß$_1$ mRNA was decreased by progestins in T-47D cells (9), but the relevance of this result for an autocrine role is unclear since TGFß receptors were not detectable. In our model we were unable to demonstrate the presence of bioactive EGF or TGFα molecules in tumor extracts, nor was there expression of TGFα in MPA-D or MPA-I tumors. On the other hand, we encountered TGFß-like polypeptides. Their synthesis in MPA-D tumors seemed to be under MPA control, being much lower in MPA-treated mice. The results obtained at the RNA level are in agreement with those at the protein level. In addition, we have demonstrated the presence of high affinity receptors for TGFß in MPA-D and MPA-I tumors.

Finally, it can be postulated that MPA could exert its proliferative effect through the regulation of at least two families of growth factors by increasing the synthesis of the mitogenic IGFs and decreasing the expression of the autocrine growth inhibitor TGFß, without any effect on the stimulatory TGFα.

References

1. Clarke CL, Sutherland RL (1990) Progestin regulation of cellular proliferation. Endocr Rev 11:266-301.
2. Lanari C, Molinolo AA, Pasqualini CD (1986) Induction of mammary adenocarcinomas by medroxyprogesterone acetate in BALB/c female mice. Cancer Lett 33:215-223.
3. Molinolo AA, Lanari C, Charreau EH, Sanjuan N, Pasqualini CD (1987) Mouse mammary tumors induced by medroxyprogesterone acetate: immunochemistry and hormonal receptors. JNCI 79:131-135.
4. Kordon E, Lanari C, Meiss R, Elizalde P, Charreau E, Pasqualini CD (1990) Hormone dependence of a mouse mammary tumor line induced in vivo by medroxyprogesterone acetate. Breast Cancer Res Treat 17:33-43.
5. Lanari C, Kordon E, Molinolo AA, Pasqualini CD, Charreau EH (1989) Mammary adenocarcinomas induced by medroxyprogesterone acetate: hormone dependence and EGF receptors of BALB/c in vivo sublines. Int J Cancer 43:845-850.
6. Elizalde PV, Lanari C, Kordon E, Tezon J, Charreau EH (1990) Transforming growth factor β activity in in vivo lines of hormone-dependent and independent mammary adenocarcinomas induced by medroxyprogesterone acetate in BALB/c mice. Breast Cancer Res Treat 16:29-39.
7. Yee D, Paik S, Lebovic GS, Marcus RR, Favoni RE, Cullen KJ, Lippman MA, Rosen N (1989) Analysis of insulin-like growth factor I gene expression in malignancy: evidence for paracrine role in human breast cancer. Mol Endocrinol 3:509-517.

8. Osborne CK, Coronado EB, Kitten LJ, Arteaga CI, Fuqua SAN, Ramasharma K, Marshall M, Li CH (1989) Insulin-like growth factor II (IGF II): a potential autocrine-paracrine growth factor for human breast cancer acting via the IGF I receptor. Mol Endocrinol 3:1701-1709.
9. Murphy LC, Dotzlaw H (1989) Regulation of transforming growth factor α and transforming growth factor β messenger ribonucleic acid abundance in T-47D human breast cancer cells. Mol Endocrinol 3:611-617.

15

The Influence of Steroid Hormones and Antihormones on the Growth and Differentiation of Normal Human Breast Cells in Culture

Frederique Kuttenn, Anne Gompel, Catherine Malet,
Etienne Leygue, Nicole Baudot, Geneviere Plu,
Jean-Christophe Thalabard, and Pierre Mauvais-Jarvis

Introduction

Breast cancer still remains the most frequent cancer in women, occurring in 1 out of 9 women, whereas advances in therapeutics have not led to a decrease in mortality. Only a policy of early screening in high-risk populations and of prevention based on a clear pathophysiological understanding could lead to a decrease in the mortality due to this cancer.

Risk factors for breast cancer are now well-known. Besides the genetic risks, hormonal factors are the most frequently incriminated. In particular, the possibility that an "unopposed estrogen effect," mainly due to progesterone (P) insufficiency during the luteal phase, might be involved in the promotion of breast cancer remains a persistent hypothesis. Estradiol (E_2) seems to be involved as a "promoter" of carcinogenesis both in epidemiological studies and in experimental studies on animals. It will take many years for epidemiologists to verify this hypothesis and evaluate its implementation in terms of prevention. It is therefore important to collect data on the action of E_2 and the potential role of its antagonists—both natural (progesterone) and synthetic (progestins and triphenylethylenic antiestrogens)—in the control of breast cell growth and differentiation. A better understanding of the action of E_2 and its antagonists would help to define the basis of a policy of breast cancer prevention by acting before the transformation of normal cells into cancer cells.

Hormone Dependence of Normal Human Breast Cells in Culture

In our laboratory, we routinely obtain cultures of normal human breast cells established from surgical specimens of reductive mammoplasty (1), which enable separate studies of epithelial cells and fibroblasts. Our studies have especially concerned epithelial cells, considered to be the principal target of steroid hormones.

We will first present data on the antagonism between E_2 and progestogens, concerning ultrastructure, cell growth, markers of differentiation: the enzyme 17β-hydroxysteroid dehydrogenase (E_2DH), ER, PR,..., and the protooncogene c-*myc* expression. We will then discuss results concerning the inhibitory effect of triphenylethylenic antiestrogens on normal human breast epithelial (HBE) cell growth.

Estradiol-Progesterone Interactions

(a) Ultrastructural characteristics of normal human breast epithelial (HBE) cells have been examined by both scanning (SEM) and transmission (TEM) electron microscopy (2-4).

On SEM, the control cells exhibit a homogeneous pattern: they are large, polygonal, and flattened. Under E_2 treatment, cells appear young, extensively protruding, with numerous bunches and blebs. However, with the addition of R5020, the bunches and blebs disappear: the cells look like control cells. With higher magnification, the microvilli appear short and rare in control cells. Under E_2 treatment, microvilli increase markedly in number and density: they are short, thick and compact. With the addition of R5020 to E_2, cells are flattened without blebs, microvilli are sparse but longer. Parallel transmission electron microscopy shows extensive Golgi apparatus and secretory activity under R5020 treatment.

(b) Growth studies were carried out on secondary cultures (5×10^5 cells replated/T25 flasks) under various hormonal conditions: E_2 (10^{-9} to $10^{-6}M$), R5020 (10^{-8} to $10^{-6}M$) with or without E_2 ($10^{-8}M$). Cell growth was evaluated by daily cell counting providing an Histometric Growth Index (HGI), and DNA assay + ^{3}H-thymidine incorporation into DNA at the most representative days of cell growth, i.e., those corresponding to the exponential growth and slowing down phases, respectively (5,6).

E_2 stimulated cell growth (Fig. 1) in a dose-dependent manner, but this E_2 effect could only be observed when the cells were cultured in a medium minimally supplemented with serum, insulin, and EGF (5,6). In contrast, R5020 inhibited cell growth either in the presence or absence of E_2. The inhibition by R5020 was dose-dependent (6; Fig. 2).

The action of the antiprogesterone RU486 was also examined in HBE cells. It is interesting to note that RU486 also has an inhibitory effect on cell growth but to a lesser extent than R5020, thus exhibiting a progesterone agonistic effect (6). In human breast epithelial cells, it therefore seems that E_2 stimulates, whereas progesterone and progestins slow down cell multiplication.

Interesting and comparable results on estradiol/progesterone interaction on cell multiplication were recently obtained *in vivo* by Dr. Barrat's group (7): 32 patients were percutaneously treated with either (1) estradiol, or (2) progesterone, or (3) placebo, locally applied to the breast during the follicular phase prior to surgery for benign breast diseases. The number of mitoses was counted in epithelial cells of the normal part of the breast. After E_2 administration, both E_2 concentration in breast tissue and the number of mitoses were found to be high; whereas after progesterone administration, progesterone concentration in breast tissue was high, but the number of mitoses was low. These data support an antimitotic effect of progesterone.

(c) Mechanisms of E_2 and progesterone antagonism in HBE cells. Two mechanisms of progesterone regulation of E_2 action, first demonstrated in the endometrium (8), have been characterized in normal mammary cells. (1) P stimulates the enzyme 17β-dehydrogenase (E_2DH) which converts E_2, the active estrogen into E_1, its less active metabolite. (2) P decreases the estradiol receptor (ER) content.

We had first studied these mechanisms in breast fibroadenoma (FA), considered to be a good model since it offers a rich epithelial cell concentration still closely resembling normal tissue (9,10). We then demonstrated these mechanisms in human breast cells in culture.

1. E_2DH activity has been measured as the production of E_1 by the cells incubated with $^3H\text{-}E_2$. It is high in the epithelial cells, yielding a 30% conversion of E_2 to E_1 in 4 hrs; and it is stimulated by progestin (Fig. 3). In

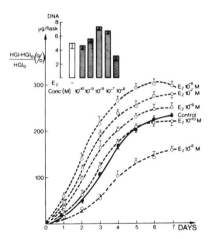

Fig. 1. Stimulatory dose-dependent effect of estradiol (E_2) on the growth of normal human breast epithelial (HBE) cells in secondary culture. The study of cell growth was based on daily cell counting and determination of a histometric growth index (HGI); the results were expressed as percentage increase in HGI as compared to its value on day 0 (HGI_0). Inset, DNA values on day 7 (mean of triplicate flasks; bars, SD) Reprinted, with permission, from Ref. 11.

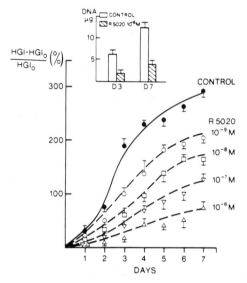

Fig. 2. Inhibitory effect of the progestin promegestone (R5020) on the growth of normal HBE cells in culture. HGI: see legend Fig. 1; Inset, DNA values on days 3 and 7 in control cell cultures (no hormone addition) and cells cultured in the presence of R5020 ($10^{-6}M$) (mean $\pm$ SD of determinations in triplicate flasks) Reprinted, with permission, from Ref. 6.

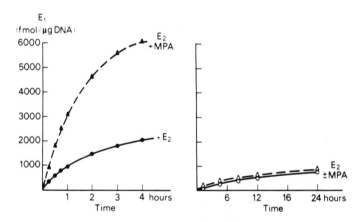

Fig. 3. Time course of E_1 formation after incubation of $[^3H]E_2$ (incubation medium 5 ml, final concentration $= 2nM$) in normal human breast epithelial cells (left panel) or fibroblasts (right panel) cultured in the presence of either E_2 ($10^{-8}M$) alone (no difference from control), or E_2 + Medroxy-progesterone acetate (MPA $10^{-8}M$) Reprinted, with permission, from Ref. 6.

contrast, E_2DH activity is very low in fibroblasts (only 4% of E_2 metabolized after 24 h) and not stimulated by P (Fig. 3) (1,6). Consequently E_2DH has been proposed as a marker of epithelial cells as well as P dependency and also PR operativity.

It therefore seemed interesting to simultaneously compare progestin action on E_2DH activity and DNA content of HBE cells: the addition of R5020 lowers DNA content and stimulates E_2DH activity. Therefore, it slows down cell multiplication and favors cell differentiation.

2. Steroid receptors are difficult to study in cultured normal breast cells due to lower levels than in cancer cells (11), requiring large amounts of cells when using the classical biochemical methods for receptor assay. However, immunocytochemical studies using monoclonal antibodies have enabled the characterization of ER and PR in these cells.

Immunostaining specific for ER has been observed in epithelial cells: it is nuclear, varying from cell to cell in positivity and intensity (11,12). Moreover, it is enhanced in E_2-treated cells. In contrast, it decreases after addition of the progestin R5020 (12). The progesterone receptor (PR) was also visualized with antibodies provided by Geoffrey Greene. It is also hormone-modulated: stimulated by E_2 and lowered by R5020 (12).

Thus, in normal breast epithelial cells, E_2 stimulates both its receptor and PR, whereas the progestin R5020 lowers both ER and PR content.

3. C-*myc* protooncogene expression in HBE cells. It has been observed in breast cancer cell lines that the stimulatory effect of E_2 on cell growth could act, in part, through the stimulation of protooncogene expression (13-15) and growth factor production (16).

The protooncogene c-*myc* is involved in the stimulation of cell replication (17) and can itself be stimulated by numerous mitogens, including E_2. E_2 stimulation of c-*myc* was demonstrated in human breast cancer cell lines (13-15) and also in noncancerous E_2-dependent target tissues (uterus, chick oviduct) (18-20). In contrast, progestins (21) and triphenylethylenic antiestrogens (15) inhibit c-*myc* expression.

We are exploring these possibilities in normal breast cells, and we have obtained preliminary results with immunocytochemical studies of the c-*myc* protein (22). The expression of the c-*myc* protein is exclusively nuclear. It is heterogeneous and the intensity of staining varies from cell to cell. The control staining with normal serum (IgG fraction) demonstrates the absence of background staining. In addition, c-*myc* expression is hormone-modulated: the number of cells and intensity of staining increase in cells treated by E_2; they decrease after the addition of R5020 to E_2.

Preliminary results from Northern blot studies seem to confirm E_2-interaction with c-*myc* expression: early stimulation of mRNA occurred 30 minutes after E_2 treatment followed by subsequent stimulation at 24 h. Interactions of progestins and c-*myc* are now being explored.

Role of E_2 and Progestins in the Two-Step Scheme for Carcinogenesis According to Moolgavkar (23)

Further studies are needed to elucidate relationships between estrogens—oncogene expression—and growth factor production. However, considering the effects of E_2 and progestins on cell growth and differentiation, we can try to define their respective roles in the process of carcinogenesis.

If we consider Moolgavkar's scheme for carcinogenesis (23), there are two steps in the evolution of normal cells to cancer cells .

A normal cell has 2 possibilities: either it divides into new cells ("a1") or it matures, differentiates ("$\beta1$" cell), and finally dies. However, if the normal cell is subjected to an initiator of carcinogenesis, it can evolve ($\mu1$) into an "intermediate" (precancerous) cell.

"Intermediate cells" can also either divide (a2) or differentiate ($\beta2$) and die. But if a second process of initiation intervenes ($\mu2$), the cell definitely evolves into a cancer cell.

Cell division is a vulnerable phase for the cells with risks for errors of replication, oncogene activation, and exogenous carcinogen intervention.

• By stimulating cell multiplication, estrogens increase the risk for error at the time of replication. In this way, they can act as "promoters" of carcinogenesis.

• By orienting cells toward maturation, progesterone and progestins exclude them from the pool of vulnerable dividing cells and could be protective.

Any endogenous or exogenous situation of estrogen-progesterone imbalance leading to an "unopposed estrogen effect" should therefore be avoided and/or corrected.

Rationale for a Progestogen Treatment of Benign Breast Diseases

Considering (1) the antiestrogenic effect of progesterone and progestins and (2) progesterone insufficiency resulting in an "unopposed estrogen effect," frequently observed in patients with Benign Breast Diseases (BBD), a progestogen treatment has been proposed. Among all the treatments proposed in BBD, it is the only one to treat both the cause, progesterone insufficiency, and the consequence, epithelial hyperplasia.

A question remains: can progesterone and progestins have a protective effect in the long term and thus reduce the risk for breast cancer?

A long-term epidemiological study has been conducted in our department on the risk for breast cancer in 1,012 patients, treated or not with progestogen, in order to try to answer this question. The patients have been followed-up for 10 years; 425 patients receiving progestogen treatment (lynestrenol) have been compared to 587 patients with BBD but untreated, and matched for the other risk factors. Six breast cancers occurred in the group with progestogen treatment vs. 22 in the untreated group. These results are being analyzed (G. Plu, J.C. Thalabard, manuscript in preparation), but we can already say that progestogen treatment does not favor breast cancer, as has been suggested (24,25), but rather seems to be protective.

Triphenylethylenic Antiestrogen Action on Normal Human Breast Epithelial Cells

Triphenylethylenic antiestrogens (tamoxifen and its derivatives) are competitive inhibitors of E_2 binding to its own receptor (26). They are known to slow down breast cancer cell growth (27) and are used as hormonal adjuvant therapy in breast cancer. They have also been proposed for the prevention of breast cancer (28-31).

It was thus important to also study their effects on normal, nontransformed cells. The action of tamoxifen (Tam) and 4-hydroxy-tamoxifen (4OHTam) was studied on (a) the ultrastructural aspects of the cells, (b) cell growth, and (c) c-*myc* protein expression.

Scanning Electron Microscopy. At low magnification, the cells that exhibit high proliferative activity under E_2 treatment return to a quiescent aspect very similar to that of control cells when Tam, or even better 4OHTam, is added. At high magnification, microvilli, which were numerous and thick in E_2-treated cells, are less dense and thinner with Tam. This effect is still more marked with 4OHTam.

Cell growth (Figs. 4 and 5). Tam slows down HBE cell growth at the highest concentrations (10^{-7} and $10^{-6}M$) (11). Trans-4OHTam is 100-to-150-fold more efficient than Tam, with a clear-cut dose-effect, still obvious at $10^{-9}M$. This effect was observed in the presence of E_2 and also—but to a lesser extent—in the absence of E_2. Most of the data in the literature indicate that these compounds interact with estrogens at the level of ER. An explanation of the inhibitory effect of antiestrogens on HBE cell growth, even in the absence of E_2 addition, could be the persistence of low concentrations of E_2 in the nonstripped serum added to the medium even under conditions of minimal supplementation (6).

The inhibitory effect of Tam and 4OHTam on HBE cell growth is of the same order of magnitude as in breast cancer cell lines. It corresponds to their relative affinity for the estradiol receptor (32).

It was also important to study the *cis*-isomer of 4OHTam in parallel with the *trans*-isomer since an isomerization has been observed *in vivo* between the two forms, and since the *cis*-isomers of the triphenylethylene compounds have been shown to have a weak estrogen agonist effect (33). Despite its isomeric configuration, no agonistic effect of *cis*-4OHTam was observed in terms of cell growth stimulation; *cis*-4OHTam has a greater inhibitory effect on HBE cell multiplication than *trans*-Tam. At similar concentration, *cis*-4OHTam has 30 to 40% of the inhibitory activity of its *trans*-isomer.

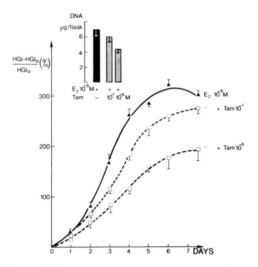

Fig. 4. Effect of the addition of TAM on estradiol (E_2) stimulated cell growth. HGI was measured every day in triplicate flasks for each hormonal condition: $10^{-8}M$ estradiol alone, compared with $10^{-8}M$ estradiol added with $10^{-7}M$ or $10^{-6}M$ TAM. The results were expressed as percentage increase in HGI as compared to its value on day 0 (HGI_0); bars, SD. Inset, DNA values assayed on day 7 under the same hormonal conditions. Reprinted, with permission, from Ref. 11.

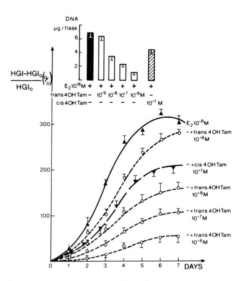

Fig. 5. Dose-dependent inhibitory effect of *trans*-40HTAM on estradiol (E2) stimulated cell growth and comparison of the potency of the *cis*- and *trans*-40HTAM isomers. See legend Fig. 4. Reprinted, with permission, from Ref. 11.

Antiestrogen action and c-myc expression. The action of the antiestrogens has been examined on the c-*myc* protein by immunocytochemistry. The immunostaining of the c-*myc* protein stimulated by E_2 decreases markedly after antiestrogen treatment.

Consequences of Oral Administration of Tamoxifen

It has been suggested, and it is now repeatedly proposed, that the cytostatic effect of Tam could be used for the prevention of breast cancer (28-31). However, it should be underlined that orally administered antiestrogens have three types of action:

1. Competitive inhibition of E_2 binding at the target cell level: this is highly appropriate when it inhibits cell multiplication.

2. Competitive inhibition of E_2 binding at the hypothalamic level. LH therefore increases and stimulates plasma E_2 (34) up to very high levels $\approx$ 1,000 to 2,000 pg/ml. It is therefore impossible to use it in premenopausal women, except when it is combined with a nonestrogen antigonadotropic agent, such as a progestin.

3. Partial estrogen agonistic action at the target cell level: this is desirable when it stimulates the progesterone receptor level, but detrimental when it induces endometrial hyperplasia and seems to favor endometrial carcinoma (35).

Percutaneous Administration of 4OHTam

Considering the possible adverse effects of orally administered tamoxifen, it has been proposed that *trans*-4OHTam, the active metabolite of Tam, be percutaneously applied onto the breast. It was demonstrated that 4OHTam penetrates through the skin and can therefore bind to ER in the breast tissue (36). This route of administration of 4OHTam avoids enterohepatic recirculation, the extensive metabolism of the first hepatic pass, thus allowing the use of much lower doses and yielding an optimal ratio of local/systemic effect.

This should offer an alternative treatment in case of benign breast disease and in women at risk for breast cancer. It constitutes a potential arm in a policy of breast cancer prevention.

Conclusion

Normal human breast epithelial (HBE) cells remain hormone-dependent in culture and constitute a useful tool for investigating hormone-dependence of the normal human mammary gland. In this culture system, E_2 stimulates whereas progestins and triphenylethylenic antiestrogens inhibit HBE cell growth. In addition, progestins favor cell differentiation. By stimulating cell proliferation, E_2 can act as a "promoter" of carcinogenesis. Any condition of estrogen-progesterone imbalance with an "unopposed estrogen effect" should therefore be avoided and/or corrected. The inhibitory effects of E_2 antagonists—progestins and antiestrogens—should be taken into account in the definition of a policy of hormonal prevention in patients considered at high risk for breast cancer because of family history of breast cancer, benign breast disease, or prolonged hyperestrogenism.

Acknowledgments

Studies in our laboratory have been supported by grants from Inserm, la Faculté Necker-Enfants Malades, and l'Association pour la Recherche sur le Cancer. We gratefully acknowledge this support.

References

1. Prudhomme JF, Malet C, Gompel A, Lalardrie JP, Ochoa C, Boue A, Mauvais-Jarvis P, Kuttenn F (1984) 17β-hydroxysteroid dehydrogenase activity in human breast epithelial cell and fibroblast cultures. Endocrinology 114:1483-1489.
2. Chomette G, Gompel A, Malet C, Tranbaloc P, Kuttenn F, Mauvais-Jarvis P (1985) Les cellules épithéliales du sein humain normal en culture. Aspects ultrastructuraux et leurs variations sous l'effet d'actions hormonales (estradiol, prolactine). Arch Anat Cytol Path 33:32-38.
3. Gompel A, Chomette G, Malet C, Spritzer P, Pavy B, Kuttenn F, Mauvais-Jarvis P (1985) Estradiol-progestin interaction in normal human breast cells in culture. Ultrastructural studies. Breast Diseases 1:149-156.
4. Chomette G, Auriol M, Tranbaloc P, Gompel A, Malet C., Kuttenn F (1986) Effect of estradiol and the synthetic progestin promegestone (R5020) on human breast cell cultures. An ultrastructural study. Path Res Pract 181:273-279.
5. Malet C, Gompel A, Spritzer P, Kuttenn F, Mauvais-Jarvis P (1986) Effect of estradiol and the synthetic progestin promegestone (R5020) on the proliferation of human epithelial mammary cells in culture. In: Endocrinology of the Breast. Basic and Clinical Aspects. Ann N.Y. Acad Sci 464:489-492.
6. Gompel A, Malet C, Spritzer P, Lalardrle JP, Kuttenn F, Mauvais-Jarvis P (1986) Progestin effect on cell proliferation and 17β-hydroxysteroid dehydrogenase activity in normal human breast cells in culture. J Clin Endocrinol Metab 63:1174-1180.
7. Barrat J, Lignieres B de, Marpeau L, Larue L, Fournier S, Nahoul K, Linares G, Giorgi H, Contesso G (1990) Effet in vivo de l'administration locale de progesterone sur l'activité mitotique des galactophores humans. J Gynecol Obstet Biol Reprod 19:269-274.
8. Tseng L, Gusberg SB, Gurpide E (1977) Estradiol receptor and 17β-dehydrogenase in normal and abnormal human endometrium. Ann NY Acad Sci 286:190-198.

9. Fournier S, Kuttenn F, Cicco N de, Baudot N, Malet C, Mauvais-Jarvis P (1982) Estradiol 17β-hydroxysteroid dehydrogenase activity in human breast fibroadenomas. J Clin Endocrinol Metab 55:428-433.
10. Kuttenn F, Fournier S, Durand JC, Mauvais-Jarvis P (1981) Estradiol and progesterone receptors in human breast fibroadenomas. J Clin Endocrinol Metab 52:1225-1229.
11. Malet C, Gompel A, Pritzer P, Bricout N, Yaneva H, Mowszowicz I, Kuttenn F, Mauvais-Jarvis P (1988) Tamoxifen and hydroxytamoxifen isomers vs. estradiol effects on normal human breast cells in culture. Cancer Res 48:7193-7199.
12. Malet C, Gompel A, Yaneva H, Crew H, Fidji N, Mowszowicz I, Kuttenn F, Mauvais-Jarvis P (1991) Estradiol and progesterone receptors in cultured normal human breast epithelial cells and fibroblasts: Immunocytochemical studies. J Clin Endocrinol Metab, June, in press.
13. Dubik D, Dembinski TC, Shiu RP (1987) Stimulation of c-myc oncogene expression associated with estrogen proliferation of human breast cancer cells. Cancer Res 47:6517-6521.
14. Dubik D, Shiu RPC (1988) Transcriptional regulation of c-myc oncogene expression by estrogen in hormone responsive human breast cancer cells. J Biol Chem 263:12705-12708.
15. Santos GF, Scott GK, Lee WMF, Liu E, Benz C (1988) Estrogen-induced post-transcriptional modulation of c-myc protooncogene expression in human breast cancer cells. J Biol Chem 263:9565-9568.
16. Lippman ME, Dickson RB (1989) Mechanisms of growth control in normal and malignant breast epithelium. Rec Prog Horm Res 45:383-435.
17. Studzinsky GP, Brelvi ZS, Feldman SC, Watt RA (1986) Participation of c-myc protein in DNA synthesis of human cells. Science 234:467-470.
18. Murphy LJ, Murphy LC, Friesen HG (1987) Estrogen induction of N-myc and c-myc protooncogene expression in rat uterus. Endocrinology 120:1882-1888.
19. Weisz A, Bresciani F (1988) Estrogen induces expression of c-fos and c-myc protooncogenes in rat uterus. Mol Endocrinol 2:816-824.
20. Odom LD, Barrett JM, Pantazis CG, Stoddard LD, Mc Donough PG (1989) Immunocytochemical study of ras and myc protooncogene polypeptide expression in the human menstrual cycle. Am J Obstet Gynecol 161:1663-1668.
21. Fink KL, Wieben ED, Woloschak GE, Spelberg TC (1988) Rapid regulation of c-myc protooncogene expression by progesterone in the avian oviduct. Proc Natl Acad Sci 85:1796-1800.
22. Gompel A, Leygue E, Gol R, Malet C, Baudot N, Mowszowicz I, Kuttenn F, Mauvais-Jarvis P (1991) Estradiol and antiestrogen interactions with c-myc expresssion in normal human breast epithelial (HBE) cells. 73th Ann Meet Am Endoc Soc, Washington, Abstract 595.

23. Moolgavkar SH, Day NE, Stevens RC (1980) Two-stage model for carcinogenesis: epidemiology of breast cancer in females. J Natl Cancer Inst 45:559-569.
24. Pike M, Henderson B, Krailo M et al (1983) Breast cancer in young women and use of oral contraceptives: possible modifying effect of formulation and age at use. Lancet ii:926-930.
25. Bergkvist L, Adami M, Persson I, Hoover R, Schairer C (1989) The risk of breast cancer after estrogen and estrogen-progestin replacement. N Engl J Med 321:293-297.
26. Lerner LF, Jordon VC (1990) Development of antiestrogens and their use in breast cancer: Eight Cain Memorial Award Lecture. Cancer Res 50:4177-4189.
27. Bardon S, Vignon F, Derocq D, Rochefort H (1984) The antiproliferative effect of tamoxifen in breast cancer cells: mediation by the estrogen receptor. Moll Cell Endocrinol 35:89-96.
28. Cuzick J, Wang DY, Bulbrook RD (1986) The prevention of breast cancer. Lancet i : 83-86.
29. Fentiman IS (1989) The endocrine prevention of breast cancer. Br J Cancer 60:12-14.
30. Powles TJ, Hardy JR, Ashley SE, Farrington GM, Cosgrove D, Davey JB, Dowsett M, Mc Kinna JA, Nash AG, Sinnett HD, Tyllier CR, Treleaven JG (1989) A pilot trial to evaluate the acute toxicity and feasibility of tamoxifen for prevention of breast cancer. Br J Cancer 60:126-131.
31. Love RR (1990) Prospects for antiestrogen chemoprevention of breast cancer. J Natl Cancer Inst 82:18-21.
32. Eckert RL, Katzenellenbogen BS (1982) Effects of estrogens and antiestrogens on estrogen receptor dynamics and the induction of progesterone receptor in MCF-7 human breast cancer cells. Cancer Res 42:139-144.
33. Katzenellenbogen BS, Norman MJ, Eckert RL, Peltz SW, Mangel WF (1984) Bioactivities, estrogen receptor interactions and plasminogen activator-inducing activities of tamoxifen and hydroxytamoxifen isomers in MCF-7 human breast cancer cells. Cancer Res 35:89-96.
34. Sherman BM, Chapler FK, Crickard K, Wycoff D (1979) Endocrine consequences of continuous antiestrogen therapy with tamoxifen in premenopausal women. J Clin Invest 64:398-494.
35. Fornander T, Cedermark B, Mattsson A et al. (1989) Adjuvant tamoxifen in early breast cancer: Occurrence of new primary cancers. Lancet i, 117-119.
36. Mauvais-Jarvis P, Baudot N, Castaigne D, Banzet P, Kuttenn F (1986) Trans-4-hydroxytamoxifen concentration and metabolism after local percutaneous administration to human breast. Cancer Res 46:1521-1525.

PART 5. GROWTH FACTORS AND ONCOGENES

INTRODUCTION

Molecular Mechanisms of Hormonal Carcinogenesis

J. Carl Barrett

Mechanisms of Hormonal Carcinogenesis

Hormones play an important role in a number of human cancers. For example, estrogens influence the incidence of mammary, endometrial, and ovarian cancers in women (1). Estrogens are also carcinogenic in animals. The natural estrogen 17β-estradiol increases the incidences of mammary, pituitary, uterine, cervical, vaginal, and lymphoid tumors, and interstitial-cell tumors of the testes in mice; it also increases the incidences of mammary and pituitary tumors in rats and renal tumors in hamsters (2). Similarly, the synthetic estrogen diethylstilbestrol increases the incidences of mammary tumors, lymphoid tumors, interstitial-cell tumors of the testes, cervical tumors, and vaginal tumors in mice; pituitary, mammary, bladder tumors in rats; and renal tumors in hamsters (2).

Three possible mechanisms have been proposed for the carcinogenic activity of estrogenic carcinogens.
  (1) Hormonal stimulation of cell proliferation
  (2) Heritable reprogramming of cellular differentiation
  (3) Induction of genetic changes in target cells either by
      (a) induction of nondisjunction and aneuploidy via microtubule alterations or
      (b) induction of mutations following activation to DNA reactive intermediates.

It has been proposed that estrogens are carcinogenic due to their ability to stimulate cell proliferation. The hormonal dependence of transplantable tumors is consistent with this proposed mechanism of action. This hypothesis is also supported by experimental observations of tumor-promoting effects of estrogens on carcinogen-initiated mammary cancers, liver cancers, and vaginal tumors (2, 3). Analyses of the influence of hormonal factors on human breast cancers also indicate an effect on a late stage in the carcinogenic process, consistent with a promotional effect (4). Therefore, there is strong evidence from several systems in support of the hypothesis that estrogens are epigenetic carcinogens acting via a promoting effect related to stimulation of proliferation of estrogen-responsive cells. Prenatal exposure to DES induces irreversible changes in differentiation of the cervicovaginal epithelium (5,6). Thus, DES "initiation" may also arise by a heritable epigenetic mechanism.

Despite the convincing evidence that estrogens have epigenetic effects on carcinogenesis, there are observations which indicate that estrogens induce mutational changes that do not involve the classical estrogen receptor. DES can induce tumors in humans and experimental animals following single or short-term prenatal exposure (2,7). The offspring of treated animals have increased tumor incidences even though not exposed to further treatment. Newbold et al. (7) have shown that DES treatment of neonatal mice from days 1-5, a time period that corresponds to late prenatal human development, results in a high incidence (90%) of uterine adenocarcinoma at 18 months. In the neonatal mouse few of the uterine epithelial cells are positive for estrogen receptor at the time of treatment; in contrast, treatment of adult animals, when all the cells are estrogen-receptor positive, does not result in DES-induced uterine cancers.

There is also evidence that estrogenic activity is not sufficient to explain the carcinogenic activity *in vivo* of estrogens in certain target tissues. In the hamster kidney model, renal tumors are induced by a variety of estrogens, and the tumors that form are estrogen-dependent (8), indicating an important epigenetic mechanism in the genesis and maintenance of this tumor (3). However, not all estrogens are active in inducing these tumors. Tumors are induced by both DES and 17β-estradiol (E_2), but ethynyl estradiol has only weak carcinogenic activity even though it competes equally well with DES and E_2 for estrogen receptors and has activity similar to carcinogenic estrogens in inducing renal progesterone receptor and serum prolacting levels (8). Similarly, 2-fluoroestradiol does not induce renal clear-cell carcinomas in hamsters despite its estrogenic potency (9).

Further evidence for a direct estrogen-induced effect on target cells is provided by studies of neoplastic transformation of Syrian hamster embryo (SHE) cells by DES, E_2, and other estrogens. We observed that DES and E_2 can induce morphological and neoplastic transformation of SHE cells, which is indistinguishable from that induced by other chemical carcinogens such as benzo[a]pyrene (10,11).

In an attempt to understand DES-induced cell transformation, we examined the ability of DES to induce a variety of genetic changes in SHE cells. We have shown that treatment of these cells with DES alone induces cell transformation without causing gene mutations, unscheduled DNA synthesis, sister chromatid exchanges, or structural chromosome aberrations (12, 13). Thus, DES can induce cell transformation in the absence of detectable DNA damage. However, under these conditions, DES does induce a specific type of genetic change, aneuploidy. DES binds to microtubules and disrupts tubulin assembly (14). Treatment of cells in mitosis with doses as low as 10 nM DES results in aneuploidy induction via nondisjunction (12). The evidence supporting the hypothesis that aneuploidy is involved in DES-induced cell transformation has

Table 1. Two classes of genes involved in carcinogenesis.

Protooncogenes	Tumor Suppressor Genes
1. Involved in cellular growth and differentiation	1. Function unknown, but possibly involved in cellular growth and differentiation (Negative regulators of cell growth?)
2. Family of genes exists	2. Family of genes exists
3. Must be activated (quantitatively or qualitatively) in cancers	3. Must be inactivated, lost, and/or mutated in cancers
4. Mutational activation by point mutation, chromosome translocation, or gene amplification	4. Mutational inactivation by chromosome loss, chromosome deletion, point mutation, somatic recombination, or gene conversion
5. Little evidence for involvement in hereditary cancers	5. Clear evidence for involvement in hereditary and nonhereditary cancers

been reviewed (14,15). In addition, in the presence of certain metabolizing systems, DES can be activated to DNA reactive, mutagenic intermediates (14).

In conclusion, it is clear that hormones affect carcinogenesis by epigenetic mechanisms such as stimulation of cell proliferation of estrogen-dependent target cells and possibly reprogramming of cellular differentiation. In addition, significant evidence exists that certain estrogens can also cause genetic alterations by mechanisms not involving the classical estrogen receptor. These findings indicate that hormonal carcinogenesis is most likely a result of the interplay of both genetic and epigenetic factors.

Molecular Alterations in Hormonal Carcinogenesis

Carcinogenesis is a multistep process involving alterations in at least two distinct classes of genes, protooncogenes and tumor suppressor genes (Table 1). Protooncogenes are a family of cellular genes with at least 40 members, which appear to be involved in normal cellular growth and development; activation or inappropriate expression of these genes results in proliferative signals involved in neoplastic growth (16). On the other hand, tumor suppressor genes are less well defined, but the function of these genes may also be in the control of normal cell division and possible differentiation. For a tumor cell to emerge, these suppressor genes must be inactivated or lost. The number of tumor suppressor genes is unknown, but multiple genes are likely to exist (16).

For common adult cancers in humans (e.g., breast, lung, and colon), multiple genetic alterations in these two classes of genes have been identified. For example, in human breast cancer eight mutations have been identified (17,18). Alterations (gene amplification and overexpression) of three different oncogenes (c-*myc*, *erb*B-2 and *int*-2) have been reported. In addition, losses of multiple tumor suppressor genes are indicated by the findings of loss heterozygosity on six chromosomes (1, 3, 11, 13, 17, and 18). Cytogenetic analyses (19) of primary breast tumors have documented frequently deletions and translocations on chromosomes 1p, 1q, 2q, 3p, 5, 6q, 8p, 8q, 11p, 11q, 12, 13q, 14a, 16, 17p, and 17q. In some cases specific genes have been implicated, e.g., RB on chromosomes 13q and p53 and NM23 on chromosome 17 (18).

These findings illustrate the molecular complexity of hormonal carcinogenesis. Further analysis of the molecular basis for hormonally induced cancers should lead to a better understanding of how hormones influence the development of these tumors. Given the multistep, multigenic, and multifactorial nature of human cancers, multiple mechanisms are undoubtedly involved.

References

1. Preston-Martin S, Pike MC, Ross RK, Jones PA, and Henderson BE. Increased cell division as cause of human cancer. Cancer Res. 50:7415-7421, 1990.
2. International Agency for Research on Cancer, Evaluation of carcinogenic risk of chemicals to humans, sex hormones (11). Vol. 21, IARC, Lyon, 1979.
3. Barrett FC and Huff J. Cellular and molecular mechanisms of chemically induced carcinogenesis. Renal Failure. In press.
4. Kaldor JM and Day NE. Interpretation of epidemiological studies on the context of the multistage model of carcinogenesis. In Barrett JC (ed): Mechanisms of environmental carcinogenesis, Vol. II, CRC Press: Boca Raton, Florida, pp. 21-57, 1987.
5. Forsberg JG. Developmental mechanism of estrogen-induced irreversible changes in the mouse cervicovaginal epithelium. Natl Cancer Inst Monogr 51:41-56, 1979.
6. McLachlan JA, Newbold RR and Bullock RC. Long-term effects on the female mouse genital tract associated with prenatal exposure to diethylstilbestrol. Cancer Res 40:3988-3999, 1980.

7. Newbold RR, Bullock BC and McLachlan JA. Uterine adenocarcinoma in mice following developmental treatment with estrogens: a model for hormonal carcinogenesis. Cancer Res 50:7677-7681, 1990.

8. Li JJ, Li SA, Oberley T. Estrogen carcinogenicity: hormonal morphologic and chemical interactions. In Politzer P. & Martin Jr J.F. (eds): Chemical carcinogens. Activation mechanism, structural and electronic factors, and reactivity, New York: Elsevier, 312-321, 1988.

9. Liehr JG. 2-Fluoroestradiol: separation of estrogenicity from carcinogenicity. Mol Pharmacol 23:278-281, 1983.

10. Barrett JC, Wong A and McLachlan JA. Diethylstilbestrol induces neoplastic transformation without measurable gene mutation in two loci. Science 212:1402-1404, 1981.

11. McLachlan JA, Wong A, Degen GH and Barrett JC. Morphological and neoplastic transformation of Syrian hamster embryo cells by diethylstilbestrol and its analogs. Cancer Res. 42:3040-3045, 1982.

12. Tsutsui T, Maizume H, McLachlan JA, and Barrett JC. Aneuploidy induction and cell transformation by diethylstilbestrol: a possible chromosome mechanism in carcinogenesis. Cancer Res 3814-3821, 1983.

13. Tsutsui T, Degen GH, Schiffmann D, Wong A, Maizumi H, McLachlan JA, and Barrett JC. Dependence of exogenous metabolic activation for induction of unscheduled DNA synthesis in Syrian hamster embryo cells by diethlstilbestrol and related compounds. Cancer Res 44:184-189, 1984.

14. Barrett JC. Relationship between mutagenesis and carcinogenesis. In Barrett JC (ed): Mechanisms of environmental carcinogenesis, Vol. I. CRC Press: Boca Raton, Florida, pp. 129-142, 1987.

15. Barrett JC, Oshimura M, Tanaka N, and Tsutsui T. Genetic and epigenetic mechanisms of presumed nongenotoxic carcinogens. In Butterworth B. & Slaga TJ (eds): Nongenotoxic mechanisms in carcinogenesis, New York: Cold Spring Harbor Laboratory, pp. 311-324, 1987.

16. Boyd JC and Barrett JC. Genetic and cellular basis of multistep carcinogenesis. Pharmacol Ther 46:469-486, 1990.

17. Callahan R and Campbell G. Mutations in human breast cancer: An overview. J Natl Cancer Inst 81:1780-1786, 1989.

18. Dickson RB and Slamon . New insights into breast cancer: The molecular biochemical and cellular biology of breast cancer. Cancer Res 50:4446-4447, 1990.

19. Mars WM and Saunders GF. Chromosomal abnormalities in human breast cancer. Cancer Metastasis Rev 9:35-43, 1990.

16

The v-*raf* and Ha-*ras* Oncogenes Inhibit Transcription from the Beta-Casein Gene Promoter by Suppression of a Mammary Gland Specific Transcription Factor

Nancy E. Hynes, M. Caitriona NicMhuiris, Urs Stiefel,
Daniela Taverna, Roland Ball, Brigitte Happ,
Michael Schmitt-Ney, and Bernd Groner

Introduction

Under the influence of pregnancy, the epithelial cells of the mammary gland undergo a complex pattern of growth and differentiation. Multiple steroid and peptide hormones cooperate in this process that ultimately leads to the production of the milk proteins. In order to study these processes at the molecular level we have simplified the complexity of the interactions by developing an *in vitro* cultured cell system. The HC11 cell line was isolated from mid-pregnant mammary gland cells of Balb/c mice (1). The cells display a normal phenotype and have retained some characteristics of mammary epithelial cell differentiation. After treatment with the lactogenic hormones prolactin and glucocorticoids, the HC11 cells express the milk protein beta-casein. It has been shown that the hormones act in a synergistic fashion to regulate transcription from the beta-casein promoter (2).

Various oncogenes have been implicated in human and rodent mammary tumor development (3-5). Normal signals controlling cell growth and differentiation are disturbed during the transformation process. We have used the HC11 cells to study the influence of oncogene expression upon cell growth and differentiation. We have previously shown that the introduction of vectors expressing an oncogenic c-*erb*B-2 (neu) protein, an activated Ha-*ras* protein, or a transforming growth factor (TGF)-alpha protein, into the HC11 cells results in their transformation. But only the expression of TGF-alpha and Ha-*ras* led to an inhibition of the lactogenic hormone induced beta-casein gene expression (6). This suggests that in the HC11 cells different signal transduction pathways are activated by these different proteins. In the results presented in this paper we have tested other oncogenes for their effects upon HC11 cell growth and differentiation. In addition, we have analyzed nuclear proteins that specifically bind the beta-casein gene promoter. We have observed that one nuclear protein, the mammary gland factor (MGF), which is important for lactogenic hormone-induced beta-casein transcription, appears to be altered in oncogene transformed HC11 cells that have lost their lactogenic hormone responsiveness. This suggests that certain oncogenes have specific effects upon this mammary gland specific transcription factor.

Material and Methods

Growth and Lactogenic Hormone-Induced Differentiation of the HC11 Cells

The HC11 cells were grown and induced for beta-casein expression by the addition of the lactogenic hormones dexamethasone, prolactin, and insulin (DIP) as previously described (6). The cells were transfected with plasmids expressing various oncoproteins using the calcium phosphate precipitation technique. The precipitate contained 0.5 μg of pSV2neo (7), and 5-10 μg of each individual expression plasmid. The transfected cells were selected by growth for 10-14 days in medium containing 200 μg/ml G418. The following oncogene expression plasmids were transfected into the HC11 cells: pKSV-v-*src* 3.9, which encodes the v-*src* protein; pS-*abl*2 which encodes the v-*abl* protein; pF4 3611-MSV which expresses the v-*raf* protein from a proviral genome (8) (all three obtained from Dr. N. Lydon, Basel); pGR (9) which expresses the v-*fgr* from a proviral copy of the GR-FSV; pSP1 which expresses the int-2 protein (10); and pHa-*ras* which expresses an activated human Ha-*ras* protein (11).

Electrophoretic Mobility Shift Assay for Detection of the MGF Protein

Nuclear extract from HC11 cells treated with either insulin alone or with the DIP lactogenic hormone mix was prepared essentially as described in reference 12. An electrophoretic mobility shift (bandshift) assay was performed as described in reference 13. A ^{32}P-labeled probe of 30 nucleotides from the rat beta-casein promoter (nucleotides -75 to -104) (14) was used in the assay.

Results

Oncogene Introduction into HC11 Cells and Analysis for Beta-Casein Protein Expression

The HC11 mammary epithelial cells retain important features of differentiation and hormonal responsiveness (1,2). Confluent cultures of HC11 cells express the milk protein beta-casein in response to the lactogenic hormones prolactin and glucocorticoids. The cells can be efficiently transfected, thus making it possible to test the effect of an exogenously introduced oncogene upon their differentiation. We have previously shown that expression of the TGF-alpha or Ha-*ras* oncoproteins leads to an inhibition of lactogenic hormone-induced differentiation. In contrast, HC11 cells expressing an activated c-*erb*B-2 (neu) oncogene respond optimally to lactogenic hormones (6). In the TGF-alpha transformed cells the mechanism of inhibition involves an autocrine activation of the EGF receptor. This suggests that, although the EGF and c-*erb*B-2 receptors are structurally very similar (15), the intracellular pathways activated by the two receptors in the HC11 mammary epithelial cells are partially distinct.

Additional oncogenes and growth factors were transfected into the HC11 cells to test for their effect upon lactogenic hormone-induced beta-casein gene expression. Table 1 lists the oncogene expression plasmids that were cotransfected together with the selectable plasmid pSV2neo into the HC11 cells. Transfected HC11 cells were selected in G418, and the clones were pooled and tested for beta-casein protein production following incubation with the lactogenic hormone mix. The results of these analyses, together with our previous results (6), are summarized in Table 1. The v-*src*, v-*fgr*, and v-*abl* proteins are all members of the *src* family of cytoplasmic protein tyrosine kinases (16). The expression of these proteins in the HC11 cells did not interfere with the lactogenic hormone-induced expression of the beta-casein protein. The int-2 protein is a member of the fibroblast growth factor (FGF) family (17). Expression of the int-2 protein in the HC11 cells leads to activation of one of the members of the FGF receptor family (10, T.Venesio, D.Taverna, and G.Merlo, unpublished). The expression of the int-2 protein in the HC11 cells does not interfere with DIP-induced beta-casein protein expression. The v-*raf* protein is a member of the serine/threonine protein kinase family (18). In contrast to the *src* family members and the int-2 protein, expression of the v-*raf* in the HC11 cells inhibits the lactogenic hormone-induced beta-casein protein expression. An immunoblotting analysis for the detection of the beta-casein protein in v-*src*, v-*fgr*, and v-*raf* transfected HC11 cells is shown in Figure 1.

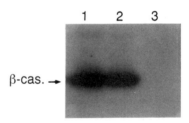

Fig. 1. Western immunoblot analysis of beta-casein in lactogenic hormone-induced HC11 transfectants. Cell lysates prepared from: v-*src* (lane 1), v-*fgr* (lane 2), and v-*raf* (lane 3) transfected HC11 cells, were electrophoressed and electroblotted, and the beta-casein protein was detected using a specific antibody followed by ¹²⁵I-labeled protein A treatment.

Table 1. Lactogenic hormone-induced beta-casein induction in transfected HC11 cells.

Transfected plasmid[a]	ß-casein induction[b]
pSV2neo	+
v-*src*	+
v-*abl*	+
v-*fgr*	+
int-2	+
c-*erb*B-2/neu	+
v-*raf*	-
Ha-*ras*	-
TGF-alpha	-

(a)   HC11 cells were cotransfected with pSV2neo and various oncogene expression plasmids. Clones of transfectants were pooled.

(b)   Transfectants were treated with the lactogenic hormones DIP and beta-casein protein levels were determined by an immunoblot analysis.

The Ha-*ras* and v-*raf* Oncogenes Inhibit Binding of the MGF Protein to the Beta-Casein Gene Promoter

The HC11 cells contain a nuclear factor (MGF) that binds specifically to the beta-casein gene promoter in lactogenic hormone-stimulated cells. MGF is also found in lactating mammary gland cells, and it appears to be a mammary epithelial cell transcription factor whose presence is essential for hormone-induced beta-casein gene transcription (19). An example of an electrophoretic mobility shift (bandshift) assay using a labeled 30 nucleotide fragment from the beta-casein promoter (-75 to -104) is shown in Figure 2. The fragment was incubated with nuclear extracts prepared from confluent cultures of HC11 cells treated for four days with the DIP lactogenic hormone mix (lane 2) or with insulin alone (lane 1). The results show that MGF binds to the beta-casein gene promoter fragment only in the DIP-induced cells. Results from site-directed mutagenesis experiments have shown that the binding of MGF to the promoter is necessary for DIP-induced beta-casein gene transcription (19). Thus, we decided to test the possibility that HC11 cells transformed by the Ha-*ras* and v-*raf* oncogenes had alterations in the MGF transcription factor that made them insensitive to the lactogenic hormones. Nuclear extracts were prepared from DIP-induced HC11 cells transformed by the Ha-*ras*, and v-*raf* oncogenes, and a bandshift analysis using the beta-casein gene promoter fragment described in Figure 2 was performed. Nuclear extract prepared from int-2 transfected cells, which maintain their responsiveness to lactogenic hormone, served as a control.

The results from the bandshift analyses are summarized in Table 2. We were not able to detect MGF transcription factor binding in the Ha-*ras* or in the v-*raf* transformed cells, whereas int-2 transformed cells displayed MGF binding activity.

Discussion

The transformation of a normal cell to a cancer cell involves both genetic and epigenetic changes that invariably lead to alterations in gene expression. It is likely that the accumulation of changes are responsible for the transformed phenotype. In order to understand the process of transformation it will be necessary to describe the changes at the transcriptional level. The HC11 mammary epithelial cells are an appropriate system for studying effects of oncogenes upon gene expression. We have used these cells to show how transformation effects transcription of a differentiation-specific gene product, the beta-casein gene. The MGF mammary cell specific nuclear transcription factor

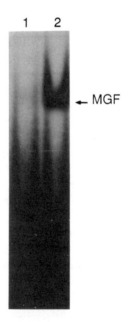

Fig. 2. Binding of the MGF transcription factor within the beta-casein gene promoter. A bandshift assay was performed using a ^{32}P-labeled fragment from the beta-casein gene promoter (-75 to -104). Nuclear extracts were prepared from confluent cultures of HC11 cells treated 4 days with: insulin (lane 1), or with the lactogenic hormone mix, DIP (lane 2).

Table 2. Detection of the MGF transcription factor in oncogene-transfected HC11 cells.

Transfected plasmid[a]	MGF transcription factor[b]
none	+
int-2	+
Ha-*ras*	-
v-*raf*	-

(a)   As in Table 1

(b)   The MGF factor binding to the beta-casein gene promoter was tested in a bandshift assay using nuclear extract prepared from lactogenic hormone-treated HC11 transfectants.

is not detectable in HC11 cells transformed by the v-*raf*, and Ha-*ras* oncogenes. It is also likely that the MGF is altered in HC11 cells transformed by autocrine expression of TGF-alpha, because there is no detectable MGF binding activity in HC11 cells treated simultaneously with EGF and the DIP lactogenic hormone mix (data not shown). Since the bandshift assay measures MGF binding to the beta-casein gene promoter, there are two explanations for these results. The oncogene transformed cells have lost the MGF protein or it has been altered in a way that prevents it from binding to the beta-casein gene promoter. These possibilities can be addressed once the protein is purified and molecular probes are available.

The HC11 cells provide a novel system for studying intracellular signal transduction pathways (20). Since activation of the EGF receptor is incompatible with DIP induced beta-casein expression, oncogenes that cause an inhibition of beta-casein expression may be linked to the EGF receptor signal transduction pathway. The *raf* protein appears to play a central role in signal transduction. The *raf* protein is a cytoplasmic serine/threonone kinase that when activated translocates to the nucleus where it can either directly or indirectly effect gene transcription. In fibroblasts the c-*raf* protein appears to integrate signals generated by the activation of many different members of the receptor tyrosine family, including the EGF receptor (18). In addition, in NIH/3T3 fibroblasts the c-*raf* protein appears to act downstream of the *ras* protein. Inhibition of *raf* kinase activity blocks the transformation of these cells by members of the *ras* family (21). The results that we have obtained with the HC11 cells also suggest that the EGF receptor, Ha-*ras*, and c-*raf* are part of one signal transduction pathway. Activation of any one of these proteins leads to an inhibition of beta-casein transcription.

Oncogenes of the *src* family, as well as activation of the c-*erb*B-2 receptor and activation of the FGF receptor by autocrine expression of the int-2 protein, had no effect upon lactogenic hormone-induced beta-casein expression. This suggests that these proteins are part of other signal transduction pathways. The EGF and c-*erb*B-2 receptors are structurally very similar, and in fibroblasts the activation of each leads to an increase in DNA synthesis. In HC11 cells these two receptors appear to activate different signaling pathways. The HC11 cells should be useful in characterizing specific substrates for members of the receptor tyrosine kinase family.

References

1. Ball RK, Friis RR, Schoenenberger CA et al (1988) Prolactin regulation of ß-casein gene expression and of a cytosolic 120-kd protein in a cloned mouse mammary epithelial cell line. EMBO J 7:2089-2095.
2. Doppler W, Groner B, Ball RK (1989) Prolactin and glucocorticoid hormones synergistically induce expression of transfected rat ß-casein gene promoter constructs in mammary epithelial cell line. Proc Natl Acad Sci USA 86:104-108.
3. Berger MS, Locher GW, Saurer S et al (1988) Correlation of C-*erb*B-2 gene amplification and protein expression in human breast carcinoma with nodal status and nuclear grading. Cancer Res 48:1238-1243.
4. Sukumar S, Notario V, Martin-Zanca D et al (1983) Induction of mammary carcinomas in rats by nitroso-methylurea involves malignant activation of H-*ras*-1 locus by single point mutations. Nature 306:658-661.
5. Perroteau I, Salomon DS, De Bortoli M et al (1986) Immunological detection and quantitation of alpha-transforming growth factors in human breast carcinoma cells. Breast Cancer Res Treat 7:201-210.
6. Hynes NE, Taverna D, Harwerth I-M et al (1990) Epidermal growth factor receptor, but not c-*erb*B-2, activation prevents lactogenic hormone induction of the ß-casein gene in mouse mammary epithelial cells. Mol & Cell Biol 10:4027-4034.
7. Southern PJ, Berg P (1982) Transformation of mammalian cells to antibiotic resistance with a bacterial gene under control of the SV40 early region promoter. J Mol Appl Genet 1:327-341.
8. Rapp UR, Goldsborough MD, Mark GE et al (1983) Structure and biological activity of v-*raf*, a unique oncogene transduced by a retrovirus. Proc Natl Acad Sci USA 80:4218-4222.
9. Ball RK, Ziemiecki A, Schönenberger CA et al. (1988) V-*myc* alters the response of a cloned mouse mammary epithelial cell line to lactogenic hormones. Molec Endocrinol 2:133-142.
10. Merlo GR, Blondel BJ, Deed R et al (1990) The mouse int-2 gene exhibits basic fibroblast growth factor activity in a basic fibroblast growth factor-responsive cell line. Cell Growth and Different 1:463-472.
11. Shih C, Weinberg RA (1982) Isolation of a transforming sequence from a human bladder carcinoma cell line. Cell 29:161-169.
12. Gorski K, Carneiro M, Schibler U (1986) Tissue specific *in vitro* transcription from the mouse albumin promoter. Cell 47:767-776.

13. Carthew RW, Chodosh LA, Sharp PA (1985) An RNA polymerase II transcription factor binds to an upstream element in the adenovirus major late promoter. Cell 43:439-448.
14. Yoshimura M, Oka T (1989) Isolation and structural analysis of the mouse beta-casein gene. Gene 78:267-275.
15. Ullrich A, Schlessinger J (1990) Signal transduction by receptors with tyrosine kinase activity. Cell 61:203-212.
16. Hanks SK, Quinn AM, Hunter T (1988) The protein kinase family: conserved features and deduced phylogeny of the catalytic domain. Science 241:42-52.
17. Goldfarb M (1990) The fibroblast growth factor family. Cell Growth and Different. 1:439-445.
18. Morrison DK (1990) The raf-1 kinase as a transducer of mitogenic signals. Cancer Cells 2:377-382.
19. Schmitt-Ney M, Doppler W, Ball RK et al (1992) Beta-casein gene promoter activity is regulated by the hormone mediated relief of transcriptional repression and a mammary specific nuclear factor. Mol.Cell Biol. In press.
20. Taverna D, Groner B, Hynes NE (1991) Epidermal growth factor receptor, platelet-derived growth factor receptor and c-*erb*B-2 receptor activation all promote growth but have distinctive effects upon mouse mammary epithelial cell differentiation. Cell Growth and Different. 2:145-154.
21. Kolch W, Heidecker G, Lloyd P et al (1991) Raf-1 protein kinase is required for growth of induced NIH/3T3 cells. Nature 349:426-428.

17

Functional Aspects of EGF-Like Peptides in Ovarian-Steroid Responsive Organs

Richard P. DiAugustine, Suzanne M. Snedeker, and Gloria D. Jahnke

Introduction

The sequence of mouse epidermal growth factor (EGF) was reported about two decades ago. During the interim, at least three EGF-like peptide growth factors were discovered, as well as a proto-oncogene (neu or HER-2) that has significant homology to the EGF receptor. Research defining the biological functions of the EGF-like peptides has emphasized identifying their mitogenic or transforming potential. This limited perspective may have obscured determining the full spectrum of their biological functions. The fact that one cell contains receptors for different growth factors suggests that cellular homeostasis is controlled by more than one growth factor receptor pathway. Cell behavior may be regulated by a coordination of tissue-specific stimulatory and inhibitory signals mediated locally by growth factors.

Investigators have long suspected that some of the actions of ovarian steroids are produced by proteins or polypeptides. There is now compelling evidence that members of the EGF family and their cognate receptors are synthesized by ovarian steroid target organs. We now seek to determine whether there are convergent aspects of sex steroid action and pathways regulated by these growth factors.

Biochemical Properties of the EGF Family of Growth Factors

Epidermal Growth Factor

EGF is a 53 amino acid polypeptide originally isolated from the submandibular gland of the male mouse, where it is synthesized in epithelial granulated convoluted tubule cells (1). The mature peptide is a potent mitogen for a variety of epithelial cells and mesenchymal cells (2). EGF derives from a single-chain precursor protein that is about 20 times ($\sim 1{,}200$ amino acids) the size of the mature growth factor (3). The EGF sequence (Fig. 1) occurs near the C-terminal region of the precursor (residues 976-1029). A 20 amino acid transmembrane domain is located between the C-terminal end of the EGF sequence and the C-terminal end of the precursor. Experimental data support that the N-terminal and EGF regions reside in the ectodomain of the precursor. Epithelial cell membranes of the murine kidney (distal tubule), uterus, and lactating gland (alveolar cells) contain EGF in this precursor form. EGF is known to originate from only one precursor protein, but tissue-specific differences exist in the post-translational processing of this protein (4). The significance of these differences with regard to the functional properties of the precursor is not known, although it is conceivable that a membrane-bound precursor might have a receptor-like function. Eight other peptides in the ectodomain contain EGF-like disulfide bond motifs, but it is not known whether these peptides are elaborated during processing (3).

Transforming Growth Factor-α

TGF-α, a 50 amino acid polypeptide, was originally isolated from conditioned medium of retrovirus transformed 3T3 cells and conditioned medium of human carcinoma cells (5). Even though the mature peptide has only about 35% sequence homology with EGF (Fig. 1), it binds to the EGF receptor and exerts similar biological effects *in vitro* and *in vivo*. It is assumed that the actions of TGF-α are conferred *in vivo* through interaction with EGF receptors, since an alternate specific receptor has not been identified. TGF-α is synthesized from a 4.8-kb mRNA as a 160 (human) or 159 (rat) amino acid precursor, which is glycosolated and palmitoylated (6,7). As with the EGF precursor, a transmembrane domain exists a short distance downstream from the growth factor sequence. Species of TGF-α varying from 6 KDa to 20 KDa are found depending on the cells in culture. The unprocessed or partially processed TGF-α precursor, including membrane bound forms, can bind to and activate the EGF receptor. Epidermal tumors and tumor cell lines express TGF-α, but generally

```
hEGF       1    NSDSECPLSHDGYCLHDGVCMYIEALDKYACNCVVGYIGERCQYRDLKWWELR
hTGF-α     1    VVSHFNDCPDSHTQFCFH-GTCRFLVQEDKPACVCHSGYVGARCEHADLLA
hAR       41    KKKNPCNAEFQNFCIH-GECKYIEHLEAVTCKCQQEYFGERCGEK
hHB-EGF   36    KKRDPCLRKYKDFCIH-GECKYVKELRAPSCICHPGYHGERCHGLSL....
```

Fig. 1. Comparison of sequences of members of the EGF family of growth factors isolated from human cells or fluids. The sequences have been aligned to provide overlap of the six cysteine residues in each peptide. Dashes are gaps introduced to maximize homology. Boxes indicate residues conserved in at least three of the four peptides. EGF and TGF-α are shown as complete mature forms, whereas only the EGF-like domain is shown for AR and HB-EGF. The numbers give the actual residue assignment of the first amino acid (reading left to right) according to the sequence reported for the mature forms.

not EGF, and the constitutive synthesis and secretion of a TGF-α peptide in the presence of sufficient receptors may contribute to tumor growth and development of malignancies. More recent studies have established that TGF-α originates from normal as well as malignant cells. TGF-α-specific transcripts or polypeptides have been detected in low abundance in such organs as the pituitary gland, skin, liver, ovary, and mammary gland (5).

Amphiregulin and Heparin-Binding EGF-Like Peptide

Investigation of factors that might be responsible for phorbol acetate inhibition of growth of the human breast adenocarcinoma cell line MCF-7 led to the discovery of a novel single-chain 84 amino acid glycoprotein termed amphiregulin (AR). A truncated 78 amino acid form of AR was the major form extracted from the conditioned medium of the phorbol acetate-treated cells. The C-terminal half of AR (residues 46-84) has the characteristic cysteine residue spacing pattern of the EGF family as well as some of the conserved animo acids (Fig. 1). AR derives from the middle portion of a 252 amino acid protein with a transmembrane domain downstream from the EGF-like region. A 1.4-kb AR transcript was prominent in human placenta and ovaries, but much less abundant in breast tissue (8). Limited studies have revealed that AR can bind to the EGF receptor but with a lower affinity than EGF. AR can replace EGF/TGF-α in stimulating murine keratinocyte growth, but unlike these peptides, it cannot stimulate anchorage-independent growth of NRK fibroblasts in the presence of TGF-β. AR also inhibits growth of some tumor cells that proliferate in response to EGF/TGF-α.

A 22-KDa heparin-binding EGF-like growth factor (HB-EGF) was recently isolated from a phorbol ester-treated human histiocytic lymphoma cell line U-937. A 208-residue HB-EGF primary translation product predicted from a cDNA clone revealed an EGF-like domain (Fig. 1). HR-EGF resembles AR in that it has a hydrophilic stretch upstream from the EGF-like domain that includes a putative nuclear targeting signal (KRKKK). A 2.5-kb HB-EGF transcript was detected by Northern analysis of human macrophage RNA. HB-EGF binds to EGF receptors and is mitogenic for BALB-3T3 fibroblasts and smooth muscle cells, but is not mitogenic for endothelial cells (9).

Synthesis and Functional Aspects of EGF-Like Growth Factors in Ovarian-Steroid Target Organs

The mechanism by which ovarian steroids, such as 17β-estradiol, influence the cell cycle in target organs is not known. With the discovery of numerous growth factors, it was reasonable to speculate that one or more growth factors mediate estrogen-induced proliferation, for instance, and thereby fulfill the roles of the elusive "estromedins." An assessment of whether an EGF receptor pathway is critical for estrogen-induced growth can be made along the same line of inquiries of any putative mediator of systemic hormone action. These include (1) evaluation of target cells for cognate receptors and functional changes in the presence of the growth factor. Growth of epithelial cells in the rodent mammary gland, uterus, vagina, and ovary is stimulated by EGF *in vitro*, and in some cases, *in vivo*. (2) The capacity of target or opposing cells to synthesize the growth factor should be determined along with (3) a study of how both positive and negative systemic stimuli influence local synthesis and secretion of the growth factor. (4) Agents that can specifically inhibit availability of the growth factor, e.g., specific antisera, or inhibit activation of receptors, e.g., tyrosine kinase inhibitors, should be evaluated for their effects on hormone action.

Mammary Gland

The secretion of ovarian estrogens initiates rapid (allometric) growth of the mouse mammary gland at about four weeks of age. This is manifested by the formation of multilayered terminal end buds (TEBs) that serve as growth points for ductal morphogenesis. Ovariectomy prevents ductal growth, which can be restored by treatment with estrogens (10). Implantation of small pellets containing ~1 nmol of EGF or TGF-α near the ductal tips of the regressed gland in castrates stimulates reappearance of TEBs (11,12). These findings suggest that availability of an EGF-like peptide can mimic normal estrogen-induced ductal growth and that responsive EGF receptors exist in the apparent absence of ovarian steroids. Binding of ^{125}I-EGF was shown *in situ* to occur along the TEB stem cell (cap cell) layer. Immunoreactivity for EGF was detected in cells of the inner layers of the TEB and in ductal cells of the subadult female mouse (12). In contrast, TGF-α immunoreactivity was present in the TEB cap cell layer and in stromal fibroblasts along the base of the TEB. Transcripts for both growth factors were detected in the developing gland. This led us to postulate that TGF-α is synthesized in the proliferating cap cells and serves as a positive growth regulator at this site (12). However, it is not known how estrogens, acting directly or indirectly, integrate with a local growth factor pathway. The stimulus for ductal growth may originate in stromal cells, since the proliferating cap cells are apparently devoid of estrogen receptors (10).

Gene expression of EGF in the mammary gland may be regulated by lactogenic hormones (13), and, in this context, elevations in serum level of growth hormone (a lactogen) in the peripubertal mouse may account for detection of EGF in the epithelium during mammary gland development. The high levels of mature EGF in mouse milk is compatible with the fact that the lactating gland exhibits widespread localization of EGF immunoreactivity in alveolar cells and a relative abundance of prepro-EGF mRNA (13). Since both EGF-specific transcripts and immunoreactivity were markedly reduced in the glands of pregnant or adult virgin mice, it is unlikely that this factor contributes to lobuloalveolar growth.

Western blot analysis of membrane preparations of the lactating gland and the pattern of immunostaining with EGF antisera suggest that milk EGF originates from proteolytic processing of the membrane-bound EGF precursor (13). We are currently investigating whether kallikrein-type proteases can function in cleaving EGF from the precursor. These enzymes have compatible substrate specificity in that they cleave Arg-X bonds and are present in a wide variety of organs. EGF precursor cognate peptides containing N- and C-terminal cleavage sites were hydrolyzed at Arg-Asn and Arg-His sites when incubated with various purified murine kallikreins. Northern analysis of lactating mammary gland RNA with a kallikrein cDNA probe revealed a band at ~1 kb characteristic for this class of proteases. Sequencing was then performed on an enzymatically amplified segment of mammary gland kallikrein cDNA. Although this segment embraced variable regions for members of the kallikrein family, a sequence was obtained that exhibited complete homology with the corresponding region of mGK-6, a known kallikrein in the murine kidney. We could not detect transcripts of mGK-9 by a primer-specific polymerase chain reaction; mGK-9 binds EGF and was proposed as the specific kallikrein that processes the EGF precursor (14). A kallikrein was detected in the milk whey fraction by both enzymatic activity and Western blot analysis. Cleavage of the ectodomain of the membrane-bound EGF precursor may be attributed to secretion of mGK-6 kallikrein. Such studies may provide a basis for understanding how other transmembrane growth factors of the EGF family are processed to bioactive peptides at the cell surface.

Uterus

Estrogens stimulate *in vivo* proliferation of the single layer of epithelial cells of the immature and adult rodent uterus. Two separate laboratories have shown that estrogens can also stimulate levels of prepro-EGF mRNA in the mouse uterus (15,16). The abundance of EGF-specific transcript was considerably less than that reported for submandibular glands or kidney (15,16). EGF was localized to the luminal and glandular epithelia. In adult ovariectomized mice, estrogen stimulated epithelial EGF immunoreactivity, which was detected first in the luminal epithelium between 12 and 24 hours, and then in the glandular epithelium by 48 hours; this response did not occur following treatment with progesterone (16). Appearance of epithelial EGF also occurred in intact females in late proestrus, estrus, and early on day 1 of pregnancy. Labeling/immunoaffinity experiments revealed only mature EGF on SDS-PAGE, which led to the proposal that little EGF precursor accumulates in the uterus (16). However, since peptides for affinity isolation were obtained in this study by acid extraction, a large or membrane-bound form of EGF could have escaped recovery. The data suggest that estrogens elaborate bioactive EGF that can recognize cognate receptors on uterine epithelial cells or, alternatively, on the conceptus (17). The contributions of other growth factors, such as TGF-α, must also be evaluated in this context.

Vagina

The stratified squamous epithelium of the vagina responds to estrogens by division and progressive differentiation of cells in the basal layer to form a cornified layer. *In situ* studies with ^{125}I-EGF revealed binding sites mostly along the basal aspect of this epithelium (18), and indicated that functional EGF receptors might be utilized in the proliferative response. Using EGF-specific antiserum, we have found immunolocalization in the stratum granulosum (nonproliferating) in the vagina of estrogen-treated ovariectomized mice. Immunostaining was not observed in untreated mice (Figs. 2 A, B, & C). Diffuse localization of TGF-α was observed throughout the epithelial layers (Fig. 2D), similar to that reported for this growth factor in the stratified skin epithelium (19). Nuclei were also stained in cells along the basal layer. As with end buds of the mammary gland, the different pattern of localization for these

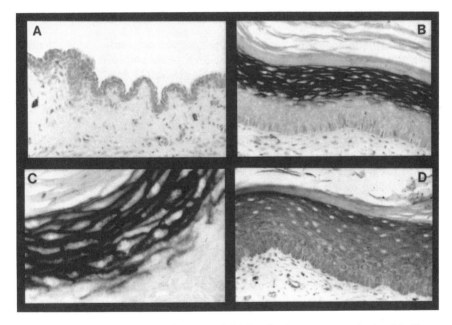

Fig. 2. Immunolocalization of EGF and TGF-α in the mouse vaginal epithelium. (A) EGF immunoreactivity is not detected in the vagina of castrates (x). (B) By contrast, EGF immunoreactivity occurs in the stratum granulosum of estrogen-treated mice (x). (C) A higher magnification of the positively stained layer reveals staining along cell borders (x). (D) Positive staining for TGF-α is observed throughout the epithelial layers in estrogen-treated mice (x). Negligible staining was observed in castrates. Adult castrated female CD-1 mice received sesame oil (controls) or 1 μg estradiol s.c. in sesame oil once a day for three days. Vaginal tissue was obtained 18 hours after the last injection. The double peroxidase-antiperoxidase method was used for immunostaining.

two growth factors suggests that they have distinct functions, and that TGF-α, and not EGF, may provide the mitogenic signal in response to ovarian estrogens.

Ovary

The detection and functional properties of EGF-like peptides in the ovary have been previously reviewed.(20) In one study, TGF-α transcripts and peptide were found in theca cells but not in granulosa cells (21). Both cell populations exhibit high-affinity binding sites for EGF and proliferate *in vitro* in the presence of EGF-like growth factors. EGF/TGF-α can also influence steroidogenesis in these cells (20). Transcripts for EGF and AR have also been detected in the ovaries of mice and humans, respectively, indicating that multiple members of the EGF family function in follicular homeostasis (4,8).

Functions in Oncogenesis and Tumor Cell Growth

The oncogenic potential of growth factors has received considerable attention since protooncogenes were found that code for proteins with sequence homology to known growth factors or growth factor receptors (22,23). One of the first relevant findings was the strong amino acid homology of the *erb*B transforming protein of avian erythroblastosis virus with that of the EGF receptor (24). EGF and TGF-α were shown to be oncogenic when corresponding expression vectors were transfected into fibroblasts (25,26). Specific antiserum to the growth factor in each case inhibits the transformation phenotype. This indicates that interaction of the growth factor with cell surface receptors is important in the sequence of events leading to transformation. This should not rule out the possibility that some products of growth factor genes influence intracellular events.

Several breast carcinoma cell lines have been shown to produce TGF-α, and estrogen treatment of hormone-responsive cell lines leads to an increase in TGF-α immunoreactivity in the conditioned medium (27). These data suggest that the growth promoting effects of estrogens may be mediated, at least in part, by TGF-α. Introduction of a recombinant retroviral vector containing the TGF-α gene into immortalized mammary epithelial cells results in enhanced growth and colony formation in soft agar, which could be inhibited by anti-TGF-α or anti-EGF receptor-blocking antibodies (28). TGF-α expression may be an intermediary event in the cellular response to some protooncogenes, since transfection of the same mammary cells with c-Ha-*ras* increases TGF-α transcript and secreted TGF-α peptide.

It is important to note that expression of TGF-α per se in breast carcinomas is neither an ectopic nor a tumor-specific event in the mammary gland, since this growth factor is produced by normal human mammary epithelial cells *in vitro* (29) and by the proliferating cap cells during ductal morphogenesis, as described above. The conditions imposed by cell culture to promote cell growth may select for cells with TGF-α and cognate receptor expression in surviving cells. In contrast EGF, whose expression we attribute to the differentiated (lactating) mammary gland, is not generally expressed by breast cancer cell lines (27).

The cumulative findings underscore the importance of evaluating the oncogenic potential of growth factor overexpression *in vivo* within the normal cell microenvironment. In this regard, female transgenic mice containing human TGF-α cDNA under the control of the MMTV enhancer/promoter exhibit overexpression of TGF-α in the mammary epithelium (alveoli and small ducts) (30). Hyperplasia was observed in virgin animals and a range of hyperplastic and neoplastic abnormalities occurred in mammary glands of multiparous transgenic mice. It is likely that transgene expression of TGF-α *in vivo* requires additional activation of one or more protooncogenes prior to formation of mammary carcinomas. We should seek then to understand how perturbations of the cell cycle caused by constitutive expression of growth factor predispose the mouse mammary gland to cancer. Such studies should provide some insight as to how ovarian steroids contribute to human breast cancer.

Conclusions

The capacity of ovarian steroid hormones, such as estradiol, to increase cancer risk in target organs, such as the mammary gland and uterus, may originate in perturbations of growth factor pathways. Different protooncogenes code for proteins that are involved in cell cycle control. These proteins include growth factors, growth factor receptors, and signal transduction elements. This underscores the importance of understanding normal cell growth and homeostasis. Members of the EGF family, such as TGF-α or EGF, and their cognate receptors, are synthesized by epithelial cells of the murine mammary gland, uterus, and vagina, and may provide a proliferative stimulus in these organs in response to estradiol. Ovarian estrogens are required for ductal morphogenesis in the mammary gland, but in ovariectomized subadult animals, TGF-α or EGF delivered locally *in vivo* appears to stimulate the normal growth pattern. Members of the EGF family may also have nonproliferative functions in these target organs, since synthesis of EGF occurs in lactating alveolar cells of the mammary gland and in cells of the vaginal stratum granulosum. Understanding how ovarian steroids influence local growth factor pathways may explain some of the actions of these hormones and help to determine early events that predispose target organs to uncontrolled proliferation.

References

1. Carpenter G, Cohen S (1979) Epidermal growth factor. Ann Rev Biochem 48:193-216.
2. Fisher DA, Lakshmanan J (1990) Metabolism and effects of epidermal growth factor and related growth factors in mammals. Endocrine Rev 11:418-442.

3. Scott J, Urdea M, Quiroga M, et al (1983) Structure of a mouse submaxillary messenger RNA encoding epidermal growth factor and seven related proteins. Science 221:236-240.

4. Rall LB, Scott J, Bell GI, et al (1985) Mouse prepro-epidermal growth factor synthesis by kidney and other tissues. Nature (London) 313:228-231.

5. Derynck R, (1988) Transforming growth factor α. Cell 54:593-595.

6. Derynck R, Roberts AB, Winkler ME et al (1984) Human transforming growth factor-α: precursor structure and expression in *E. coli*. Cell 38:287-297.

7. Lee DC, Rose TM, Webb NR et al (1985) Cloning and sequence analysis of a cDNA for rat transforming growth factor-α. Nature 313:489-491.

8. Plowman GD, Green JM, McDonald VL et al (1990) The amphiregulin gene encodes a novel epidermal growth factor-related protein with tumor-inhibitory activity. Mol Cell Biol 10:1969-1981.

9. Higashiyama S, Abraham JA, Miller J et al (1991) A heparin-binding growth factor secreted by macrophage-like cells that is related to EGF. Science 251:936-939.

10. Daniel CW, Silberstein GB, Strickland P (1987) Direct action of 17β-estradiol on mouse mammary ducts analyzed by sustained release implants and steroid autoradiography. Cancer Res 47:6052-6057.

11. Coleman S, Silberstein GB, Daniel CW (1988) Ductal morphogenesis in the mouse mammary gland: evidence supporting a role for epidermal growth factor. Dev Biol 127:304-315.

12. Snedeker SM, Brown CF, DiAugustine RP (1991) Expression and functional properties of transforming growth factor α and epidermal growth factor during mouse mammary gland ductal morphogenesis. Proc Natl Acad Sci USA 88:276-280.

13. Brown CF, Teng CT, Pentecost BT et al (1989) Epidermal growth factor precursor in mouse lactating mammary gland alveolar cells. Mol Endocrinol 3:1077-1083.

14. Drinkwater CC, Evans BA, Richards RI (1987) Mouse glandular kallikrein genes: identification and characterization of the genes encoding the epidermal growth factor binding proteins. Biochemistry 26:6750-6756.

15. DiAugustine RP, Petrusz P, Bell GI et al (1988) Influence of estrogens on mouse uterine epidermal growth factor precursor protein and messenger ribonucleic acid. Endocrinology 122:2355-2363.

16. Huet-Hudson YM, Chakraborty C, De SK et al (1990) Estrogen regulates the synthesis of epidermal growth factor in mouse uterine epithelial cells. Mol Endocrinol 4:510-523.

17. Simmen FA, Simmen RCM (1991) Peptide growth factors and proto-oncogenes in mammalian conceptus development. Biol Reproduct 44:1-5.

18. Bossert NL, Nelson KG, Ross KA et al (1990) Epidermal growth factor binding and receptor distribution in the mouse reproductive tract during development. Dev Biol 142:75-85.

19. Coffey RJ, Derynck R, Wilcox JN et al (1987) Production and auto-induction of transforming growth factor-α in human keratinocytes. Nature 328:817-820.
20. May JV, Schomberg DW (1989) The potential relevance of epidermal growth factor and transforming growth factor-alpha to ovarian physiology. Seminars in Reproductive Endocrinol 7:1-11.
21. Skinner MK, Coffey RJ (1988) Regulation of ovarian cell growth through the local production of transforming growth factor-α by theca cells. Endocrinol 23:2632-2638.
22. Goustin AS, Leof EB, Shipley GD et al (1986) Growth factors and cancer. Cancer Res 46:1015-1029.
23. Cross M, Dexter TM (1991) Growth factors in development, transformation and tumorigenesis. Cell 64:271-280.
24. Downward J, Yarden Y, Mayes E et al (1984) Close similarity of epidermal growth factor receptor and v-*erb*-B oncogene protein sequences. Nature 307:521-527.
25. Stern DF, Hare DL, Cecchini MA et al (1987) Construction of a novel oncogene based on synthetic sequences encoding epidermal growth factor. Science 235:321-324.
26. Rosenthal A, Lindquist P, Bringman TS et al (1986) Expression in rat fibroblasts of a human transforming growth factor-α cDNA results in transformation. Cell 46:301-309.
27. Perroteau I, Salomon D, DeBortoli M et al (1986) Immunological detection and quantitation of alpha transforming growth factors in human breast carcinoma cells. Breast Cancer Res Treat 7:201-210.
28. Ciardello F, McGeady ML, Kim N et al (1990) Transforming growth factor-α expression is enhanced in human mammary epithelial cells transformed by an activated c-Ha-*ras* protooncogen, and overexpression of the transforming growth factor-α complementary DNA leads to transformation. Cell Growth & Differentiation 1:407-420.
29. Zajachowski D, Band V, Pauzie N et al (1988) Expression of growth factors and oncogenes in normal and tumor-derived human mammary epithelial cells. Cancer Res 48:7041-7047.
30. Matsui Y, Halter SA, Holt JT et al (1990) Development of mammary hyperplasia and neoplasia in MMTV-TGFα transgenic mice. Cell 61:1147-1155.

18

Androgen Regulation of Growth Factor and Early Growth Repsonse Gene Expression in Hamster DDT1-MF2 and Human Prostate LNCAP Cells

Stephen E. Harris, Zeng X. Rong, Jeffrey A. Hall,
Murray A. Harris, James S. Norris, Roy G. Smith,
Dennis B. Lubahn, Elizabeth M. Wilson, and
Frank S. French

Introduction

The Syrian hamster DDT-1 cell line was originally derived from an estrogen/androgen-induced ductus deferens tumor and has served as a model for analyzing androgen-induced growth (1). Likewise a human prostate carcinoma cell line, LNCAP, has served as a human-derived model for analyzing a stage of androgen-induced growth and may represent human prostate cancer before development of hormone autonomy (2). The mechanism of hormone-regulated growth is thought to reside in the control of PDGF-B and FGF family of growth factors, important autocrines in a wide variety of cancers. Earlier results indicate that a PDGF-B-like mRNA and acidic FGF mRNA are made by DDT-1 cells in response to androgens (3,4). In the LNCAP system, it has been demonstrated that androgens, as well as estradiol 17β, can increase aFGF mRNA levels. Therefore, the purpose of this article is to present (1) recent finding on the nature of the PDGF-B-like mRNA and gene in DDT-1 cells, (2) evidence using sense and antisense PDGF/v*sis* constructions that the DDT-1 v*sis* mRNA is important for growth of these cells, (3) data on androgen induction of the early growth response gene, Nur 77 mRNA, and (4) findings on the structure of the aFGF gene. Finally, the nature of androgen-induced early growth response gene expression and aFGF expression in LNCAP cells will be addressed, as well as the possible mechanism of why LNCAP cells are growth responsive to not only androgens, but progestins, estradiol 17β, and antiandrogens.

PDGF/v*sis*-Like mRNA in DDT1 Cells

Structure of DDT1 v*sis* mRNA

A 4.2 kb cDNA homologous to PDGF-B was isolated and sequenced from a DDT-1 MF2 cDNA library (4). Figure 1 represents the unusual structural organization of the mRNA. This PDGF-like mRNA, referred to as DDT1 v*sis* mRNA, appears to be a chimeric mRNA with a rearranged SSV gnome. Parts are identical to SSV and other regions identical to different retroviral regions or hamster DNA. The LTR structure is quite unique in that the 3' most LTR is an inverted copy of the SSV 5' LTR. It is as if the 5' part of a SSV-like virus region has been inverted and ligated to the 3' end of DDT1 v*sis* mRNA structure. The reverse transcriptase (RT) region is not like SSV but more like the RT region of Molony-MLV. This suggests a unique origin for this v*sis* mRNA.

Sense and Antisense v*sis* 3.9 cDNA Transfection

A 3.9kb v*sis* CDNA was placed between the SV-40 enhancer/promoter and the neocassette of parent pSV2-Neo, such that the 3.9 kb v*sis* CDNA would be

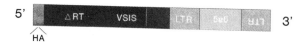

Fig 1. Diagram of the 4.2 kb v*sis* mRNA isolated from a λgt11-DDT1 cDNA library. RT, MO MLV-like RT region; v*sis*, identical to v*sis* in SSV; ha, hamster sequence; LTR, identical to the LTR sequences in SSV; gag, identical to gag region in SSV (4).

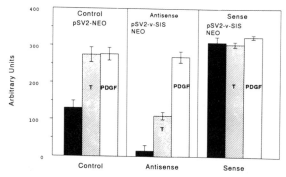

Fig 2. DDT1 cells transfected with control pSV2-Neo, pSV2-v*sis* antisense-neo, and pSV2-v*sis*-Sense-Neo plasmids. 18-35 Neo^R clones were pooled and analyzed for growth properties. Porcine PDGF-B, 40 ng/ml; T, $10^{-7}M$ (4).

forcedly transcribed in any Geneticin- or G418-resistant colonies. Stable transfected DDT1 cells with either the sense or antisense constructions were analyzed for their growth properties and the results are summarized in Figure 2 (4).

The control DDT1 cell clones transfected with the parent vector, pSV2-neo, have retained their androgen and PDGF responsiveness. However, the clones transfected with antisense vsis (pSV2-vsis-Antisense-Neo) grow much slower, and androgens do not stimulate growth to the extent of control cells. PDGF-B added to the antisense DDT1 cells restores the growth rate to the level of androgen or PDGF treated control DDT1 cells.

The DDT1 cells transfected with the sense construction (pSV2-vsis-Sense-Neo) have lost all androgen or PDGF-B responsiveness and are growing at a near-maximum rate. Added PDGF-B has little effect.

vsis mRNA Expression in Control, vsis^A, vsis^s DDT1

Control DDT1 cells, vsis^A DDT1, and vsis^s DDT1 cells were grown on collagen-coated dishes to high density ($10^7/135^{cm2}$) and then withdrawn from androgens for 3 days. To the cultures, T at $10^{-7}M$ was added for 3 days. vsis expression was then analyzed using ^{32}P-cRNA probe to the 434bp PstI/SmaI vsis fragment. The results are presented in Figure 3.

Testosterone stimulates a 4.2 kb and 3.5 kb sis mRNA in control cells. In the vsis^A DDT1 cells, less 4.0 kb and 3.5 kb sis mRNAs are observed. In the vsis^s DDT1, extensive overexpression of a 3.0 kb mRNA is observed. These results suggest overexpression of vsis mRNA plays a role in the loss of androgen responsiveness and rapid growth. On the other hand, expression of the vsis^A mRNA appear to be blocking expression or translation of the DDT1 sis mRNA, resulting in growth retardation and attenuated responsiveness to T.

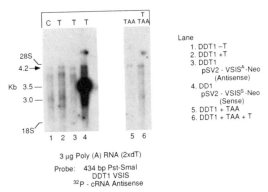

3 µg Poly (A) RNA (2xdT)

Probe: 434 bp Pst-SmaI
DDT1 VSIS
^{32}P - cRNA Antisense

Fig 3. Expression of sis mRNA is DDT1, vsis^A DDT1, or vsis^s DDT1 cells. Poly(A) RNA was analyzed using ^{32}P-cRNA from 434bp Pst/SmaI fragment (4). Cells were grown to high density on collagen-coated dishes in DFITS media plus T. They were "withdrawn" for 3 days in DFITS media without T. T was then added for 48 hrs (4).

DDT Cell v*sis* Gene

When DDT1 DNA and normal Syrian hamster DNA are probed using a DDT1 Pst/SmaI 434 bp fragment, several unique and amplified PDGF related bands are noted in DDT1 DNA (not shown). There is a 1.0 kb Pst/SmaI fragment in DDT1 DNA not observed in liver DNA but most of the remainder of the bands are identical, at least at this level of resolution. This suggest that (1) the v*sis* specific gene is amplified in DDT1 cells, and (2) since a 1.0 kb Pst/SmaI fragment was observed, and not an intronless 434 bp fragment, the v*sis* DDT1 gene may have introns and could have arisen by homologous recombination of a rodent SSV-like virus with the normal endogenous C*sis* gene. Activation of a endogenous v*sis* like gene in normal tissues as a result of hormonal treatment of the original hamsters is also considered a reasonable hypothesis.

aFGF and NUR 77 Expression in DDT1 Cells

aFGF

Figure 4a presents analysis of poly (A$^+$) RNA from DDT1 cells grown on collagen, "withdrawn" from T in serum-free media (4) for 3 days and then challenged with T and TAA for 48 hrs. There is a major 0.8 kb aFGF mRNA and a larger mRNA at 4.0 kb. Both aFGF mRNAs are androgen induced and glucocorticoids (TAA) do not prevent T induction. Cycloheximide given the last 4 hrs of the 48 hr T treatment blocks aFGF mRNAs expression, suggesting aFGF mRNA is rapidly turning over and requires continued protein synthesis.

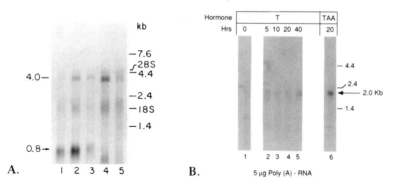

Fig 4. aFGF mRNA and Nur 77 expression in DDT1 cells. Cells were stimulated and withdrawn as in Fig 3. (a) T and TAA were added at $10^{-7}M$ for 48 hrs. Cycloheximide at 10 μg/ml was added the last 4 hrs of the culture. Lane 1, -T; 2, +T, 3; T+cycloheximide; 4, T+TAA; 5, +TAA. Probe: 700 bp DDT1 aFGF cRNA. (b) Testesterone at 10^{-7} was added to withdrawn DDT1 cells as Fig. 3. After the indicated time, RNA was collected and processed. Lane 1, control 0 hrs; 2, 5 hrs; 3, 10 hrs; 4, 20 hrs; 5, 40 hrs; 6, TAA for 20 hrs.

T + TAA appears to stabilize the 4.0 kb mRNA, as suggested earlier by *in situ* hybridization analysis in low-density cultures (5).

Nur 77

Nur 77 belongs to the class of early growth response genes mRNAs, originally isolated by Lau, et al. (6) and subsequently cloned under a variety of names (5). Nur 77 is a classical orphan receptor and early growth response gene (6,7).

Using the human Nur 77 probe, the level of Nur 77 mRNA induction in DDT1 was analyzed. The results are presented in Figure 4b. It is clear that T applied to "withdrawn" DDT1 cells on collagen can induce a transient increase and decrease in Nur 77 expression. The nature of the response is most likely due to the fact that the "withdrawn" DDT1 cultures are slowly growing and asynchronous with respect to the cell cycle. The results do imply that the mechanism of early androgen induced growth responses may be very similar to those seen with FGF, PDGF, EGF, other growth and serum factors using synchronized NIH 3T3 serum-starved/GF activated cell systems (6,7).

Structure and Function of the aFGF Gene from DDT1

aFGF Gene

Using a DDT1 cosmid and a λ genomic library and a DDT1 aFGF probe, two overlapping cosmid clones and several λ clones were isolated and mapped. The gene is divided into three coding exons and a 5'-noncoding exon (Figure 5a). The transcription unit is over 60 kb and the DDT1 5'-noncoding exon has not been colinearized with Exons 2-4. By RNase protection experiments, a major transcription start site has been identified approximately 200 bp upstream of the 72 bp 5'-noncoding exon region identified in the aFGF cDNA (3).

A 7.0 kb PstI fragment of the aFGF gene, including exon 1 and some 3,000 bp of 5'-flanking region were cloned into pBL3CAT and transfected into DDT1 cells. The results (Figure 5b) indicate that androgens can increase CAT activity, but the strength of the response suggests that it is not direct and may involve many other factors and possible early growth gene activity for function.

LNCAP/ADEP Express aFGF mRNA and Early Growth Response Genes Egr1 and NUR 77 in Response to Androgens and Estradiol 17B

A variety of steroids and steroid analogs stimulate LNCAP cell growth in a serum-free medium (2). The LNCAP cells are stimulated to grow with T, E_2, PROG, HOFLU, and CY (8).

aFGF mRNA

LNCAP cells were grown to high density in a serum-free media supplemented with EGF (5 ng/ml) and T at $10^{-7}M$ (8). The cells were then "withdrawn" from T for 8-10 days and subsequently challenged with T or E2. At 96 hrs, the RNA was collected, poly (A) RNA prepared and analyzed. Figure 6a demonstrates that several aFGF mRNA species are induced by T or E2.

Nur 77 and Egr-1 mRNA

In a similar manner, "withdrawn" LNCAP cell cultures were challenged with T and expression of the early growth response genes Egr-1 and Nur 77 were analyzed. Egr1 belongs to the class of early growth response gene transcription factors containing three Cys_2-His_2 type of Zn^{++} fingers (9). Egr-1 most likely plays an important role in regulation of Nur 77, since the 5'-flanking region of Syrian hamster and mouse Nur 77 contain two closely spaced Egr-1 response DNA elements (7,8).

Figure 6b demonstrates that androgens alone can induce Egr-1 by 5 hrs. This is a much slower process than that observed with serum- or GF-induced Egr-1 in the NIH 3T3 synchronized cell system (6,9). Egr-1 mRNA is regulated at multiple levels. At the transcription level, it is positively regulated through AP-1/fos-jun elements and is negatively regulated through the SRE in the NIH 3T3 system (9). How androgens activate Egr-1 mRNA in LNCAP is unknown, but most likely involves androgen regulation of the fos-jun complex (9).

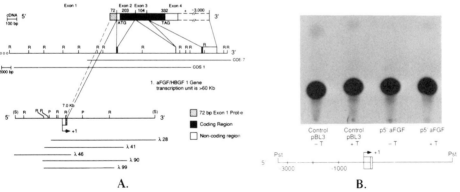

A.   B.

Fig 5. Structure and function of the DDT1 aFGF gene. (a) ■, coding region; □, 72bp 5'-noncoding or exon 1 region and probe; □, noncoding region. A major transcription start site was mapped 280 bp upstream of the 72 bp region by RNase protection assay. (b) The 7.0 kb Pst 1 fragment encompassing exon 1 and 3,300 bp of 5' flanking region of aFGF gene was placed in pBL3 CAT vector and transvected into DDT1 cells. They were plated on collagen-coated dishes. The cells were treated with T at $10^{-7}M$ for 3 days and CAT activity measured (8).

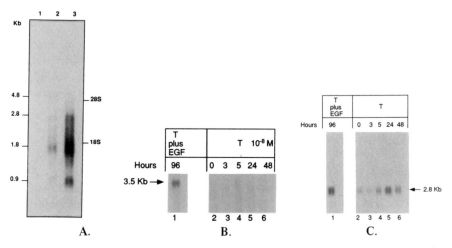

Fig 6. Expression of aFGF, Nur 77, and Egr-1 in mRNA LNCAP/Adep cell. LNCAP/Adep cells were grown to high density (10^7 cells/135CM²) in DFITS + 0.2% charcoal-stripped FCS+EGF (5 ng/ml) +T at $10^{-8}M$. They were then withdrawn from T and GF for 8-10 days, and then challenged with GF and/or T or E2 at $10^{-7}M$. 5 μg poly (A)RNA/Lane. (a) aFGF. Lane 1, Control-T; 2, +T for 4 days; 3, +E2 for 4 days. Probe: ha 700 bp aFGF ^{32}P-cRNA. (b) Egr-1. Lane 1, T+EGF 96 hrs; 2, 0 hrs; 3, 3 hrs +T; 4, 5 hrs +T; 5, 24 hrs +T; 6, 48 hrs +T. Probe: ^{32}P-3.5 kb cDNA to mouse Egr-1 mRNA. (c) Nur 77. Lane 1, T+EGF 96 hrs; 2, 0 hrs; 3, 3 hrs +T; 4, 5 hrs +T; 5, 24 hrs +T; 6, 48 hrs +T. Probe: 2.1 kb cDNA to human Nur 77 (8).

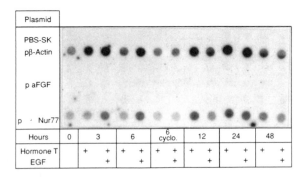

Fig 7. Nuclear run-on assay of LNCAP Nur 77 transcription. Cells were grown and withdrawn as in Fig 6 and (8). They were then stimulated with T @ $10^{-8}M$ or T plus EGF 10 ng/ml for times indicated. Nuclei were isolated and assayed as describes (8), using blue-script plasmid with the 2.1 kb cDNA Nur 77 insert, mouse β-actin insert, or control pBS-SK(-) plasmid.

As expected, Nur 77 mRNA is also up regulated by androgens and is a delayed process compared to the synchronized, serum, or GF activated NIH 3T3 system (7). This result is presented in Figure 6c and again strongly support that Egr-1 and Nur 77 are directly involved in androgen-stimulated growth.

Nur 77 Transcription Rate Is Increased by Androgens and EGF

Figure 7 presents a nuclear run-on experiment in which "withdrawn" LNCAP cell cultures ($\sim 10^7$ cells/135 cm^2) were challenged with T or T plus EGF. By 6-12 hrs androgens increase the transcription rate of the Nur 77 gene. It peaks at 24 hrs and then declines. The addition of androgen plus EGF speeds up the whole process of Nur 77 induction and decline where the peak transcription rate is 6 hrs and declines by 12 hrs. Cycloheximide (10 μg/ml) for 6 hrs blocks the increased transcription of Nur 77 by androgens or androgens plus EGF. The cycloheximide experiment suggest that prior protein synthesis is required for transcriptional activation of the Nur 77 gene by androgens or androgens plus EGF. β actin transcription was used as a control (8).

LNCAP Androgen Receptor Mutation

LNCAP AR contains a mutation that converts amino acid 877 Thr→877 Ala and allows the LNCAP AR to transactivate with antiandrogens, progesterone, estradiol 17β, as well as T (10).

Normal and LNCAP AR Expression Vector

In Figure 8 is presented a diagram of the normal and LNCAP AR expression vectors and the MMTV-CAT reporter gene used in the transfection of CV1 cells.

Figure 9a presents the CAT activity results and demonstrates that the normal AR cannot transactivate the reporter gene with E$_2$ or HOFLU, while the mutant LNCAP AR can transactivate with E$_2$ and HOFLU.

Figure 9b demonstrates the mutant LNCAP AR is also capable of steroid-induced transactivation with $10^{-9}M$ PROG, while the normal AR shows little activity.

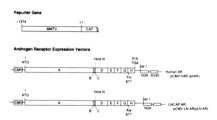

Fig. 8. Structure of the normal and the mutant LNCAP-AR expression plasmids. MMTV-CAT was used as reporter gene.

Figure 10 shows that the LNCAP AR mutation is in an important region involved in dimerization and steroid binding and now supports the reasonable hypothesis that the "aberrant" growth response of LNCAP cells to antiandrogens, PROG, E_2 can be explained by this single-point mutation.

Conclusions

DDT1 and LNCAP cells are androgen responsive. DDT1 cells produce an unusual vsis mRNA, aFGF mRNA, and early growth response gene, Nur 77 mRNA, under androgen control. The aFGF gene is >60 kb and may have multiple promoters. One of the promoters responds positively to androgens. In LNCAP cells aFGF mRNA and the early growth response gene transcription factors, Egr1 and Nur 77 are also regulated by androgens, and, at least in part, at the transcription level. A mutation in the LNCAP AR was described which may explain the positive growth response to E_2, HOFLU, and PROG.

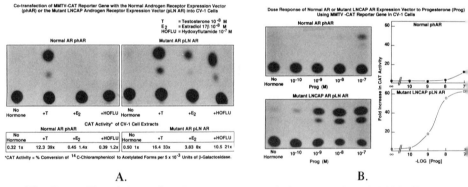

A.   **B.**

Fig 9. CAT activity using MMTV-CAT and the normal and LNCAP-AR expression plasmids transfected into CV-1 cells (10). (a) Affect of T, HOFLU, and E2 (b) Affect of PROG.

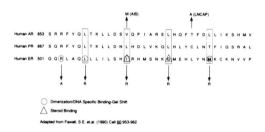

Fig 10. Comparison of the amino acid sequence of the AR, PR, and ER in a hydrophobic region forming a heptad repeat and playing an important role in dimerization and steroid-dependent transactivation. The LNCAP AR mutation is in a region homologous to an area in the ER that is important for steroid binding and transactivation.

Acknowledgments

This research was supported by NIH grant PO1 DK38639, Project 3 and an NIH/NCI Program Project. We are grateful to Dr. James Dunn, and Karen Schultz for their technical assistance and to Gloria Peché for her expert skill in the preparation of this manuscript. We also thank V. Sukhatme for the mouse Egr-1 probe and C. Chang for the human Nur 77 probe.

References

1. Smith RG, Harris SE, Lamb DJ (1991) Mechanism of growth regulation of androgen responsive cells. Mol Cell Biol Pros Can 15-26.

2. Harris SE, Harris MA, Rong Z, et al (1991) Androgen regulation of HBGF-1(aFGF) mRNA and characterization of the androgen receptor mRNA in the human prostate carcinoma cell line-LNCAP/A dep. Mol Cell Biol of Pros Can 315-330.

3. Hall JA, Harris MA, Malark M, et al (1990) Characterization of the hamster DDT1 cell aFGF/HBGF1 gene and cDNA and its modulation by steroids. J Cell Biochem 43:1-10.

4. Harris SE, Hall JA, Monk R et al. An unusual vsis/PDGF-B mRNA from DDT1 cells: Affect of sense- and anti-sense construction on androgen induced growth (unpublished data).

5. Harris SE, Smith RG, Zhou H, et al (1989) Androgens and glucocorticoids modulate heparin-binding growth factor mRNA accumulation in DDT1 cells as analyzed by *in situ* hybridization. Mol Endocrinol 3:1839-1844.

6. Lau LF, Nathans D (1985) Identification of a set of genes expressed during the Go/G1 transition of cultured mouse cells. EMBO J 4:3145-3151.

7. Ryseck RP, MacDonald BH, Mattei, MG et al (1989) Mapping and expression of a growth factor inducible gene encoding a putative nuclear hormonal binding receptor. EMBO J 8:3327-3335.

8. Rong ZX, Harris MA, Chang C, Harris SE Acidic FGF and early growth response genes, Egr-1 and Nur 77 mRNA are regulated by androgens and estradiol 17β in LNCAP/Adep cells (unpublished data).

9. Gius D, Cas X, Rauscher III F, et al (1990) Transcriptional activation and repression by *fos* are independent functions: The C terminus represses immediate-early gene expression via CArG elements. Mol Cell Biol 10:4243-4255.

10. Harris SE, Rong Z, Harris MA, Labahn DB (1990) Androgen receptor in human prostate carcinoma LNCAP/ADEP cells contains a mutation which alters the specificity of the steroid-dependent transcriptional activation region. Endocrinology Abstracts No. 275 p. 93, Atlanta, GA.

Abbreviations

T-testosterone E_2-estradiol 17β PROG-progesterone HOFLU-hydroxyflutamide CY-cyproterone acetate TAA-triamcinalone acetonide LTR-long-terminal repeat SRE-serum response DNA element [CC(A/T)$_6$GG] egr 1 RE-early growth response gene 1 response element [CGC(C/A)CCCGC] AP-1-*fos*-jun DNA element [TG(A/C)GTCA) AR-androgen receptor CAT-chloramphenicol transferase GF-growth factor aFGF-acidic fibroblast growth factor PDGF-B-platelet-derived growth factor with two β chains v*sis* mRNA-DDT1 v*sis* related mRNA SSV-simian sarcoma virus v*sis*^{A}-DDT1 cells with 3.9kb v*sis* cDNA-antisense v*sis*^{s}-DDT1 with 3.9 kb v*sis* cDNA-sense EGF-epidermal growth factor DFITS-DMEM:F12 plus insulin, transferin, selenium.

19

Estrogen Regulation of Protooncogene Expression

Salman M. Hyder, Connie Chiappetta, John L. Kirkland,
Tsu-Hui Lin, David S. Loose-Mitchell, Lata Murthy,
Claudia A. Orengo, Ulka Tipnis, and George M. Stancel

Introduction

Our basic approach to the problem of hormonal carcinogenesis has been to investigate the mechanisms by which physiologically relevant levels of estrogens regulate the growth and function of normal target tissues. This information is required to understand the mechanisms of carcinogenesis in hormone target tissues, the role of the hormone in these processes, and rational approaches to the prevent,ion and treatment of major human diseases such as prostate, endometrial, and breast cancer. The experimental system we have used for our studies is the immature rat uterus.

Treatment of immature rats (25-30 days of age) with estradiol initiates a series of events that culminates in DNA replication and division of uterine cells approximately 24 hours after treatment (1). In the immature animal, the hormone stimulates all of the major uterine cell types (luminal and glandular epithelium, stroma, and myometrium) to divide. It is important to note that the hormone itself is cleared from the tissue long before DNA synthesis occurs (1). Thus, uterine growth must involve mechanisms that amplify and propagate the signal emanating from interactions between the hormone and its receptor. This realization has prompted much research aimed at identifying uterine events that could play a role in amplifying and mediating estrogen-induced tissue growth.

Recently, several laboratories have begun to investigate the potential involvement of protooncogenes, or cellular oncogenes, in estrogen-induced uterine growth. Protooncogenes were originally identified as the normal, cellular analogs of the oncogenes present in transforming retroviruses. The different protooncogenes code for products that have a variety of biological activities, including growth factors and growth factor receptors, kinases, transcription factors, and G proteins. In most cases, regulation of the viral gene expression or its product's activity are not subject to the same regulation as the cellular analog, and this difference is thought to be important for transformation. It is important, however, to emphasize two points: (1) the protooncogenes are expressed during growth and development of normal cells, and (2) overexpression of normal, cellular protooncogenes can cause transformation in experimental systems (2). In this article, we discuss some of our results on the regulation of protooncogene expression in the immature rat uterus by estrogen.

Protooncogene Expression and Regulation in the Uterus

To date, the expression of six different protooncogenes has been observed in the rodent uterine system as illustrated in Table 1. In all cases estradiol regulates the level of the transcripts of these genes, although it is not unequivocally established in all cases that these effects are mediated at the transcriptional level.

In this chapter, we will focus on c-*fos* as the prototype of a uterine gene that is regulated by estrogenic steroids.

Regulation of Uterine c-*fos* Expression by Estrogen

The data in Figure 1 illustrate the induction of uterine c-*fos* mRNA following administration of estradiol to immature female rats. Induction is very rapid— transcript levels double within 30 minutes and peak increases of 20-40 fold are routinely observed within 2 to 3 hours. The rapidity of this increase suggested that the effect was mediated at the transcriptional level. Measurement of transcription by nuclear run-on assays (3) and the insensitivity of induction to protein synthesis inhibitors (4) provide strong support for a transcriptional

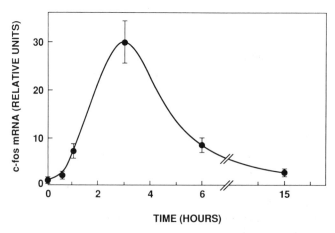

TIME (HOURS)

Fig. 1. Induction of uterine c-*fos* mRNA by estradiol. Groups of immature rats were treated with estradiol for the indicated times. Uterine tissue was removed, total tissue RNA was prepared, and analyzed by RNA blots. The levels of the 2.2 Kb *fos* transcript illustrated above were determined by densitometric analysis.

mechanism of induction. Other experiments demonstrated that this induction is dose dependent, exhibits hormonal specificity for estrogens, and is abolished by actinomycin D (4). More recent experiments have indicated that progesterone blocks the estrogen-induced increase in uterine c-*fos* mRNA and that the antiestrogen tamoxifen can also elevate uterine levels of this transcript (Kirkland et al., in preparation). In another series of studies, we determined by *in situ* hybridization that the c-*fos* message is expressed in all uterine cell types (Tipnis et al., in preparation).

Identification of a c-*fos* Estrogen-Response Element(s)

Since estrogen regulation of *fos* expression appears to be a direct transcriptional effect, we and others (5) have tried to identify the estrogen-response element (ERE) that mediates the hormonal induction. Hormone-response elements are typically found in the 5'-upstream regulatory region of target genes, and we initially examined this region of c-*fos* for an ERE. We prepared a series of *fos*-CAT constructs for transient transfections in MCF-7 and GH3 cell lines, which contain endogenous estrogen receptors. This analysis illustrated that the *fos*-CAT reporter containing the -278 to -135 region of mouse c-*fos* is induced twofold to threefold by estradiol, although we have not yet defined the specific nucleotide sequence that mediates this effect. This is a weaker induction than that typically seen in the uterus, but in these cell lines the induction of the endogenous *fos* gene is stimulated only twofold to threefold. This may suggest that the estrogen receptor functions in concert with other cell-specific transcription factors to regulate c-*fos* expression, at least in the uterus. While our studies examined the mouse gene, other workers have defined a sequence in the 5'-region of the human gene (5) that confers a threefold to fourfold inducibility to reporter constructs. It is noteworthy that neither the mouse nor human 5'-sequences contain the consensus ERE, GGTCAnnnTGACC, found in genes such as vitellogenin (6).

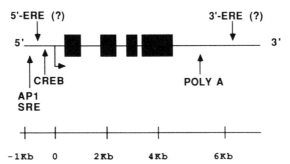

Fig. 2. Structure of the mouse c-*fos* gene. The horizontal scale is relative to the start site of transcription (taken as 0) which is indicated by the bold arrow. Elements include tentative EREs; the serum-response element (SRE); an AP-1 site; and a site that mediates cyclic AMP induction (CREB).

The above findings indicate that 5'-upstream region(s) of the *fos* gene can confer estrogen inducibility, but does not rule out the participation of other mechanisms in regulating this gene *in vivo*. To further explore this possibility we utilized CAT reporters containing other regions (exons, introns, and 3'-flanking regions) of the *fos* gene for transfection analysis. A 1.3 Kb BamH1 - Nco fragment located in the 3'-untranslated region was found to confer marked estrogen inducibility to TK-CAT and also to function as an inducible enhancer with the homologous c-*fos* promoter. The level of inducibility seen in these constructs is the same order of magnitude as that seen with vitellogenin A2-TK-CAT in our transfection studies. We have now sequenced this region, and it does not contain the palindromic consensus ERE sequence. These results on the c-*fos* ERE and other regulatory sequences of the gene are illustrated in Figure 2.

c-*fos* Regulation Is both Negative and Positive

During our studies on estrogen induction of uterine c-*fos*, we observed that the overall regulation of gene expression involves negative as well as positive control mechanisms. This became clear when we tried to reinduce *fos* mRNA after the transient rise in transcript levels illustrated in Figure 1. If a second dose of estrogen is administered between 6 and 24 hours after the initial hormone treatment, c-*fos* mRNA is not induced. In other words, the gene becomes "desensitized" or "refractory" to a second exposure to hormone. It is particularly interesting to note that if the second dose of estrogen is administered more than 24 hours after the first (i.e., after a round of hormone-induced DNA replication), the gene is again inducible. This implies that a mechanism exists to insure that estrogen-dependent *fos* expression is transient during normal cell growth.

While we have not yet defined the mechanism by which the gene becomes desensitized to estrogen induction, we have obtained some very interesting initial data (1). Desensitization is not due to the lack of available estrogen receptor. Administration of the first or second doses of estradiol leads to a comparable occupancy of estrogen receptors under the conditions of our studies. (2) Desensitization occurs at the level of transcription, since both nuclear run-on studies or measurement of mRNA levels by RNA blots yield similar results. (3) Desensitization is homologous, i.e., estradiol desensitizes the gene to subsequent induction by itself, but not to induction by other regulators, e.g., phorbol esters. This implies that desensitization is not mediated by *fos* itself.

Expression of c-*fos* in Models of Hormonal Carcinogenesis

As noted at the outset, the studies described above were performed in the uterus as a model of a normal estrogen target tissue. Given our findings on c-*fos* regulation in this normal growth model, we next explored expression of this gene in several experimental models of hormonal carcinogenesis.

c-*fos* Expression in the Syrian Hamster Kidney

One widely used model of hormonal carcinogenesis is the Syrian hamster kidney tumor. In this system, chronic administration of estrogen to male animals causes a 100% incidence of kidney tumors. We thus treated hamsters for 9 months to allow tumors to develop, separated the tumors from surrounding kidney tissue, and analyzed RNA from both for the levels of protooncogene mRNAs. In tumors, the levels of c-*fos*, c-*myc*, and c-*jun* transcripts were elevated 15-, 4-, and 6-fold, respectively, compared to levels in the kidney of control animals that did not receive steroid treatment. The levels of the three mRNAs were also elevated in the kidney tissue surrounding the tumors in the estrogen-treated animals, although the relative increases were less than those in the tumors (7). In another series of experiments, animals treated with estrogen for 5 months did not develop tumors and did not exhibit increases in the levels of the three mRNAs. These results indicate that there is a correlation between elevated protooncogene expression and tumor development, but do not yet establish the relationship between the two events.

Effect of Neonatal Estrogen on c-*fos* Expression

Another model that has been used to examine hormonal carcinogenesis is the neonatal (e.g., days 1-5 of age) administration of diethylstilbestrol (DES) to rodents. Following this treatment, both males and females develop a number of abnormalities in the reproductive tract including uterine tumors. For our initial studies, we administered 10 μg of DES once daily to rat pups on days 1-5 after birth. The animals were then allowed to grow until 20-25 days of age, at which time they were ovariectomized to remove any ovarian influences. At 30 days of age, both basal and estradiol-stimulated levels of uterine c-*fos* mRNA were determined by RNA blot analysis. The basal levels of the c-*fos* transcript are significantly elevated (fourfold to fivefold) in DES-treated vs. control animals that received vehicle alone on days 1-5 of age. Estradiol treatment produces a transient elevation of c-*fos* mRNA in both DES and control animals, and peak levels of the transcript were comparable in both cases. Thus, neonatal DES alters the basal but not estrogen-stimulated levels of gene expression (Lin et al., in preparation.)

Discussion

Estrogens induce c-*fos* mRNA in the uterus, and the data support a transcriptional mechanism for this effect. However, comparison of the large induction in the uterus (typically 20-40 fold) with the smaller (twofold to fivefold) inductions seen in GH3 and MCF-7 cells suggests that hormonal control of *fos* mRNA levels involves cell-specific effects.

Despite several uncertainties, it appears that the c-*fos* gene is not controlled by the consensus ERE originally identified for the xenopus vitellogenin A2 gene

(6). If this can be unequivocally established, it has great potential significance for hormonal carcinogenesis in the following manner. To our knowledge, the consensus ERE has only been found to control genes involved in differentiated function, e.g., the secretion of vitellogen or prolactin. The apparent absence of this sequence in the c-*fos* gene may indicate that there are several classes of EREs. For example, one sequence may be used to regulate differentiated functions that are controlled by estrogens, but a different sequence may be used to regulate genes expressed during a growth response to the hormone. While admittedly speculative, this arrangement might provide a pharmacological approach to selectively producing differentiated functions without cell growth.

The realization that *fos* expression is subject to negative as well as positive controls also has potential significance for hormonal carcinogenesis. It has been shown that overexpression of normal cellular protooncogenes such as *fos* can cause transformation. Experimentally this has been established by increasing the synthesis of the transcript, e.g., by transfection of expression vectors. However, if *fos* overexpression is important in the development of human cancers, our results suggest that this could occur in two different ways. First, by activation of a positive mechanism(s) that regulates expression of the gene (e.g., high levels of circulating estrogens), or second, by loss of a negative regulatory mechanism analogous to the one we have observed in the rodent uterus. This is an important conceptual distinction since many studies try to identify people at risk for diseases such as breast cancer by examining variables such as estrogen synthesis, estrogen-receptor levels, levels of plasma hormone-binding proteins, estrogen to progesterone ratios, etc. Endocrine studies of this nature are unlikely to identify individuals at risk because they have a predisposition to lose a negative regulatory mechanism. Thus, we must determine the exact nature of this negative control mechanism before we can evaluate the likelihood that it is involved in hormonal carcinogenesis, and if so, to develop a rational strategy for identifying individuals at risk via this route.

Another point about the possible role of protooncogene overexpression in hormonal carcinogenesis should also be noted. It is established that *fos* expression is regulated by estrogens in several systems, but it is also clear that a variety of other agents regulate expression of this gene. These include phorbol esters and other agents that activate protein kinase C, agents that elevate cyclic AMP levels, and serum and a number of peptide growth factors. It is thus conceivable that protooncogene overexpression in estrogen target tissues could be activated by estradiol, a variety of other physiological, pharmacological, or toxicological agents, or a combination of these agents and the hormone. This raises the possibility that diseases such as breast and endometrial cancer could result from *fos* overexpression even with a normal endocrine profile of estrogens. Such tumors could have similar phenotypic properties as those caused by abnormalities in estrogen synthesis or metabolism, since the signaling pathways activated by estrogenic and nonestrogenic stimuli would converge at a common point, i.e., protooncogene expression.

Table 1. Uterine protooncogenes regulated by estradiol.

Oncogene	Type	Reference
c-*fos*	Transcription Factor	Mol. Endocrinol. $\underline{2}$:816 & 946, 1988
c-*jun*	"	Ibid. $\underline{4}$:1041, 1990 & BBRC $\underline{168}$:721, 1990
c-*myc*,N-*myc*	"	Endocrinol. $\underline{120}$:1882, 1987
ras	G Protein	FEBS Lett. $\underline{196}$:309, 1986 & $\underline{211}$:27, 1987
erb B	Growth Factor Receptor	Mol. Endocrinol. $\underline{2}$:230, 1988

Finally, it is interesting to consider estrogen regulation of cell growth in the context of paradigms developed for other systems such as fibroblasts. In fibroblasts, growth is regulated by distinct factors that act at separate points in the cell cycle. For example, certain growth factors (e.g., PDGF) regulate the transition of resting cells from G_0 to G_1—these are "competence" factors since they make the cells "competent" to respond to other growth signals that regulate "progression" through G_1 to S phase. Prototype progression factors are peptides such as IGF-1 and EGF. The point is that distinct signals regulate different aspects of cell growth from the resting state through DNA replication and cell division. In contrast, estrogens may have regulatory roles in both competence and progression—like events in normal hormone target tissues. For example, estrogens very rapidly stimulate expression of protooncogenes such as *fos*, *myc*, and *jun* (see Table 1) which are usually associated with the G_0 to G_1 transition. At slightly longer times (e.g., 2-6 hours) estrogens stimulate expression of other genes such as IGF-1 (8), IGF-1 receptors (9), and EGF receptors (10) that are associated with progression through G_1 in fibroblast-like systems. This raises the possibility that hormonal carcinogenesis in some cells involves aberrations in the estrogenic regulation of the G_0/G_1 transition and in others it involves aberrations in hormonal regulation of progression through G_1 toward S. In this paradigm, alterations in estrogen synthesis or metabolism could produce tumors with very different phenotypes dependent upon which estrogen-regulated events were affected by the endocrinopathy in any specific case.

Acknowledgments

Studies in our laboratories have been supported by NIH grants HD-08615 and DK-38965 and a grant from the John P. McGovern Foundation. We gratefully acknowledge this support.

References

1. Mukku VR, Kirkland JL, Hardy M, Stancel GM (1982) Hormonal control of uterine growth: temporal relationships between estrogen administration and DNA synthesis. Endocrinology 111:480-487.
2. Herrlich P, Ponta H (1989) Nuclear oncogenes convert extracellular stimuli into changes in the genetic program. Trends in Genetics 5:112-116.
3. Weisz A, Bresciani F (1988) Estrogen induces expression of c-*fos* and c-*myc* protooncogenes in rat uterus. Mol Endocrinol 2:816-824.
4. Loose-Mitchell DS, Chiappetta C, Stancel GM (1988) Estrogen regulation of c-*fos* messenger ribonucleic acid. Mol Endocrinol 2:946-951.
5. Weisz A, Rosales (1990) Identification of an estrogen response element upstream of the human c-*fos* gene that binds the estrogen receptor and the AP-1 transcription factor.
6. Klein-Hitpass L, Schorp M, Wagner U, Ryfell GU (1986) An estrogen responsive element derived from the 5'-flanking region of Xenopus vitellogen A2 gene functions in transfected human cells. Cell 46:1053-1061.
7. Liehr JG, Chiappetta C, Stancel GM (1990) Elevation of protooncogene mRNAs in estrogen induced kidney tumors in the hamster. Proc 81st Am Assoc Cancer Res Ann Mtg 31:220.
8. Murphy LJ, Murphy LC, Friesen HG (1988) Estrogen induces insulin-like growth factor-I expression in the rat uterus. Mol Endocrinol 1:445-452.
9. Ghahary A, Murphy LJ (1989) Uterine insulin-line growth factor-I receptors: regulation by estrogen and variation throughout the estrous cycle. Endocrinology 125:597-604.
10. Lingham RB, Stancel GM, Loose-Mitchell DS (1988) Estrogen regulation of epidermal growth factor receptor messenger ribonucleic acid. Mol Endocrinol 2:230-235.

PART 6. CARCINOGENESIS RISK ASSESSMENT OF SEX HORMONES

INTRODUCTION

Receptor-Mediated Carcinogenesis: Implications for Carcinogenic Risk of Sex Hormones

George W. Lucier

Issues relevant to risk assessment for carcinogenic actions of sex hormones are difficult to evaluate because of the mechanisms responsible for hormone action in target cells. It is also difficult to select specific issues to discuss in an introduction paper. The other papers in this presentation deal with endometrial and breast cancer risks (1) and the role of synthetic estrogens in liver cancer (2), including a comparison of animal and human data. In my paper, I will focus on some of the issues involved in the effects of chemicals on hormone action, including the interactions of hormonally active chemicals with key receptor systems.

Effects of Chemicals on Hormone Action

Chemicals may interact directly with receptors leading to receptor-mediated events critical to site-specific carcinogenesis, or on the other hand, receptor occupancy may block hormone actions by mechanisms analogous to antiestrogen action. In addition, there are reports in the literature providing evidence for the contention that metabolites of some hormonally active chemicals can bind covalently to DNA. This raises the possibility that some hormonally active chemicals may possess both initiating and promoting activity, whereas others might possess promoting activity only. Chemicals may also modify hormone action by indirect means and thereby modify carcinogenic risks. For example, hormones may cause changes in hormone metabolism/clearance leading to altered hormone concentration at the target site. Also, chemical exposure might produce changes in components of receptor pathways including receptor number, activation of the ligand receptor complex and signal transduction events.

There are several reasons responsible for increased interest in hormonal carcinogenesis. One of the reasons is that nearly 40% of the chemicals that are positive for carcinogenicity in the National Toxicology Program Bioassay appear to act by nongenotoxic mechanisms (3). Nongenotoxic carcinogens do not bind covalently to DNA, do not induce DNA repair and are negative in *in vitro* and *in vivo* tests for mutagenicity. There is increasing evidence that the underlying mechanisms responsible for nongenotoxic carcinogens involve perturbations of hormone action and signal transduction pathways. These findings have stimulated regulatory agencies to develop approaches for estimating human risks from exposure to carcinogens that require receptor action. Of particular importance is the issue of cell proliferation.

There is now growing and compelling evidence that carcinogenesis is truly a multistep process (4). Figure 1 illustrates the point that more than one DNA damaging step and more than one round of increased cell replication are involved. The term tumor promotion refers to the clonal expansion of a genetically altered cell. Although tumor promotion is an operational not a mechanistic term, it is generally considered that altered hormone action is one of the mechanisms. Another frequently invoked mechanism of tumor promotion is compensatory cell proliferation caused by chemically mediated cytotoxicity.

There are a number of examples where interactions with receptor systems are thought to be a critical mechanistic event in the carcinogenic process. One is the case of environmental estrogens where interaction with estrogen receptors is thought to represent an important event in the carcinogenic process (5).

A second example is for 2,3,7,8-tetrachlorodibenzo-*p*-dioxin (TCDD) and its

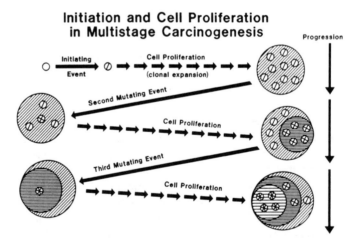

Fig. 1. Schematic of the role of cell proliferation in the initiation, promotion, and progression of carcinogenesis. The extent of clonal expansion necessary for second or third mutational events is dependent on the amount of spontaneous and chemically induced DNA damage.

Recent evidence has shown that a key step in the promotion process is interaction with protein kinase C (PKC) leading to a sustained activation of PKC (6). The phorbol esters mimic the endogenous activation of PKC by diacylglycerol, but activation by the phorbol esters produces a more protracted response.

structural analogs. TCDD is produced inadvertently during the synthesis of many organochlorine compounds, such as the herbicide agent orange, and it is an environmentally ubiquitous and biologically persistent chemical. TCDD is a potent carcinogen in animal bioassays, although it does not bind DNA covalently and is negative in tests for genetic toxicity, such as the Ames Salmonella test (7). The initial event in the toxic effects of TCDD is binding to the arylhydrocarbon receptor. This receptor system is analogous in function to receptors for steroid hormones, but TCDD does not bind to this class of receptor, and conversely, steroid hormones do not bind to the Ah receptor. Finally, a third example that interacts in signal transduction is phorbol esters, a commonly studied class of skin tumor promoters as analogs or diacylglycerol.

Risk-Assessment Approaches

One of the centerpieces of the highly controversial field of risk-assessment methodology is the use of tumor-incidence models. These models are mathematical and make numerous and frequently unsubstantiated assumptions regarding the biological basis for carcinogenic response.

The threshold model assumes that there is a dose or exposure below which no toxic effects occur. This is frequently used in risk assessments of reproductive and developmental toxicants, and in some countries, it is used to estimate carcinogenic risks in humans based on data obtained from animal experiments. The process identifies a "no effect level" of exposure in animals followed by application of a safety factor, usually 100-fold, to set human exposure limits in the workplace or from food consumption.

Statistical models are frequently used in the United States to estimate risks. These models define an acceptable risk level (1 cancer in 1,000,000 or 100,000 exposed population) and derive an acceptable daily intake level assuming a linear reltionship between exposure and dose. The most common statistical method is the linear multistage model. These methods are thought by some to be inappropriate for estimating risks from tumor promoters, because it is felt that they drastically overestimate risks to compounds that are carcinogenic but do not cause somatic mutations.

The third risk-assessment approach is termed "mechanistically based models" and is gaining proponents. This approach attempts to use statistical models that most accurately reflect mechanism of action and are tailored for individual classes of chemicals.

The method chosen to conduct a risk assessment exerts a profound influence over the derivation of an acceptable daily intake (ADI) as shown in Table 1. ADIs range from 6 to 13,000 fg/kg/day, although all ADIs were derived from the same data to estimate human risks; i.e., tumor incidence in female rat liver. The difference reflects the choice of model; either linear multistage or threshold. Data on the mechanism of action indicate that neither model is based on the generally accepted mechanisms for receptor-mediated events. Since, it is generally agreed that the Ah receptor is necessary for the carcinogenic actions

Table 1. Acceptable daily intakes for TCDD calculated by various regulatory agencies.

Agency	Method	Allowable Intake (fg/kg/day)
US Environmental Protection Agency	Linearized multistage	6
US Centers for Disease Control	Linearized multistage	28
California		
Toxic Air Program	Linearized multistage	8
Prop 65	Linearized multistage	80
US FDA	Safety factor (77)	13,000
Canada	Safety factor (100)	10,000
Netherlands	Safety factor (250)	4,000
Germany	Safety factor (1,000)	1,000

of TCDD, risk-assessment models are now being developed that are more applicable to receptor-mediated carcinogenesis than either threshold or linear multistage models (8,9).

One of the difficult components of biologically based models for carcinogens that act through receptor-mediated events is the relationship between receptor occupancy and biological response. If there is a proportional relationship between occupancy and response, then modeling can be relatively straightforward, provided that reliable data on binding properties and tissue localization of receptor are available. However, it is unlikely that such a simple relationship exists for receptor-mediated carcinogenesis. There is now considerable evidence that several steps are involved with formation of a ligand-receptor complex representing only the initial recognition event. Tissue-specific factors that act on transduction and response events must be considered when constructing mechanistically based models for risk assessment of hormonally active carcinogens. Unfortunately, the identity and characteristics of these tissue-specific factors are poorly understood.

Research Needs

There are several research needs that are relevant to issues of hormonal carcinogenesis. These are (1) elucidation of the mechanisms responsible for receptor-mediated cell proliferation in genetically altered cells (preneoplastic cells) compared to normal cells, (2) determination of the quantitative relationship between receptor occupancy and biological response, (3) identification of the factors that regulate the cellular specificity of the response following the formation of a ligand-receptor complex, (4) evaluation of critical target genes in hormonal carcinogenesis, and (5) development of approaches to determine the relevancy of using animal models to estimate human risks, i.e., are the same hormone-responsive genes activated in an animal model as in humans?

These points reflect the fact that risk assessments require reliable estimates of dose-response relationships, and the reliability of these estimates is enhanced by the judicious use of mechanistically based biomarkers. These points also reflect the need to use appropriate animal models for estimation of human risks.

References

1. Pike M (1991) Endogenous hormone levels as the major determinants of endometrial and breast cancer risk. In: Li JJ, Nandi S, and Li SA (eds), Hormonal Carcinogenesis, Springer Verlag, NY.
2. Li JJ (1991) Synthetic estrogens and liver cancer: risk analysis of animal and human data. In: Li JJ, Nandi S and Li SA (eds), Hormonal Carcinogenesis, Springer Verlag, NY.
3. Tennant RW, Margolin BH, Shelby MD, Zeiger E, Haseman JK, Spalding J, Caspary W, Resnik M, Stasiewitz S, Anderson B et al. (1987) Prediction of chemical carcinogenicity in rodent from *in vitro* genetic toxicity assays. Science 236 (4804): 933-941.
4. Swenberg JA, Richardson FC, Boucheron JA, Deal FH, Belinsky SA, Charbonneau M, Short BG (1987) High- to low-dose extrapolation: critical determinants involved in the dose response of carcinogenic substances. Environ. Health Perspect, 76: 57-63.
5. McLachlan JA (ed)(1980) *Estrogens in the Environment*, Elsevier Publishing Co., NY.
6. Fischer SM, Reiners JJJr, Pence BC, Aldaz CM, Conti CJ, Morris RJ, O'Connell JF, Rotstein JB, Slaga TJ (1988) Mechanisms of carcinogenesis using mouse skin: the multistage assay revisited. In: Langenbach, R, Elmore E, Barrett JC (eds) *Tumor Promoters: Biological Approaches for Mechanistic Studies and Assay Systems*, Raven Press, NY.
7. Huff JE, Salmon AG, Hooper NK, Zeise L (1991) Long-term carcinogenesis studies on 2,3,7,8-tetrachlorodibenzo-*p*-dioxin and hexachlorodibenzo-*p*-dioxins. Toxicol Appl Pharmacol 7(1):67-94.

8. Lucier GW (1991) Receptor-mediated carcinogenesis. In: Vanio H, Magee P, McGregor D, McMichael AJ (eds) *Mechanisms of Carcinogenesis in Risk Identification*. IARC Scientific Publication Series, International Agency for Research on Cancer, Lyon France, (in press).

9. Lucier GW, Tritscher AM, Clark G (1991) Tumor promotion in liver. In: Gallo M, Scheuplein R, Van der Heidjen C (eds) *Banbury Report on Biological Basis for Risk Assessment of Dioxin and Related Compounds*, Banbury Report, Cold Spring Harbor Laboratory, Cold Spring Harbor, NY (in press).

20

Endogenous Estrogen and Progesterone as the Major Determinants of Breast Cancer Risk: Prospects for Control by 'Natural' and 'Technological' Means

Malcolm C. Pike and Darcy V. Spicer

Introduction

Studies over the last 20 years of breast, endometrial, and ovarian cancers, and of normal breast and endometrial tissue, have now provided us with a sufficient understanding of the etiology of these cancers to allow us to envisage the practical possibility of significantly reducing their risk.

Epidemiological observations in the use of combination-type oral contraceptives (COCs) indicated that they provide very significant long-term protection against both endometrial and ovarian cancer, but no protection against breast cancer. These observations showed that a practical method of reducing female cancer rates is almost within our grasp. Only the fear that COCs may increase breast cancer rates prevents us from espousing COCs as a breakthrough in cancer prevention.

Viewing the epidemiological data on these three cancers, together with observations made on the biology of their tissue of origin, shows that the control of normal cell division rates in breast, endometrium, and ovarian tissue is at least one key to their etiology. Altering cell division rates in all three tissues is possible on the basis of present technology. Recent studies of hormone levels in certain Oriental women suggest that the control of mitotic rates through "natural" means is a realistic possibility.

Epidemiological Background

For most nonhormone dependent cancers a plot of the logarithm of incidence against the logarithm of age produces a straight line (1). In sharp contrast, the incidence of breast, endometrial, and ovarian cancer shows a significant slowing down of the rate of increase around age 50 (Figure 1); this is a direct result of menopause (natural or artificial) (1-4). The termination of ovarian function is thus anticarcinogenic for all three cancers. The effects of smaller changes in ovarian function have been more difficult to establish on these cancers, but it now appears that relatively small changes are important in the etiology of endometrial and breast cancer, but only ovulation suppression protects against ovarian cancer.

Why menopause is protective is most evident for endometrial cancer; it is the drastically reduced mitotic activity of endometrial cells after menopause. All the major endometrial cancer risk factors can be explained by considering their effect on endometrial division rates. This same reasoning can also explain all the major risk factors for ovarian and breast cancer (5). This hypothesis can be justified simply in terms of its success in describing the epidemiology of these cancers; it also has a basis in the known biology of carcinogenesis. "Initiation" is affected because the probability of DNA damage being repaired is by a more rapid cell division and "promotion" is intimately associated with cell division (6).

Endometrial Cancer

Endometrial cancer risk decreases steadily with a decreasing age at menopause, with increasing parity, and with COC use, and increases markedly with increas-

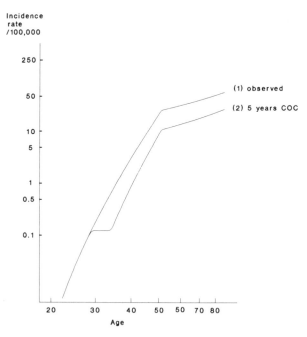

Fig. 1. Age-incidence curve of endometrial cancer (from data for West Midland Region of England, 1968-72): (1) as observed, (2) predicted with five years of COC use.

ing weight (in pre- and postmenopausal women) and steadily with estrogen replacement therapy (ERT) use (3). These risk factors can all be explained in terms of the "unopposed estrogen hypothesis" for endometrial cancer, i.e., risk is increased by exposure to estrogen that is not "opposed" by a progestogen, and this is caused by the associated increased mitotic activity. Estrogens stimulate mitosis in endometrial cells, but only in the absence of progestogens. The mitotic rate is near maximal early on in the menstrual cycle; it drops to a very low level in the face of the postovulation increase in progesterone (Pg). The maximal rate is induced by the early follicular serum estradiol (E_2) concentration (50 pg/ml). Very low E_2 concentrations (5 pg/ml) in slender postmenopausal women are associated with an atrophic endometrium. There will be a dose-response relationship between endometrial mitotic rate and serum E_2 concentration in the 5 to 50 pg/ml range.

On the mitotic rate hypothesis, early menopause reduces risk by reducing the unopposed E_2 concentration of the follicular phase to the low level of the postmenopausal period. Pregnancies reduce risk because there is no unopposed estrogen during gestation. Obesity increases risk in premenopausal women through the Pg deficiency associated with their increased anovulation; and the risk is further increased postmenopausally because of increased serum E_2 and decreased serum sex hormone binding globulin (SHBG), and thus, an increase in non-SHBG bound E_2. Serum non-SHBG bound E_2 of a woman using conjugated equine estrogens (CEE) as ERT is approximately two-thirds of the early follicular level (3). CEE contains other potent estrogens and the total mitotic activity over a 28-day period will be between 1.6 and 2.0 that of a premenopausal woman (3). Therefore, such ERT will have a major effect on endometrial cancer risk, as has been consistently observed.

COCs reduce risk because endometrial mitotic activity is near zero during COC use; COCs are a combination of an estrogen and a fairly high dose of progestogen, so that endometrial cells are exposed to unopposed estrogen only during the seven days that the COC is not taken, and the endogenous estrogen levels during these seven days are very low. The incidence curve will be very nearly flat during the use of COCs, and when COCs are stopped, the curve will increase as before (Figure 2 shows the effect of five years of COC use) (1-3). Such long-term effects of COC (and ERT) use have been observed to the extent possible in epidemiological studies.

Ovarian Cancer

The risk of developing ovarian cancer decreases with an early age at menopause, with increasing parity, and with COC use. All can be explained in terms of the mitotic activity of the ovarian surface, the tissue from which ovarian cancer arises. The major impetus to ovarian surface tissue cell replication is the repair of the ovarian surface after each ovulation. Therefore, any respite from ovulation is predicted to reduce the risk of ovarian cancer (2).

Breast Cancer

Breast cancer risk decreases with late menarche and early menopause; early first birth is associated with a long-term decreased risk, but with an increased risk for a brief period after the birth. (The complex nature of the effects of first birth appears to be due to the change in "structure" of the breast. We will not discuss this phenomenon any further here.) Obesity decreases risk in premenopausal women and increases risk in postmenopausal women. COCs either have no effect or they increase risk. ERT is associated with a relatively small increase in risk (4).

Breast cell division is concentrated in the luteal phase of the menstrual cycle (Figure 2) (7). This suggests that E_2 alone induces some cell division, but that E_2 and Pg together induce considerably more, that is, the "estrogen plus progestogen hypothesis." This interpretation is supported by animal data and by a recently published study in which a distinctly larger increase in breast cancer risk was found in women who had used a progestogen with ERT than in women who had used ERT alone (8).

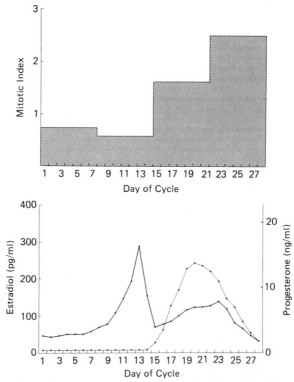

Fig 2. Breast mitotic rate by day of cycle (day 1 is first day of menses and 28-day cycle assumed with ovulation on day 14); and serum concentrations of E_2 and Pg by day of cycle.

Menopause is associated with decreased risk because the drastic reduction in both E_2 and Pg results in a very low mitotic rate in breast cells. The complex effects of obesity are explained by the increased anovulation associated with premenopausal obesity, which will decrease exposure to both E_2 and Pg, and the increased E_2 levels after menopause.

COCs work as a contraceptive by causing the ovary to effectively cease functioning. A woman on COCs is thus "postmenopausal," and if this was the sole effect of COCs, COC use should cause a large reduction in breast cancer risk. The reason that this does not happen is because the ovarian steroid loss is compensated for by the synthetic estrogen and progestogen in the COC. ERT use in the postmenopausal period causes only a small increase in breast cancer risk. This is explained by the level of estrogen achieved during ERT and by the lack of progestogen (4).

If these ideas are correct, then we should be able to explain the large difference in breast cancer rates between women in Japan and the US (1). Differences in age at first birth and age at menopause are small. Age at menarche was, however, until quite recently some two years later in Japan, and this has quite a large effect (1). Three recent studies of postmenopausal Oriental women still living in the traditional way showed a marked reduction (27%, 63%, 70%) in serum E_2 levels in the Oriental women studied compared to the Western white women, and the effect was larger than could be explained on the basis of weight alone (9-11). Three recent studies of premenopausal women also showed clearly decreased serum E_2 levels in "traditional" Oriental women: the effects were large (17%. 26%, 44%) and could not be explained by anovulation (9,10,12). These differences are more than sufficient to account for the remaining difference if the mitotic rate is related to hormone concentration in this range, which appears to be the case (4). A complete hormonal explanation of the difference between Japanese and US breast cancer rates is thus at hand.

Prevention through 'Natural' Means

The lower E_2 levels of traditional Oriental women will of course effect endometrial cancer rates as well as breast cancer rates, but the details of the magnitude of the endometrial effect remain to be worked out. The reason for these lower hormone levels in Oriental women are not yet known, but energy output and dietary composition seem likely to play important roles. There is every reason to be confident that the "natural" factors that lead to these "protective" levels of E_2 will soon be found.

Prevention through Hormonal Contraception

On the basis of the above analyses, it is clear that: (1) reducing the frequency of ovulation will reduce ovarian cancer risk; (2) reducing exposure of the endometrium to "unopposed" estrogen will reduce endometrial cancer risk; and (3) reducing exposure of the breast to "estrogen plus progestogen" will decrease

Table 1. Prototype contraceptive.

Agent	Rationale
GnRHA	Suppress ovulation
	Prevents side effects
Estrogen:	
CEE	
Progestogen:	Reverse any
MPA every	endometrial
fourth cycle	hyperplasia

breast cancer risk, certainly if the "estrogen plus progestogen" is reduced to a postmenopausal or postmenopausal plus ERT level.

COCs provide significant protection against ovarian cancer and against endometrial cancer. COCs do not, however, provide protection against breast cancer, because they deliver estrogen plus progestogen to the breast in quantities sufficient to replace the action of the natural estrogen plus progesterone of the normal menstrual cycle.

COCs have two separate and distinct functions. The first function is to stop ovulation. The reason for the lack of menopausal symptoms in women using COCs is because of the second function of COCs, i.e., their function as a form of hormone-replacement therapy (HRT). These two functions need to be clearly distinguished. The best COC formulation to stop ovulation is not necessarily the best formulation to prevent the adverse side effects of stopping ovarian function.

The reversible ovulation inhibiting function of COCs can be achieved by using a gonadotropin-releasing hormone agonist (GnRHA); this approach enables one to concentrate solely on finding the best formulation of hormones to prevent the adverse effects (hot flushes, significant bone loss, an increase in low-density lipoprotein cholesterol). Present-day COCs could be added to the GnRHA regimen to obviate these side effects, however, this would achieve nothing that has not already being obtained from COC use alone. Can a lower estrogen-progestogen formulation obviate the side effects and achieve a major reduction in breast cancer risk?

Extensive experience with estrogen-progestogen hormone preparations of lower than COC dose has been gained with HRT in postmenopausal women. On the basis of this experience, the regimen shown in Table 1 is currently undergoing test at our institution. Experience with ERT shows that the harmful side effects of GnRHA use are very likely to be eliminated by CEE use (13). Table 2 shows the predicted relative risks for breast cancer of using this regimen for 5, 10, or 15 years at premenopausal ages. These relative risks are calculated assuming that the computed effective mitotic rates of postmenopausal women on ERT would apply to a premenopausal woman taking GnRHA plus ERT. This

Table 2. Predicted relative reduction in lifetime risk for cancer with the prototype contraceptive.

	Duration of Regimen (yrs)		
	5	10	15
Breast	31%	53%	70%
Endometrium	18%	33%	45%
Ovary	41%	67%	84%

regimen is calculated to reduce lifetime breast cancer risk by nearly a third if used for only 5 years.

Table 2 also shows the predicted relative risks for ovarian cancer using the GnRHA regimen. Use of GnRHAs for only 5 years is predicted to reduce the lifetime risk for ovarian cancer by as much as 40%.

The proposed regimen is unlikely to adversely affect bone metabolism or cardiovascular disease risk and may well be beneficial. However, specific long-term studies need to be conducted (13).

There are quite firm grounds for the predicted beneficial effects of the proposed regimen in women who have had a full-term pregnancy. The regimen appears likely also to benefit young women, especially when one considers it as simply a very low dose COC.

At present, GnRHA is given in a monthly injection. However, it should soon be possible to give GnRHA as a four-monthly injection, and this will make the regimen actually useful if the price of GnRHA can be lowered to a fraction of its present level. This does not appear to be an insurmountable obstacle, since GnRHAs are relatively simple compounds.

We have not discussed the use of tamoxifen as a drug to prevent breast cancer. Trials of this are currently underway and there is every reason to be optimistic that tamoxifen will be effective in postmenopausal women (14). Tamoxifen should be considered complementary to the GnRHA approach, not as a competitor. GnRHA, for example, will be effective against ovarian cancer, a disease that tamoxifen will not affect.

References

1. Pike MC, Krailo MD, Henderson BE, et al (1983) 'Hormonal' risk factors, 'breast tissue age' and the age incidence of breast cancer. Nature 303:767-770.

2. Pike MC (1987) Age-related factors in cancers of the breast, ovary and endometrium. J Chron Dis 40, Suppl II:59-69.
3. Key TJA, Pike MC (1988) The dose-effect relationship between 'unopposed' estrogens and endometrial mitotic rate: its central role in explaining and predicting endometrial cancer risk. Br J Cancer 57:205-212.
4. Key TJA, Pike MC (1988) The role of estrogens and progestogens in the epidemiology and prevention of breast cancer. Eur J Cancer Clin Onc 24:29-43.
5. Henderson BE, Ross RK, Pike MC, et al (1982) Endogenous hormones as a major factor in human cancer. Cancer Res 42:3232-3239.
6. Preston-Martin S, Pike MC, Ross RK, et al (1990) Increased cell division as a cause of human cancer. Cancer Res 50:7415-7421.
7. Going JJ, Anderson TJ, Battersby S, MacIntyre CCA (1988) Proliferative and secretory activity in human breast during natural and artificial menstrual cycles. Am J Pathol 130:193-204.
8. Bergkvist L, Adami H-O, Persson I, et al (1985) The risk of breast cancer after estrogen and estrogen-progestin replacement. N Engl J Med 321:293-297.
9. Goldin BR, Adlercreutz H, Gorbach SL, et al (1986) The relationship between estrogen levels and diets of Caucasian American and Oriental immigrant women. Am J Clin Nutr 44:945-953.
10. Bernstein L, Yuan J-M, Ross RK, et al (1990) Serum hormones levels in premenopausal Chinese women in Shanghai and white women in Los Angeles. Cancer Causes & Control 1:51-58.
11. Key TJA, Chen J, Wang DY, et al (1990) Sex hormones in rural China and in Britain. Br J Cancer 62:631-636.
12. Shimizu H, Ross RK, Bernstein L, et al (1990) Serum estrogen levels in postmenopausal women: comparison of US whites and Japanese in Japan. Br J Cancer 62:451-454.
13. Spicer D, Shoupe D, Pike MC (1991) GnRH agonists as contraceptives agents: predicted significantly reduced risk of breast and ovarian cancer. Contraception 44:289-310.
14. Spicer D, Pike MC, Henderson BE, Groshen S (1991) Tamoxifen and estrogen replacement therapy as agents of disease prevention. J Natl Cancer Inst 83:63-64.

21

Synthetic Estrogens and Liver Cancer: Risk Analysis of Animal and Human Data

Jonathan J. Li, Hadley Kirkman, and Sara Antonia Li

Introduction

In 1971, Baum et al. (1) reported a causal relationship between estrogen exposure and hepatic tumors in women. At that time, there was little or no evidence available indicating that liver tumors could be induced following prolonged estrogen treatment in experimental animals, even at high doses (2-5). Nevertheless, over the years, epidemiologic evidence continued to accumulate that supported this initial causal association in humans following the therapeutic use of estrogens in the liver (6-13). The present report summarizes the human data, largely in women, regarding the association of liver tumor incidences and estrogen intake. In addition, we present heretofore unpublished observations concerning liver tumor incidences in male and female hamsters exposed to various natural and synthetic estrogens in the absence of any other intervening agent.

Epidemiologic Evidence

Estrogens have been implicated in the formation of both focal nodular hyperplasias (FNH) and adenomas in human livers (1,6,8,10). The frequency of case reports supporting a causal association between hepatocellular carcinomas and estrogen intake has been rising (6,7,9, 11-13). The causal relationship between estrogens and liver neoplasms is not restricted to exposure only to such synthetic estrogens as mestranol, ethinylestradiol (EE), and diethylstilbestrol (DES) (Table 1). A number of studies have also indicated similar associations following prolonged ingestion of either estradiol or Premarin, the equine conjugated estrogens (6,7,10). Regression of liver adenomas following hormone withdrawal suggest that estrogens may be involved in the etiology of these neoplasms (14,15). While liver tumors are extremely

Table 1. Estrogen-associated human liver neoplasms.

Years on OCs or Estrogen	Estrogen	Neoplasm	Source	Year
0.5-7.0	Mestranol (OC)	Adenoma	Baum (1)	1973
1.6-4.0	Mestranol/EE (OC)	FNH/Adenoma	Nissen & Kent (6)	1975
6.0	Premarin	Hepatocellular Carcin.		
9.0	Polyestradiol-PO$_4$	Heptatocellular Carcin.	Sotaniem (7)	1975
1.0-9.1	Mestranol	Adenoma	Edmundson (8)	1976
14.0	Mestranol (OC)	Hepatocellular Carcin.	Pryor (9)	1977
3.0	Premarin/ Mestranol (OC)	Adenoma	Aungst (10)	1978
4.9-6.9	Mestranol (OC)	Hepatocellular Carcin.	Vana & Murphy (11)	1979
4.5	DES-PO$_4$ (3mg/day)	Hepatocellular Carcin.	Brooks (12)	1982
3.0	DES-PO$_4$ (100mg/day)	Hepatocellular Carcin.	Endo (13)	1987

rare in U.S. women within the 15- to 45-year-old age group, it has been estimated that women who have been exposed to OCs for > 3 but < 4 years have about a 100 times greater relative risk for developing liver adenomas and for women exposed to oral contraceptives (OC) for > 7 years, the relative risk is increased 100- to 500-fold (14,16). In contrast, risk estimates for women developing hepatocellular carcinomas following estrogen exposure are much lower. For OC users the range varies from 3.8- to 7.2-fold, while 5 to 8 year OC users the relative risk increases to 13.5- to 20.1-fold (16-18). The relative risk for liver tumor development employing recent low-dose OC users, however, remains to be determined.

Animal Studies

Except for the initial administration of carcinogen (19,20), estrogen treatment alone, whether natural or synthetic, has been shown to be ineffective in inducing significant liver tumor incidences in either rats or mice (2-5, 21, 22) (Table 2). The low tumor incidences (1-21%) reported in these species may not differ appreciably from the spontaneous liver tumor incidences seen. Additionally, no

Table 2. Experimental animal models in estrogen-associated liver tumors.

Animal Model	Treatment	Incidence (%)	Source
Hamster			
Syrian			
Castrated male	EE/DES	20/5-7	Li (23)
Castrated male	EE + ANF	90-100	Li (27)
Armenian			
Intact male	DES, EE	83	Coe (24)
Intact female	DES	55	
European			
Intact male	DES	29	Reznik-Schüller (25)
Intact female		6	
Rat			
SD			
Male or female	DES, EE	0	Schardein (3) Li (23)
Holtzmann	EE	0	Schuppler (21)
SD	DEN + DES	93	Yager (19)
F-344	DEN + EE	100	Wanless (20)
Mice			
BALB/c	Enovid	0	Heston (4)
C3H			
C57BL			
CF-LP	Mestranol	0	Barrows (5)

hepatic tumors have ever been demonstrated in either primates or dogs following chronic estrogen treatment (22). In contrast, liver tumors may be induced in various subspecies of hamsters employing synthetic estrogens in the absence of any other etiologic agent (23-25). It is notable that at least for Syrian hamsters, the spontaneous adenoma and carcinoma incidence in the liver is nil or insignificant (Table 3) and this finding is consistent with the observations of Pour et al (26). Nevertheless, these liver tumor incidences in various hamster subspecies, except perhaps for the Armenian hamster, are relatively low (20-30%) employing only estrogen exposure. In the presence of EE and concomitant treatment with α-naphthoflavone (ANF), the liver tumor incidences in male Syrian hamsters approach 100% (27). The Armenian hamster may prove to be an attractive model for estrogen carcinogenesis in the liver except perhaps for its high rate of acute hepatotoxicity and hence mortality as a result of estrogen exposure (24).

Table 3. Incidence of hepatic tumors in untreated and estrogen/androgen-treated hamsters.

Tumors	Nontreated Incidence[1] (%)	Estrogen -treated Incidence[2] (%)	Androgen -treated Incidence[3] (%)	E + A -treated Incidence[4] (%)
Cholangioma	0.20	0.26	0.45	0.15
Cholangiocarcinoma	0.08	0.16	0.00	0.19
Adenoma	0.00	0.69	0.00	1.02
Carcinoma	0.02	0.42	0.45	0.54
Hemangioma	0.01	0.00	0.00	0.05
Hemangiosarcoma	0.00	0.00	0.00	0.00

[1]Incidence derived from 6,614 hamsters   [3]Incidence derived from 223 hamsters
[2]Incidence derived from 3,065 hamsters   [4]Incidence derived from 2,056 hamsters

Table 4. Incidence of liver tumors induced by natural estrogens in Syrian golden hamsters.

Treatment[a]	Duration (mo.)	Number Animals with Tumors/n	Incidence (%)	Tumor
17β-Estradiol				
Intact male	13.7	0/33	0.0	-------
Castrated male	11.2	0/12	0.0	-------
Intact female	11.4	0/12	0.0	-------
Ovx. female	8.4	0/22	0.0	-------
Estrone				
Intact male	13.6	0/21	0.0	-------
Castrated male	15.3	0/10	0.0	-------
Estriol				
Intact male	15.0	1/22	4.5	Adenoma
Castrated male	17.1	0/11	0.0	-------
Intact female	20.0	0/7	0.0	-------

[a]Hormone pellets (20 mg) were implanted subcutaneously and additional pellets added every 3.0 months.

Table 5. Incidence of liver tumors induced by natural estrogens in Syrian golden hamsters.

Treatment[a]	Duration (mo.)	Number Animals with Tumors/n	Incidence (%)	Tumor
DES				
Intact male	10.1	18/1547	1.2	Adenoma
Castrated male	10.0	1/86	1.2	Carcinoma
Intact female	9.3	10/536	1.9	Adenoma/Carcin.
Ovx. female	7.9	1/173	0.6	Adenoma/Carcin.
Intact male	10.0	1/22	4.5	Hepatobiliary[a]
Intact male	13.0	1/55	1.8	Hepatobiliary[b]
Castrated male	10.0	1/86	1.2	Hepatobiliary[c]
Ethinylestradiol				
Intact male	13.1	5/15	33.0	Adenoma
Intact male	11.7	6/27	22.2	Adenoma
Intact male	11.7	16/47	34.0	Adenoma
Intact female	12.5	1/41	2.4	Adenoma

[a]Hormone pellets (20 mg) were implanted subcutaneously and additional pellets added every 3.0 months.

Estrogen-Induced Syrian Hamster Liver Tumors

No liver tumors were detected in either male or female hamsters after 17β-estradiol or estrone treatment following chronic hormone treatment for as long as 13.7 months regardless of the endocrine status of the animal (Table 4). One intact male hamster receiving estriol pellets for 15 months developed small liver tumors resulting in an incidence of 4.5%. This liver tumor was classified as an adenoma upon histologic examination. No liver tumors, however, were observed after estriol treatment in either castrated male or intact female hamsters. On the other hand, the synthetic estrogens, DES and EE exhibited more consistent liver tumor incidences regardless of the endocrine status of the hamster (Table 5). However, DES treatment resulted in markedly lower liver adenoma/carcinoma incidences (1.2-1.9%) compared to EE (22-34%). DES treatment also resulted in a low frequency of hepatobiliary neoplasms in male hamsters. Table 3 also summarizes the different types of liver neoplasms employing estrogens, androgen (testosterone), and combinations of these two hormones.

Table 6. Possible biochemical factors for estrogens and liver cancer.

Estrogens

1. Types of synthetic estrogen (esp. DES, Ethinylestradiol)

2. Relative P-450 associated oxidative metabolism, pharmacokinetics & mitochrondrial alternations

3. Degree of hepatotoxicity toxicity and damage (repair mechanisms)

4. Hormone receptor and responsiveness (enhanced cell proliferation & adaptive hyperplasia)

5. Immune competence

6. Sex difference

Liver Tissue

Risk Assessment in the Human and Hamster

Known etiologic factors for liver cancer in humans evidently do not play a significant role in hormone- (i.e., OCs, estrogen) associated liver tumors in women. These factors include cirrhosis, alcoholic or nonalcoholic, hepatitis B virus, hepatic fibrosis, hepatocarcinogens, such as vinyl chloride, aflatoxins, etc., chronic hepatitis, α-1-antitrypsin deficiency and smoking. It is conceivable however, that OC or estrogen-induced liver cholestasis may increase carcinogenic bile acids and effect hepatic dysfunction as well. Pregnancy status may also enhance liver tumor growth, thus facilitating the carcinogenic process.

It is evident from the animal data presented herein that ethinylestradiol is the most potent liver tumorigenic hormonal agent in the hamster and is coincidentally also responsible for the majority of reported estrogen-associated liver tumors in humans. This suggests that the 17α-alkyl functional group on EE and secondarily the phenolic A ring may be involved in these neoplastic events. Table 6 summarizes possible biochemical factors that may be pertinent in the development of liver tumors by estrogen, and this suggests future avenues of research in this highly important area.

Acknowledgment

This study was supported in part by NCI, NIH grant CA41387 (Shannon Fund) of the U.S. Public Health Service.

References

1. Baum JK, Holtz F, Bookstein JJ, Klein EW (1973) Possible association between benign hepatomas and oral contraceptives. Lancet 926-929.
2. Gibson JP, Newberne JW, Kuhir WL, Elsea JR (1967) Comparative chronic toxicology of three oral estrogens in rats. Toxicol Appl Pharmacol 11:489-510.
3. Schardein JL, Kaump DH, Woosley ET, Jellema MM (1970) Long term toxicologic and tumorigenesis studies on an oral contraceptive agent in albino rats. Toxical Appl Pharmacol 16:10-23.
4. Heston WE, Vlahakis G, Desmukes B (1973) Effect of the antifertility drug Enovid in female strains of mice with particular regard to carcinogenesis. J Natl Cancer Inst 51:209-224.
5. Barrows GH, Christopherson WM, Drill VA (1977) Liver lesions and oral contraceptives steroids. J Toxicol Environ Health 3:219-230.
6. Nissen ED, Kent DR (1975) Liver tumors and oral contraceptives. Obst Gynecol 46:460-467.
7. Sotaniemi EA, Alavaikko MJ, Kaipainen WJ (1975) Primary liver cancer associated with long-term oestrogen therapy. Ann Clin Res 7:287-289.
8. Edmundson HA, Henderson B, Benton B (1976) Liver cell adenomas associated with use of oral contraceptives. New Engl J Med 294:470-472.
9. Pryor AC, Cohen RJ, Goldman RL (1977) Hepatocellular carcinoma in a woman on long-term oral contraceptives. Cancer 40:884-888.
10. Aungst CW (1978) Benign liver tumors and oral contraceptives. New York State J Med 78:1933-1934.
11. Vana J, Murphy GP (1979) Primary malignant liver tumors. Association with oral contraceptives. New York J Med 79:321-325.
12. Brooks JJ (1982) Hepatoma associated with diethylstilbestrol therapy for prostatic carcinoma. J Urology 128:1044-1045.
13. Endo H, Murakarni T, Nishimoto I, Sekine I, Yokoyamo M (1987) Multicentric hepatocellular carcinoma following phosphate diethylstilbestrol therapy for prostatic cancer. Acta Pathol Jpn 37:795-806.
14. Edmundson HA, Reynolds TB, Henderson B, Benton B (1977) Regression of liver cell adenomas associated with oral contraceptives. Ann Internal Med 86:180-182.
15. Penkava RR, Rothenberg J (1981) Spontaneous resolution of oral-contraceptive-associated liver tumor. J Computer Assisted Tomog 5:102-103.
16. Rooks JB, Ory AW, Ishak KG, Strauss LT (1979) Epidemiology of hepatocellular adenomas. JAMA 242:644-648.
17. Neuberger J, Forman D, Doll R, Williams R (1986) Oral contraceptives and hepatocellular carcinoma. Brit Med J 292:1355-1357.
18. Forman D, Vincent TJ, Doll R (1986) Cancer of the liver and the use of oral contraceptives. Brit Med J 292:1357-1361.

19. Yager JD Jr, Fifield DS Jr, (1982) Lack of hepatogenotoxicity of oral contraceptive steroids. Carcinogenesis 3:625-628.

20. Wanless, IR, Medline A (1982) Role of estrogens as promoters of hepatic neoplasia. Lab Invest 46:313-320.

21. Schuppler J, Gunzel P (1979) Liver tumors and steroidal hormones in rats and mice. Arch Toxicol Suppl 2:181-195.

22. El Etreby MF (1980) Influence of contraceptive steroids on tumor development in experimental animals and man: a short review. In: E Genzzzani et al. Ed Pharmacological Modulation of Steroid Action, Raven Press, New York p. 239.

23. Li JJ, Li SA (1990) Estrogen carcinogenesis in hamster tissues: a critical review. Endocrine Rev 11:524-531.

24. Coe JE, Ishak KG, Ross MJ (1990) Estrogen induction of hepatocellular carcinomas in Armenian hamsters. Hepatology 11:570-577.

25. Reznik-Schuller H (1979) Carcinogenic effects of diethylstilbestrol in male Syrian golden hamsters and European hamsters. J Natl Cancer Inst 62:1083-1088.

26. Pour P, Althoff J, Salmasi SZ, Stepan K (1979) Spontaneous tumors and common diseases in three type of hamsters. J Natl Cancer Inst 63:797-811.

27. Li JJ, Li SA (1984) High incidence of hepatocellular carcinomas after synthetic estrogen administration in Syrian golden hamsters fed α-naphthoflavone: a new tumor model. J Natl Cancer Inst 73:543-547.

22

Carcinogenic Risk Assessment of Steroid Hormone Exposure in Relation to Prostate Cancer Risk

Maarten C. Bosland

Introduction

Cancer of the prostate is presently the most frequently diagnosed cancer and the second most frequent cause of death due to cancer in men in many Western countries, including the US (1). The causes of prostate cancer are poorly understood, in part due to the very old age of most prostate cancer patients, which impedes epidemiological studies (1). Androgenic steroid hormones have been implicated in the etiology of prostate cancer, because many prostate carcinomas are androgen-sensitive, and a role of estrogens has also been suggested (1,2). The purpose of this paper is to attempt to apply the traditional carcinogenic risk-assessment process (3,4) to prostate cancer risk and exposure to androgenic and estrogenic hormonal agents. A major problem in this respect is that significant endogenous as well as exogenous sources of androgenic and estrogenic substances exist, while carcinogenic risk assessment is usually only applied to exogenous agents. Nevertheless, as long as essential information exists, such as dose-response data, it is possible to apply the basic elements of the carcinogenic risk-assessment process, hazard identification, analysis of dose-response data, exposure assessment, and risk characterization and evaluation (3). Risk management, i.e., prevention of prostate cancer, will only be touched upon.

Androgens

The prostate is the prototypical target organ for androgenic hormones, which are essential for the processes of development, cell death and renewal, and cellular differentiation in the prostate gland. There are anabolic substances that have the same receptor-mediated effects on the prostate as testosterone and its metabolite 5α-dihydrotestosterone. The majority of human prostate carcinomas are androgen-sensitive and respond to androgen-deprivation therapy, albeit only temporarily; relapse to a hormone-insensitive state always occurs sooner or later. The often-mentioned absence of prostate cancer in eunuchs is purely anecdotal as evidence for a causal role of androgens in the etiology of prostate cancer. However, such a relation between androgens and prostate carcinoma development is biologically very plausible, and prostate cancer could be regarded as a derangement of the mechanisms that regulate the normal balance between androgen effects on cellular differentiation and androgen effects on cell proliferation and cell death rates in the prostate (see refs. 1 and 2 for references).

Qualitative Risk Assessment: Hazard Identification

Except for one case report of prostate cancer in an individual who abused anabolic steroids (4), there are no human data that directly link androgen exposure to the development of prostate cancer. Production of prostate cancer by long-term testosterone treatment has been reported in five different rat strains (5-8), but one strain was unresponsive (9). The prostate cancer incidence found in these studies ranged from approximately 5 to 50%, and the latent period was between 8 and 16 months. Prostate carcinomas occur spontaneously only in very low incidence (between 0.03 and 0.5%) in 2.5 to 3-year-old rats (10). Prostate cancer incidences ranging from 35 to 70% have been reported resulting from chronic administration of testosterone after a single or short-term treatment with three different chemical carcinogens that can target the prostate, N-methyl-N-nitrosourea (MNU), N-nitrosobis(2-oxopropyl)amine, and 3,2'-dimethyl-4-aminobiphenyl, in four different rat strains (7-9,11-13), while one rat strain did not respond (8). These carcinogens by themselves produced either no prostate cancer or a low (3-10%) prostate cancer incidence. The latent period of the prostate carcinomas was comparable in all these studies. All thus induced prostate cancers were adenocarcinomas, and they occurred exclusively in the dorsolateral prostate, which probably has embryological homology with the human prostate (14). Interestingly, the last two mentioned carcinogens also produced neoplastic lesions in the ventral prostate, which is not homologous to the human prostate (14), but the androgen treatment did not influence this effect (7,9). Thus, chronic treatment with testosterone has, by definition, weak complete carcinogenic activity and strong tumor promotor properties for the rat prostate.

Quantitative Risk Assessment: Dose-Response Data

With one exception (8), none of the earlier mentioned studies that demonstrated the carcinogenic and tumor promotor activity of testosterone involved more than one testosterone dose, and circulating testosterone levels were supra-physiological, 5-20 times control values, in most studies (9,11-13). As yet largely unpublished data (8) from the laboratory of the author, however, showed that even a very slight elevation of circulating testosterone, twofold to threefold as compared with control values, results in a 10-15% prostate cancer incidence. This incidence was comparable to that produced by a sixfold to ninefold testosterone elevation. Both of these testosterone doses increased prostate cancer incidence to 50-60% when given after a single injection with MNU. The carcinogen treatment alone resulted in a 5-10% incidence. An even lower dose of testosterone, which did not produce a measurable testosterone elevation, induced prostate cancer in approximately 45% of MNU-treated rats, which was not statistically different from the incidences resulting from the higher testosterone doses. This low testosterone dose probably only smoothed the 24-hour circadian rhythm of circulating testosterone.

Quantitative Risk Assessment: Human Exposure Assessment

Human male populations that are at high risk for prostate cancer often, but not always, have slightly higher circulating testosterone levels than populations that have a lower risk (1,2,15,16). For example, total and free testosterone levels in young US black men have been shown to be approximately 20% higher than in age-matched white males, in the absence of differences in sex-hormone-binding-globulin levels (15). Androgen exposure of black males may already be higher than that of white men before birth, because primiparous pregnant black women have been shown to have circulating testosterone levels that are 48% higher than age-matched white women in their first pregnancy, irrespective of sex of the offspring (16). Circulating total testosterone was approximately 13% higher in aged Dutch men who are at high risk for prostate cancer than in age-matched low-risk Japanese (2). Thus, associations between exposure to endogenous testosterone and prostate cancer risk have been demonstrated, but more research is required to confirm these few studies and to determine the strength and magnitude of this association.

Testosterone substitution therapy is a standard medical treatment for conditions such as hypogonadism (17), and chronic testosterone administration is being tested as a form of male contraception (18). The serum testosterone concentrations that result from these medical applications may be as high as 1.5- to threefold normal levels (18,19). Furthermore, the nonmedical use of anabolic steroids with androgenic activity in males in the US and probably many other countries is considerable. Seven percent of US high school seniors, 10-20% of US college athletes, and as many as 30% or more of professional sportsmen are estimated to (ab) use anabolic steroids (20). The exact magnitude of anabolic steroid abuse, both in terms of numbers of exposed men and in terms of doses, is very difficult to determine and remains uncertain presently. Considerable exposure to exogenous androgenic substances is thus a reality in a significant number of males.

Risk Characterization Evaluation

There are no adequate human data that link exposure to testosterone and other androgenic substances with prostate cancer risk. However, there is limited circumstantial evidence that high circulating testosterone levels are associated with a high risk for prostate cancer from hormonal studies in healthy male populations that differ in prostate cancer risk. These studies indicate that circulating levels of testosterone can be slightly elevated (in the order of 10-20%) due to endogenous androgen production. Moderate to high levels of androgen exposure can result from medical and nonmedical (ab)use, respectively.

There is sufficient evidence that testosterone at very low doses induces and strongly promotes the formation of prostatic carcinomas in rats, which rarely develop this carcinoma spontaneously, and if so only at very old age. There is no clear dose-dependency for the carcinogenic and tumor promoting activities of testosterone in rats, and not all rat strains tested responded. However, this should not be interpreted to reduce the amount of evidence for carcinogenicity (3), because of (1) the magnitude of the response, even at physiological levels of exposure, and (2) the fact that of the five tested only one rat strain did not respond to testosterone promotion after carcinogen treatment and only one other strain did not respond to prostate cancer induction by testosterone alone.

The mechanism of the carcinogenic/tumor promoting effect of testosterone on the rat prostate remains unknown. The apparent absence of a threshold below which testosterone has no effect on prostate carcinogenesis would suggest that the hormone acts via a receptor-mediated mechanism. The very strong tumor-promoting properties of testosterone in rats may well underlie its apparent weak complete carcinogenic activity. The dose-response data in rats suggest a very steep dose-response curve for the carcinogenic and tumor promoting activities of testosterone, which reaches a maximum at low circulating testosterone levels. Thus, a very slight elevation of circulating testosterone increased prostate cancer risk in rats at least tenfold, irrespective of prior carcinogen treatment. Such a dose-response relationship would explain the large differences in prostate cancer incidence observed among human populations in the absence of equally large variations in circulating testosterone levels.

Estrogens

Although androgens are the predominant hormonal regulators of prostatic structure and function, the prostate is also sensitive to estrogens, and the presence of estrogen receptors has been demonstrated in the prostate of humans and other species. Although the exact role of estrogen in prostatic physiology and pathology is currently undefined, canine studies have shown that estrogens are involved in the regulation of prostatic cellular differentiation. As prostate cancer is typically a disease of old age, relations between prostate cancer development and changes in endocrine function have been examined. Increasing levels of circulating 17β-estradiol and/or decreases in circulating testosterone with aging have been observed, and resulting androgen/estrogen imbalances have been suggested to play a role in prostatic carcinogenesis (see ref. 1 for additional references).

Qualitative Risk Assessment: Hazard Identification

There are no human data that directly associate estrogen exposure with prostate cancer risk. However, combined exposure to 17β-estradiol or diethylstilbestrol (DES) and testosterone has been shown to produce a 75-100% incidence of preneoplastic lesions (dysplasia or intraepithelial neoplasia) and a 20-100% incidence of adenocarcinomas of the dorsolateral prostate in two different rat strains (21-24). The preneoplasia was observed as early as after 8-16 weeks of treatment, and the latent period of the carcinomas was in the order of one year. The androgen component of the treatment maintained normal concentrations of circulating testosterone, whereas circulating 17β-estradiol levels were supraphysiological (22,23).

Perinatal exposure of rodents to DES leads to structural abnormalities of the male genital tract, including the accessory sex glands. In mice, prenatal DES exposure resulted in a 25% incidence of "nodular enlargements" of the coagulating gland, ampullary gland, and colliculus seminalis, and a 4% incidence of "early carcinoma" in this area when mice were sacrificed at an age of 9 to 10 months (25). Of mice that died between 20 and 26 months of age, 25% had carcinomas of the seminal vesicle or the coagulating gland, which is the anterior prostate lobe (14), and 25-38% had hyperplastic or squamous metaplastic lesions of the coagulating gland, ventral prostate, and/or seminal vesicle (26,27). In 19% of neonatally DES-treated mice, adenocarcinomas were observed in the area of the dorsolateral prostate (28). Castrated rats neonatally treated with DES developed a 100% incidence of papillary hyperplastic and squamous metaplastic lesions of the coagulating gland and colliculus seminalis and an 18% incidence of squamous cell carcinoma in the area of the dorsolateral prostate and coagulating gland (27). Squamous metaplasia was also found in intact DES-treated rats, but hyperplastic and neoplastic lesions did not occur.

Squamous metaplasia of the prostatic utricle and prostatic ducts occurred in 65 and 55%, respectively, of a group of 31 DES-exposed male infants that died perinatally (29). Unspecified prostate problems were reported in 15% of a group of 94 DES sons, as compared with a 0.3% incidence in men under 45 years of age from the 1985 National Health Interview Survey (30).

In conclusion, 17β-estradiol and DES are carcinogenic for the androgen-supported rat prostate, and perinatal DES exposure is carcinogenic for the rodent prostate and other accessory sex glands, and it causes squamous metaplasia in the prostate and prostatic utricle in male infants. The reported "prostate problems" in DES sons suggest that prenatal DES exposure can have long-term effects on the human prostate.

Quantitative Risk Assessment: Dose-Response Data and Human Exposure Assessment

There are no dose-response data from animal studies concerning prostate effects resulting from perinatal or chronic exposure to estrogens.

Considerable occupational exposure to estrogens, leading to clinical effects such as gynecomastia, has been documented in workers in the pharmaceutical industry (31). Chronic, low-level exposure to estrogenic substances may occur in humans from intake of foods contaminated with phytoestrogens, estrogenic mycotoxins, estrogenic growth promoting chemicals used in animal production, and estrogens from other environmental sources (32-34). Prenatal exposure has occurred in an estimated 0.5 to 1.5 million men in the USA alone (35). Thus, significant perinatal, chronic, or episodic exposure to estrogens may occur or has occurred in human populations. The magnitude of this exposure, although known in some cases, is generally uncertain.

Risk Characterization Evaluation

There are no adequate human data that relate estrogen exposure to prostate cancer risk. However, there is sufficient evidence that estrogens can cause prostate carcinomas in rats when coadministered with androgens, and that perinatal DES exposure causes accessory sex gland carcinomas in rodents. The evidence that perinatal DES administration causes adenocarcinomas specifically of the prostate in rodents should be considered limited. There is limited evidence that prenatal DES exposure causes prostatic squamous metaplasia in male infants, and inadequate evidence that this exposure has long-term effects on the human prostate. Substantial human prenatal exposure and considerable occupational exposure to DES have occurred, and chronic, low-dose human exposure can occur via intake of foods contaminated with a wide variety of environmental estrogens.

The mechanism whereby estrogens cause prostate cancer development in the androgen-supported rat prostate and whereby they might cause human prostate cancer is unknown. Among the possible mechanisms are direct or indirect genotoxicity, estrogen-receptor-mediated effects, and influences on prostatic cellular differentiation and/or androgen metabolism.

Concluding Remarks

Testosterone and other androgenic substances should be regarded as probable human prostate carcinogens, because there is sufficient evidence that testosterone is carcinogenic for the prostate gland in experimental animals. There is circumstantial, and therefore inadequate, evidence that testosterone is carcinogenic for the human prostate. Based on data available up to 1987 on androgens and risk for all types of cancer, the IARC has classified androgenic (anabolic) steroids as probable carcinogens (group 2A of its classification system) (4). The data on androgens and prostate cancer risk summarized in this paper further strengthen the classification of androgens in group 2A.

Consequently, testosterone substitution therapy should be used with reluctance, and with as low a dose as clinically possible. Furthermore, human studies on testosterone as a male contraceptive method should be halted for the time being, until more information about long-term risks of such medical use of testosterone is available. Further efforts should be put in place to abolish the abuse of anabolic steroids in sports and other settings. To determine the actual carcinogenic risks of androgens in human populations, retrospective epidemiological studies of long-term effects of medical and nonmedical use of androgenic steroids should be stimulated.

Men that have been prenatally exposed to DES are currently entering their fourth decade of life. They are possibly at increased risk for cancer of the prostate or other accessory sex gland structures. It is thus advisable that all known DES-exposed men undergo regular screening for prostate cancer using state-of-the-art methods from age 40. It is highly unlikely that a possible increased occurrence of prostate cancer among these men will be easily detected because of the high "spontaneous" incidence of prostate cancer. Therefore, prospective cohort studies are highly warranted of men prenatally exposed to DES.

Acknowledgments

This work was supported in part by Grants No. CA43151, CA48084, and CA13343 from the National Cancer Institute and EPA grant No. CR813481.

References

1. Bosland MC (1988) The etiopathogenesis of prostatic cancer with special reference to environmental factors. Adv Cancer Res 51:1-106.
2. Schröder FH (1990) Androgen and carcinoma of the prostate. In: Nieschlag E, Behre HM (eds) Testosterone-Action, Deficiency, Substitution. Springer-Verlag, Berlin, pp 245-260.
3. Hart RW, Hoerger FD (eds) (1988) Carcinogen Risk Assessment: New Directions in the Qualitative and Quantitative Aspects. Cold Spring Harbor Laboratory, Cold Spring Harbor.
4. International Agency for Research On Cancer (1987) Overall Evaluations of Carcinogenicity: An Updating of IARC Monographs Volumes 1 to 42. IARC Monographs on the Evaluation of Carcinogenic Risks to Humans, Suppl 7. IARC, Lyon.
5. Noble RL (1982) Prostate carcinoma in the Nb rat in relation to hormones. Int Rev Exp Pathol 23:113-159.
6. Pollard MP, Luckert PH, Schmidt MA (1982) Induction of prostate adenocarcinomas in Lobund Wistar rats by testosterone. Prostate 3:563-568.

7.   Pour PM, Stepan K (1987) Induction of prostatic carcinomas and lower urinary tract neoplasms by combined treatment of intact and castrated rats with testosterone propionate and N-nitrosobis(2-oxopropyl)amine. Cancer Res 47:5699-5706.

8.   Bosland MC, Scherrenberg PM, Ford H, Dreef-van der Meulen HC (1989) Promotion by testosterone of N-methyl-N-nitrosourea-induced prostatic carcinogenesis in rats. Proc Am Assoc Cancer Res 30:272.

9.   Shirai T, Tamano S, Kato T, Iwasaki S, Takahashi S, Ito N (1991) Induction of invasive carcinomas in the accessory sex organs other than the ventral prostate of rats given 3,2'-dimethyl-4-aminobiphenyl and testosterone propionate. Cancer Res 51:1264-1269.

10. Bosland MC (1987) Adenocarcinoma, prostate, rat. In: Jones TC, Mohr U, Hunt RD (eds) Genital System. Springer-Verlag, Berlin, pp 252-260.

11. Pollard M, Luckert PH (1986) Production of autochthonous prostate cancer in Lobund Wistar rats by treatment with N-nitroso-N-methylurea and testosterone. J Natl Cancer Inst 77:583-587.

12. Pollard M, Luckert PH (1987) Autochthonous prostate adenocarcinomas in Lobund-Wistar rats: A model system. Prostate 11:219-227.

13. Hoover DM, Best KL, McKenney BK, Tamura RN, Neubauer BL (1990) Experimental induction of neoplasia in the accessory sex organs of male Lobund-Wistar rats. Cancer Res 50:142-146.

14. Price D (1963) Comparative aspects of development and structure in the prostate. Natl Cancer Inst Monogr 12:1-25.

15. Ross R, Bernstein L, Judd H, Hanisch R, Pike M, Henderson B (1986) Serum testosterone levels in healthy young black and white men. J Natl Cancer Inst 76:45-48.

16. Henderson BE, Bernstein L, Ross R, Depue RH, Judd HL (1988) The early in utero oestrogen and testosterone environment of blacks and whites: Potential effects on male offspring. Br J Cancer 57:216-218.

17. Nieschlag E, Behre HM (1990) Pharmacology and clinical uses of testosterone. In: Nieschlag E, Behre HM (eds) Testosterone-Action, Deficiency, Substitution. Springer-Verlag, Berlin, pp 92-114.

18. World Health Organization Task Force on Methods for the Regulation of Male Fertility (1990) Contraceptive efficacy of testosterone-induced azoospermia in normal men. Lancet 336:955-959.

19. Matsumoto AM (1990) Effects of chronic testosterone administration in normal men: Safety and efficacy of high dosage testosterone and parallel dose-dependent suppression of luteinizing hormone, follicle-stimulating hormone, and sperm production. J Clin Endocrinol Metabol 70:282-287.

20. Yersalis CE, Anderson WA, Buckley WE, Wright JE (1990) Incidence of the non-medical use of anabolic-androgenic steroids. In: Lin GC, Erinoff L (eds) Anabolic Steroid Abuse. National Institute on Drug Abuse Research Monograph 102. US DHHS Publ No (ADM)90-1720. NIDA, Rockville, pp 97-112.

21. Drago JR (1984) The induction of Nb rat prostatic carcinomas. Anticancer Res 4:255-256.

22. Leav I, Ho S-M, Ofner P, Merk FB, Kwan PW-L, Damassa D (1988) Biochemical alterations in sex hormone-induced hyperplasia and dysplasia of the dorsolateral prostates of Noble rats. J Natl Cancer Inst 80:1045-1053.

23. Ofner P, Bosland MC (1992) Differential effects of diethylstilbestrol and 17β-estradiol in combination with testosterone on rat prostate lobes. In press.

24. Bosland MC, Ofner P, Leav I. Unpublished observations.

25. McLachlan JA, Newbold RR, Bullock B (1975) Reproductive tract lesions in male mice exposed prenatally to diethylstilbestrol. Science 190:991-992.

26. McLachlan JA (1981) Rodent models for perinatal exposure to diethylstilbestrol and their relation to human disease in the male. In: Herbst AL, Bern HA (eds) Developmental Effects of Diethylstilbestrol (DES) in Pregnancy. Thieme-Stratton, New York, pp 148-157.

27. Arai Y, Mori T, Suzuki Y, Bern H (1983) Long-term effects of perinatal exposure to sex steroids and diethylstilbestrol on the reproductive system of male mammals. Int Rev Cytol 84:235-268.

28. Newbold RR, Bullock BC, McLachlan JA (1988) Prostatic cancer in developmentally estrogenized mice. Proc Am Assoc Cancer Res 29:239.

29. Driscoll SG, Taylor SH (1980) Effects of prenatal maternal estrogen on the male urogenital system. Obstet Gynecol 56:537-542.

30. Wingard DL, Turiel J (1988) Long-term effects of exposure to diethylstilbestrol. Western J Med 149:551-554.

31. Zaebst DD, Tanaka S, Haring M (1980) Occupational exposure to estrogens - Problems and approaches. In: McLachlan JA (ed) Estrogens in the Environment. Elsevier North Holland, New York, pp 377-388.

32. Setchell KDR (1985) Naturally occurring non-steroidal estrogens of dietary origin. In: McLachlan JA (ed) Estrogens in the Environment II. Influences on Development. Elsevier, New York, pp 69-83.

33. Knight WM (1980) Estrogens administered to food-producing animals: Environmental considerations. In: McLachlan JA (ed) Estrogens in the Environment. Elsevier North Holland, New York, pp 391-401.

34. Bulger WH, Kupfer D (1985) Estrogenic activity of pesticides and other xenobiotics on the uterus and male reproductive tract. In: Thomas JA, Korach KS, McLachlan JA (eds) Endocrine Toxicology. Raven Press, New York, pp 1-33.

35. Heinonen OP (1972) Diethylstilbestrol in pregnancy. Frequency of exposure usage patterns. Cancer 31:573-577.

CLOSING REMARKS

Hormonal Carcinogenesis—Future Perspectives

Gerald C. Mueller

Introduction

In this symposium we have been treated to a smorgasbord of progress in the subject area defined as "hormonal carcinogenesis." Each speaker, an expert in his field, has presented his most recent achievements and in varying degrees has also laid out his own particular interpretation or perspective as to where we are going from here. It has been an exciting experience—and I am sure that the future will be even more provocative and productive. In fact, with respect to my particular assignment—"Future Perspectives on Hormonal Carcinogenesis" much of the turf has already been covered in the specialized topic areas. However, I shall take it as my responsibility to speak a bit panoramically—providing a cell biological framework that, hopefully, will be useful in interpreting ongoing experiments and making productive choices among the many future directions that are currently possible or are likely to soon arise. In particular, I shall try to point out some areas of cell and molecular biology where new knowledge is greatly needed if we are to reap the ultimate benefits from research in the field of hormonal carcinogenesis—a route to the prevention of these types of cancer or the development of an effective therapy for dealing with the human disease.

Some Parameters of the Problem

Progress in the understanding of cancer in general has been very rapid in the last few years. For example, we have come to know that cancer in general terms reflects either the overexpression of genes that predispose a cell to have a replicative advantage (i.e., the oncogenes)—or the underexpression of genes that limit replication and/or favor terminal differentiation (i.e., the suppressor genes and the cell-destruct genes). In fact, as chronicled in studies of the initiation and progression of colon cancer (1), both situations may contribute to the malignant state—with a disastrous outcome for the patient. The most important message from these studies is that the establishment of the malignant phenotype reflects mutational events that occur initially in single cells—and that successive mutations can also occur and actually be selected for in the progeny of the initial transformants.

237

A number of oncogenes code for growth factors or growth factor receptors—whereas others code for proteins such as *myc, fos, ras*, etc., whose levels are intimately involved in the nuclear replicative processes (2,3). The actual mechanisms of their effects, however, is not well defined as yet - except that they frequently interact with or modify the function of transcription complexes for specific genes (2).

With respect to the cellular roles of the opposing gene set (i.e., the suppressor genes), we have even less information. However, recent studies have highlighted the ability of the retinoblastoma susceptibility gene product and the wild-type *p*53 proteins to form physical complexes with the oncogenic protein from the SV40 virus, the SV40 large T antigen, to make it inactive as a triggering factor for nuclear replication (4-7). In addition, a cellular protein (i.e., a 46-20K protein) has been described recently that mimics the action of the SV40 large T antigens (8). Presumably, similar situations will soon surface for the expanding list of new suppressor genes.

Recent research from many laboratories has also shown that the mutagenic events leading to the derangement or imbalance in the expression of genes leading to the cancer state can be induced by an oncogenic chemical (a carcinogen), an oncogenic virus, or a genetic accident arising during chromatin replication. In each case the significant change appears to be site-specific, irreversible, and selectively integrated into the behavioral state of the affected cell—as it lives interactively with its other cell cohorts in the tissue of reference. It is important to appreciate, however, that for every alteration in the genome, there is automatically a resetting of the regulatory events that determine the balance of genes promoting cell replication and genes leading to blocked replication and/or terminal differentiation—a situation that reflects the roles of new protein states and their interactions with the genes of interest.

To understand the problem of hormonal carcinogenesis and to identify the role of the hormone in this process—we must find answers for the following two sets of questions:

1. What is the role of the hormone in the oncogenic process? Is the hormone itself a carcinogenic chemical in that it or a metabolite can directly attack genetic material—or does it act through an existing receptor mechanism to regulate genes that in turn implement the production of oncogenic chemicals, facilitate the interaction of an oncogenic virus with the cell's genome—or contribute to a cellular state that makes the cell prone to a genetic accident during chromatin replication?
2. Is the hormone required for the continued expression of the malignant state—or is it involved only in initiating an oncogenic process? The role of hormones as initiators of malignancy must be distinguished in particular from their actions as supporters of malignant cell growth. For a given hormonally induced malignancy, what is the identity of the major mutated gene or genes? Do they belong to or affect the oncogene set that promotes cell replication—or do they rank with the suppressor genes, cell-destruct genes or their

regulation mechanisms—functioning either to limit replication or favor terminal differentiation?

In addressing the first set of questions, we are actually querying the role of the hormone itself in the initiation of the malignant state. For peptide hormones, there seems to be little reason to postulate that the hormone functions as an oncogenic chemical in the analogy of carcinogenic chemicals that directly damage the cell genome. This class of hormones, in most cases operating through specific receptor proteins localized in the cell membrane, appear to set in motion specific cascades of phosphorylation and dephosphorylation. Their effects on oncogenesis are most likely to reflect the altered gene expressions that ensue from the associated enzymology. Thus the peptide hormones do not appear as logical mediators of genotoxic chemistry directly.

While this possibility has not been totally excluded for hormones belonging to the steroid, aromatic amines, or fatty acid derivative classes, it appears to this investigator that the latter are also more likely to function as hormones, using again their specific receptor mechanisms, to induce or activate metabolic processes that indirectly might lead to the production of genotoxic chemicals *in situ* or make the cell more prone to a genetic accident during cell replication process. If an oncogenic chemical were to be produced, this product would then be expected to effect the oncogenic change in a manner not too different from the way exogenous carcinogenic chemicals act. For example, point mutations might well be anticipated with a direct genotoxic metabolite of a hormone. If this proves to be the case, the prophylaxis of hormonal carcinogenesis might be achieved by selectively regulating the activation pathways. Recent research has already well documented the fact that individuals, both humans and lower animals, vary dramatically in their abilities to induce the pathways leading to carcinogen activation and the processes that can metabolically side-track or reduce the level of the carcinogenic hazards.

Conversely, if the action of the hormone is to facilitate the action of an oncogenic virus or to predispose to genetic accidents during replication, genetic translocations and chromosomal derangement would be indicators. Early loss of chromosomes and aneuploidy have in fact been a frequent correlation in certain hormonal carcinogenesis experiments.

Some insight into the potentials of this area are provided in the properties of the receptors themselves. In this connection, steroid hormone receptors are best understood examples at this time. Perhaps their most striking property is that they are highly adaptive molecules—responding conformationally to an incoming steroid ligand, a complementary protein surface, or the response element in a DNA chain. This property permits them to act like mechanical transducers in the mediation of the sequential assembly of multiprotein complexes at the regulatory sites in a steroid-sensitive gene.

To demonstrate this phenomenon in action, our laboratory has devised a technology that clearly shows this role for the estrogen receptor (9). Briefly, one introduces both Budr and 32P into the DNA of interest by nick translation using the respective nucleotide triphosphates. When this DNA is put in contact with the soluble proteins (nuclear + cytosolic) from a target tissue, proteins assemble on the DNA sequences in specific molecular complexes. A brief irradiation with ultraviolet light 313-20-nM cross-links the Budr-sensitized DNA to the proteins that are clustered about this DNA. Subsequent digestion of the cross-linked products with nucleases releases proteins with very short 32P labeled DNA tags. Electrophoresis of the products in SDS gels yields bands of 32P-labeled proteins —showing the sizes of the proteins that resided initially in the crosslinking reaction zone of interest. Using cold DNA to dilute out DNA segments of lesser interest identifies only those proteins that are associating as molecular complexes with the DNA of interest.

Using two estrogen-sensitive genes, the PS2 and prolactin genes, one finds that the assembly of proteins around the 5' regulatory sequences is estrogen-receptor and ligand dependent. If an antiestrogen such as HO-tamoxifen or ICI is used, the spectrum of proteins participating in the assembly is distinctly different. In addition, while some proteins are used in both assemblies, some of these components are different depending on the particular gene. An important feature of the assembly process is that the accessory proteins are brought in close physical proximity to the estrogen receptor, in fact, an antibody to the estrogen receptor retrieves these assemblies as molecular complexes—even after the DNA has been digested with nucleases. Since such complexes contain the estrogen receptor, we have named them receptorsomes.

Experiments using this technology show that estrogen receptors, and presumably other steroid receptors acting in like manner, guide the assembly of proteins around regulatory segments of the hormone-sensitive genes. The character of such assemblies determines in turn the transcriptional performance of a target gene. In addition to showing the steroid receptor in action, the protocol also marks the participating proteins by size—and provides an important identifier for the isolation and characterization of the participating proteins.

These findings have relevance for hormonal carcinogenesis, as in the near future, it will be important to identify the accessory proteins for all receptors and genes that are involved in the hormonal carcinogenesis process, since the ease with which such multiprotein complexes are assembled depends on the relative concentrations of these proteins, as well as the presence of a functional receptor. Any mutations or regulatory defects impacting on the state or numerical availability of any one of these proteins has the potential to play an important role in gene expression and ultimately will impact on the phenotypic character of the target cell. An oncogenic process could easily be one that affects the level of such a protein and thus contributes to the malignant phenotype.

To answer the second set of questions there is simply no substitute for the in-depth genetic analysis of each type of hormone-related malignancy—one by one. What genes are mutated and what role do they play in the tumor cell's growth advantage? In this quest, two areas of replication control appear important to survey for possible oncogenic derangement and/or altered responsiveness to hormonal control: (1) those genes contributing to the start and assembly of a functional DNA replicate system; and (2) the genes that code for events leading to terminal differentiation.

In considering the first area one should appreciate that the duration of the G1 interval is the major determinant of replication frequency in most mammalian cells. This interval can vary from minutes—to hours—to days, or even years, yet despite its importance only recently have we begun to get clues as to the fundamental processes that affect the regulation. We now know that the action begins with a "start" gene—and ends with the assembly and function of a DNA replicase system. Once started, the actual process of DNA replication carried out in a chromatin setting (as described below), proceeds in a manner that is difficult to stop. The events leading up to this transition, however, are most important in the growth of organized tissues and are likely to be the targets of an oncogenic change that leads to more frequent cell replication. For example, they are clearly involved in growth factor action—and are the responders to any mutational event affecting the level or function of such components. Insight into this area of replication biology has been slow to develop, but in the last few years there has been a remarkable burst of progress—coming out of studies of cell cycle mutants in yeast and the regulation of processes leading to mitosis and meiosis of sea urchin and clam eggs (10). The CDC-2 gene product and its equivalent in other species has been identified as a protein kinase, which on activation performs critical and essential phosphorylation events leading to mitosis in both the eggs and yeast cells; most remarkably, however, is that it is also tightly tied to the progression of mammalian cells through the G1 interval into S phase reactions. The level of this enzyme remains rather constant throughout the cell cycle; however, it is only activated when the level of cyclin proteins rises to a triggering level. On formation of a complex between these entities, the CDC-2 kinase proceeds to phosphorylate proteins critically needed for S-phase events, the accumulated cyclins are then degraded acutely to a basal level—only to once again start accumulating due to resynthesis. This whole progression and its oscillatory nature appears to be dependent on the balance of timely phosphorylations and dephosphorylations that are slowly becoming better defined (10).

The likelihood is high that the growth factor mechanisms impinge rather directly on the balance of these rate processes. In addition, there are other proteins—working through molecular complexing—that seem as well to impact on the oscillations of the CDC-2 kinase/cyclin system. Their identities as well as the manner in which growth promoting hormones and factors influence their levels and function constitute a timely subject for investigation with respect to the problem of hormonal carcinogenesis.

The second important area of inquiry has to be the identification of the genes that lead to terminal differentiation and cell death. Cells of different types have separate and different mechanisms for dying. An oncogenic process that decreases their influence on cell survival will lead to cell accumulation even if replication frequency is only minimally stimulated. In this connection it is important to recognize that oncogenically transformed cells—in most cases still retain functional genes leading to terminal differentiation—but their expression is blocked in the malignant phenotype. Experiments with phorbol esters, dimethylsulfoxides, retinoic acid, and certain antigrowth factors, however, can frequently superinduce these genes—and cell death ensues. The processes that underlie such progressions [i.e., heme production in erythroid cells (11), chromatin fragmentation in certain lymphoid cells, the activation of cell membrane damage in keratinocytes, and the release of cell surface proteoglycans in colon cancer (12)] need to be identified and investigated specifically for hormone-related malignancies. Most important, ways have to be discovered or invented to selectively activate these pathways in the cancer cell. The relationship of hormone action to such processes could be very important in both the hormonal carcinogenesis events and the ensuing growth of a resulting tumor.

Finally, a few comments should be made concerning the actual process of chromatin replication and how it might impact on the production or stabilization of a particular differentiation state. As we have heard several times in this symposium, hormonal pretreatment can yield "remembered" states in which exogenous chemical carcinogens or endogenous oncogenic processes are facilitated. Some insight into the potentials in this area emanate from studies of replication mechanisms themselves.

In our earlier studies in nuclei of S phase synchronized Hela cells, we showed that DNA replication in a chromosomal setting required the cooperation of specific sets of soluble proteins and that worked as combinations of proteins with a specificity for the DNA that was undergoing replication at the time (i.e., early, middle, or late S-phase DNA). This requirement for the combinatorial action of proteins was further correlated with the observation that as the replication fork advanced these proteins entered into physical complexes with the newly replicated DNA—giving an immature form of chromatin. In the absence of the right proteins or an inadequate concentration of some particular units, the replication fork failed to advance. However, with the optimal concentrations of the needed proteins, an immature chromatin was formed that was 30% richer in protein than the normal interphase state of this chromatin. This transitory immature chromatin state changed *in vivo*, however, when the depositions of histones took place. Our interpretation of these findings was that the incoming histones displaced those chromatin complexes that were unstable due to deficiency or a functional inadequacy of some key protein in the complex. In this way competitive events influencing the concentrations or activity states of critical proteins might impact on the phenotype of a cell without altering genotype—i.e., a remembered differentiation event.

Since it is the character of the chromosomal complexes that ultimately determines the phenotype of a cell (i.e., its transcriptional responsiveness to hormones and other inducing agents) it is postulated that this aspect of chromatin replication provides a way for the cell to sense its recent inductive past in a manner that also results in a directed stabilization or alteration of phenotype. Since hormone action prior to a replication event can induce massive changes in the concentrations of specific proteins, it follows that hormones naturally have the mechanisms for massively influencing the phenotype of cells coming out of a replication experience. I submit in principle that this situation provides a basis for altering the specific sensitivity of certain genes by hormonal treatment during chemical carcinogenesis.

With respect to answering both sets of the above questions, I am optimistic that we now have the tools to make dramatic progress in resolving the stated problems. By far the most powerful approaches reside in the realm of molecular genetics. For example, we are now able to test given pathways for their normalcy in a given malignant state in that we can literally create test systems by genetic engineering and transgenic mechanisms in which specific gene functions are either amplified or depressed. This technology makes it possible to assess in quantitative terms the relative importance of a given gene in the establishment and perpetuation of a particular hormone-related malignancy. In addition to answering such questions directly, we can also assess the role of combinatorial actions between different gene sets that may operate interactively in a given malignant state. I am also optimistic that the answers will go a long way in controlling problems of hormonal carcinogenesis—and in devising therapies for hormonally regulated malignancies.

References

1. Fearson ER, Vogelstein B (1990) A genetic model for colorectal tumorigenesis. Cell 61:759-767.
2. Lewin B (1991) Oncogenic conversion by regulatory changes in transcription factors. Cell 64:303-312.
3. Cantley LC, Auger KR, Carpenter C, Duckworth B, Graziani A, Kapeller R, Soltoff S (1991) Oncogenes and signal transduction. Cell 64:281-302.
4. Friedman PN, Kern SE, Vogelstein B, and Prives C (1990) Wild-type, but mutant, human p53 proteins inhibit replicative activities of simian virus 40 large tumor antigen. Proc Natl Acad Sci USA 87:9275-9279.
5. Hu Q, Dyson, Harlow E (1990) The regions of the retinoblastoma protein needed for binding to adeno E1A or SV40 large T antigen are common sites for mutation. EMBO J 9:1147-1155.
6. Ludlow JW, Shon J, Pipas JM, Livingston DM, and DeCaprio JA (1990) The retinoblastoma susceptibility gene product undergoes cell cycle-dependent dephosphorylation and binding to and release from SV40 large T. Cell 60:387-396.
7. Offringa R, Gebel S, Dam HV, Timmer M, Smits A, Zwart R, Stein B, Bos JL, Eb AV, Herrlick P (1990) A novel function of the transforming domain of E1a: repression of AP-2D1 activity. Cell 62:527-538.
8. Huang S, Lee WH, Lee EYHP (1991) A cellular protein that competes with SV40 T antigen for binding to retinoblastoma gene product. Nature (in press).
9. Schuh TJ, Mueller GC (1991) Use of photo-crosslinking to demonstrate receptor-dependent, ligand modulated assembly of multi-protein complexes on the rat prolactin gene. (Manuscript submitted)

10. Lewin B (1990) Driving the cell cycle: M phase kinase, its partners and substrates. Cell 61:743-752.
11. Lo SH, Aft R, Mueller GC (1981) Role of nonhemoglobin heme accumulation in the terminal differentiation of Friend erythroleukemia cells. Cancer Res 41:864-870.
12. McBain JA, Pettit GR, Mueller GC (1990) Phorbol esters activate proteoglycan metabolism in human colon cancer cells en route to terminal differentiation. Cell Growth Different. 1:281-291.

COMMUNICATIONS

Cytogenetic Changes in Renal Neoplasms and During Estrogen-Induced Renal Tumorigenesis in Hamsters

Sushanta K. Banerjee, Snigdha Banerjee, Sara Antonia Li, and Jonathan J. Li

Summary

Cytogenetic changes have been implicated in tumor development. Such changes were studied in male Syrian hamster kidneys after chronic exposure to either diethylstilbestrol(DES) or 17β-estradiol(E_2). The frequency of aneuploidy and micronuclei was elevated in estrogen-induced renal tumors. The frequency of aneuploidy in DES- and E_2-induced tumors was 8.5-fold and 8.0-fold higher than in untreated kidneys, respectively. The number of micronuclei also increased 3.8- to 4.3-fold in these estrogen-induced tumors. Nonrandom numerical chromosomal abnormalities were +1, +2, +3, +11, +13, +16, +20, +21, and -8, -19, -20 in the DES- and 1, +2, +3, +6, +11, +16, +20, +21, +X and -14,-20 in the E_2-induced tumors. Structural changes were observed only in E_2-induced tumors. Endomitosis, telomeric associations, and breaks were also seen in these kidney tumors. The frequency of chromosomal abnormalities was higher in 3.5 months estrogen-treated hamster proximal tubules after culture. The findings suggest that chronic estrogen exposure induces genetic instability in the hamster kidney and it may be associated with renal tumorigenesis. (NCI, NIH. CA22008)

Introduction

Both synthetic and natural estrogens (e.g., DES and 17β-E_2) are carcinogenic in human and animals (1-5). Multiple bilateral renal tumors can be induced by estrogens in both intact and castrated male Syrian hamsters with an incidence approaching 100%. Furthermore, these tumors are dependent on estrogens for continuous growth, and tumor regression occurs when estrogen is withdrawn or when estrogen antagonists are provided (5). The exact role of these hormones in the induction of kidney tumors in the hamster is not clear. Basic questions regarding the mechanisms of induction and progression of renal tumorigenesis in hamsters remain unanswered. One pertinent question is whether estrogens elicit any genetic alterations or abnormalities in the kidney of the hamster that may be involved in events leading to neoplastic transformation.

As a prelude to studying possible nonrandom chromosomal changes induced by estrogen in renal tumorigenesis, we have undertaken cytogenetic studies of estrogen-dependent renal tumors. Since no data are available concerning the changes in renal tumors of the hamster, these studies may open a new approach to understand the possible genetic mechanisms of estrogen-induced renal tumorigenicity in the Syrian hamster kidney. Preliminary results are also presented regarding early cytogenetic changes in the kidney after three months of estrogen treatment.

Results

A high frequency of cytogenetic abnormalities in renal tumors and during estrogen-induced renal tumorigenesis in Syrian hamsters was observed. These findings indicated that all of the DES- and E_2-induced renal tumors examined exhibited karyotypic and other cytogenetic alterations. In untreated cultured proximal tissues, the majority of metaphases had $2n = 44$ chromosomes ($92.1 \pm 1.16\%$). The frequency of near diploid (i.e., 40 to 43 and 45 to 48) was $5.7 \pm 0.9\%$ and near tetraploid (i.e., > 50) was $1.7 \pm 0.7\%$. But in DES-induced tumors, the near diploid was $51.4\% \pm 4.2\%$ and in E_2 it was $46.3 \pm 3.7\%$. The frequency of near tetraploid was also very high in both estrogen-induced renal tumors. It was $9.0 \pm 1.9\%$ in DES-induced tumors and $14.1 \pm 3.6\%$ in E_2-induced tumors. Moreover the frequency of aneuploidy increased in 3.5 months estrogen-treated kidney of hamsters.

Furthermore, the numerical and structural chromosomal changes in the tumors were studied. A summary of these observations is shown in Table 1. There were no structural abnormalities in DES-induced tumors, but numerical changes were found. For example, chromosomes 1, 3, 11, 13, 16, and 21 were consistently overrepresented and chromosomes 8 and 19 were underrepresented in most of the observed tumors (i.e., 75 to 100%). On the other hand in E_2-induced tumors both numerical and structural changes were found. Chromosomes 1, 2, 3, 7, 11, 16, 21, and X were overrepresented and 14 was underrepresented in 64 to 100% of observed tumors. Chromosome 20 exhibited both consistent gains and losses in both DES- and E_2-induced tumors. Structural changes were only found in two of E_2-induced tumors. Chromosomes $1q^+$ was found in one tumor and $3q^+$ in the other. Numerous marker chromosomes of unknown origin were found in both DES- and E_2-induced tumors. Present findings indicate that more or less the same chromosomes were consistently shown to be either overrepresented or underrepresented in both tumors.

The frequency of chromosomal aberrations (i.e., breaks, micronuclei formations, endoduplication, and telomeric associations) in these tumors and during the estrogen-induced tumorigenesis is shown in Table 2. The frequency of chromosomal aberrations was significantly increased in both these tumors and in DES-treated nonneoplastic kidney proximal tubules compared to control.

Table 1. Chromosomes involved in numerical and structural changes in estrogen-induced hamster kidney tumors.

Estrogens[1]	Treatment Month	Numerical Changes[2]	Structural Changes
DES	9.0	+1, +2, +3, +11 +13, +16, +20 +21, + Mar -8, -19, -21	
E	9.0	+1, +2, +3, +7, +11, +16, +20, +21 +X, +Mar -14, -20	dup: 1q, 3q

[1]DES, Diethylstilbestrol; E, 17β-Estradiol
[2]Only consistent changes (i.e., two cells with the same chromosome gain or structural rearrangements and three with same loss; according to the 1985 ISCN nomenclature) that were observed in most of the tumors were considered for present experiment.

Table 2. Cytogenetic analysis of untreated, DES-treated, and estrogen-induced tumors in Syrian hamster kidneys.

Cytogenetic Changes (%)	Age-matched control kidney (3.5 months)	DES-treated kidney (3.5 months)	Age-matched control kidney (9 months)	DES-induced tumor	E-induced tumor
Micronuclei	1.0 ± 0.4	3.1 ± 0.8	1.6 ± 0.3	6.7 ± 0.4	6.4 ± 0.26
Endomitosis	0.0	6.5 ± 5.4	0.0	6.0 ± 7.6	9.0 ± 13.2
Breaks					
Chromatid	1.3 ± 0.4	10.3 ± 2.0	3.4 ± 3.1	16.2 ± 5.3	15.9 ± 3.3
Chromosome	0.2 ± 0.2	5.1 ± 0.9	0.0	10.0 ± 2.8	6.0 ± 17
Telomeric association	0.2 ± 0.2	8.5 ± 1.6	0.0	38.6 ± 10.6	27.7 ± 10.7

Data are expressed as mean ± SE.

Conclusion

In conclusion, our studies have demonstrated that a high frequency of aneuploidy with specific chromosome gains or losses and other cytogenetic aberrations were consistently observed in estrogen-induced tumors. Furthermore, aneuploidy and chromosomal aberrations were also found in culture proximal tubules after 3.5 months of estrogen treatment of male Syrian hamsters. Present findings suggest that aneuploidy and specific chromosomal changes and chromosomal aberrations may be associated with tumorigenesis in hamster.

References
1. IARC Group (1979) IARC Monogr Eval Carcinog Risk Chem Hum 21:139-362.
2. Persson, I (1985) The risk of endometrial and breast cancer after estrogen treatment. A review of epidermiological studies. Acta Obstet Gynec Scand (Suppl) 130:59-66.
3. Whitehead, MI and Fraser, D (1987) Controversies concerning the safety of estrogen replacement therapy. Am J Obstet Gynec 156:1313-1322.
4. Li, JJ and Nandi, S (1990) Hormones and carcinogenesis: Laboratory studies. Principle and practice of endocrinology and Metabolism. (Ed. Becker, KL) JB Lippincott Co. Philadelphia, USA.
5. Li, JJ and Li, SA (1990) Estrogen Carcinogenesis in hamster tissues: A critical review. Endocrine Rev 11:524-531.

Pituitary Regulation of Sex-Differentiated Promotion of Rat Liver Carcinogenesis

Agneta Blanck, Jan-Åke Gustafsson, and Inger Porsch-Hällström

Summary

Promotion of diethylnitrosamine(DEN)-induced hepatic lesions with 2-acetylaminofluorene (2-AAF) and partial hepatectomy (PH), with dietary deoxycholic acid (DCA) or a choline-deficient (CD) diet gave rise to a faster growth rate of enzyme-altered foci in male than in female rat livers. "Feminization" of the secretory pattern of growth hormone (GH) in males by continuous administration of bovine GH or implantation of ectopic pituitary grafts (PG) decreased the growth rate to that in females. The faster focal growth in males was accompanied by a GH-regulated increase in hepatic c-*myc* expression during treatment with all promoters. A marked mitoinhibition in response to PH was observed in males treated with 2-AAF/PH in the resistant hepatocyte model (RH-model) and during CD promotion. GH-treated or PG-bearing males regenerated at a higher rate, similar to that of females. DCA treatment stimulated liver regeneration in rats of both sexes. These data suggest that GH is a major determinant of sex-differentiated promotion of rat liver carcinogenesis.

Introduction

Sex differences in promotion of rat liver carcinogenesis have been observed with a number of different regimens, including treatment according to the RH-model (1) and promotion of DEN-initiated hepatic lesions with a diet containing the secondary bile acid DCA or a CD diet (2). With all these regimens, putatively initiated hepatic lesions, detected as foci of enzyme-altered cells, grew faster in male than in female rat livers. We have previously demonstrated that GH-secretion, which is sex differentiated in the rat, seems to be responsible for the sexual dimorphism resulting after carcinogen treatment in the RH model. The present study was undertaken to investigate whether GH is responsible for the sex differences in focal growth rate observed with DCA and CD diets, as well as to establish whether a sex-differentiated expression of the c-*myc* protooncogene, previously demonstrated in the RH model ($\delta > \female$) (3), is also present in these models. Since selective mitoinhibition has been suggested to be of importance for promotion in the RH-model, the regenerative response in livers from rats treated with different promotion regimens was also investigated.

Results

Following treatment of DEN-initiated male, female, and "feminized" male rats with three different promotion regimens (Fig. 1), the area per focus at the end of the experiments was markedly larger in livers from males than from females.

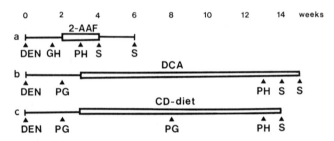

Fig. 1. Rats ($\delta, \female$) initiated with DEN (200 mg/kg, i.p.) were treated with diets containing 2-AAF (0.02%, w/w)(a), DCA (0.5%, w/w)(b) or with a CD diet (c). Feminization of male rat liver was performed either by GH-infusion (5 μg/h) or by implantation of two PG:s under the kidney capsule once (b) or twice (c) during promotion. Liver material was collected at the time of PH and at sacrifice (S).

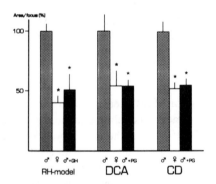

Fig. 2. Mean size of enzyme-altered hepatic foci stained for γ-glutamyltrans-ferase (2,3) activity (RH model) or immunohistochemical staining for the placental form of glutathione-S-transferase (3) (DCA and CD) at the end of each experiment. Values are presented as percent ± S.E.M. of intact male rats ($n=5$-11). *Significantly different from intact males (Wilcoxon rank sum test; $p<0.05$).

Males receiving either GH infusion or PG:s under the kidney capsule during promotion, lead to feminization of hepatic function in male rats (Fig. 2). Expression of the c-*myc* gene was measured by hybridization of RNA in the total nucleic acid (TNA) fraction of the samples to cRNA probes in solution (3). Two days post-PH in the RH model and at the time of PH in rats fed the DCA or CD diets, c-*myc* expression was markedly higher in male than in female and feminized male rat livers (data not shown). Livers from male rats treated in the RH model were more mitoinhibited one week after PH than the livers of female or GH-treated rats. A similar pattern of mitoinhibition was observed one week after PH in CD-treated rats. Rats fed DCA did not show any sex differences in regenerative capacity following PH, although a general stimulatory effect of DCA was found compared with initiated rats fed standard diet (data not shown).

Conclusions

The present study supports the view that GH secretion is a major determinant of sex-differentiated promotion of hepatocarcinogenesis in the rat. In contrast to the sex-differentiated mitoinhibitory effects on liver regeneration seen in the RH model and with CD promotion, DCA treatment exerted a general stimulatory effect on liver regeneration in rats of both sexes. Although the influence of GH and PG give rise to a similar response in terms of focal growth and c-*myc* expression, the differences in regeneration indicate that more than one mechanism for promotion might be influenced by GH.

References

1. Blanck A, Hansson T, Eriksson LC, Gustafsson J-Å (1987) Growth hormone modifies the growth rate of enzyme-altered hepatic foci in male rats treated according to the resistant hepatocyte model. Carcinogenesis 8:1585-1588.
2. Cameron RG, Blanck A, Armstrong D (1990) Sex differences in response to four promotion regimens in spite of common first cellular steps in the hepatocellular cancer process initiated by diethylnitrosamine. Cancer Letters 50:109-113.
3. Porsch-Hällström I, Gustafsson J-Å and Blanck A (1989) Effects of growth hormone on the expression of c-*myc* and c-*fos* during early stages of sex-differentiated rat liver carcinogenesis in the resistant hepatocyte model. Carcinogenesis 10:2339-2343.

Modulation of Estrogen Metabolism by Inducers of P-4501A2: Possible Application to the Chemoprevention of Breast Cancer

H. Leon Bradlow, Michael Osborne, Jon J. Michnovicz, and Nitin T. Telang

Summary

In these studies we have demonstrated that noninvolved mammary tissue obtained from a breast containing a tumor showed increased FTP binding activity of *ras*-P21 and increased 16α-hydroxylation of estradiol relative to the level in normal breast tissue. In addition, a hyper response in the levels of both parameters was observed following treatment of the tumor-related breast tissue in organ culture with benzopyrene and/or fatty acids. The results suggest that the apparently normal breast tissue from a cancerous breast is biochemically different from breast tissue taken from a normal breast (mammoplasty). The shifts in these parameters after both treatments are in the direction associated with increased cancer risk.

Introduction

The aim of these studies is to examine the validity of a molecular and an endocrine biomarker for breast cancer risk in noninvolved breast tissue taken from subjects undergoing mammoplasty and from patients undergoing mastectomy. For this purpose we have measured the FTP binding activity of *ras*P21 (an indirect measure of *ras* gene expression), and 2- and 16α-hydroxylation of estradiol from explant cultures of mammary terminal duct lobular units (TDLU). In addition, the modulation of the two biomarkers was examined in response to *in vitro* treatment of the cultures with a prototype carcinogen, benzo(a)pyrene(BP) and selected dietary fatty acids.

Methods

TDLU were dissected from breast tissues after staining with methylene blue and maintained in organ culture (1). TDLU derived from noncancerous breast (mammoplasty) were designated as low-risk LR-TDLU, while those from cancerous breasts (mastectomy) were designated as high risk TDLU-HR (2). Binding of GTP to P21 was measured by uptake of a-GTP-^{32}P as previously described (3). Protein or DNA was determined conventionally, and all results were normalized per unit protein or DNA.

Results

We have demonstrated that GTP binding of *ras* P21 and estradiol 16α-hydroxylation are markedly elevated in TDLU-HR relative to TDLU-LR (Table 1, Figure 1). We have further shown that TDLU-HR are hyperresponsive to treatment with BP or fatty acids relative to TDLU-LR (Table 2). The TDLU-HR show a further increase when the explants are additionally treated with linoleic (LNA) or arachidonic acid (APA) added to the media. The response is blocked when W-3 fatty acids are added. BP depresses 2-hydroxylation along with stimulation of 16α-hydroxylation (Table 3).

Discussion

These studies were designed to demonstrate direct responses of noninvolved human mammary tissue from "low-risk" mammoplasty or "high-risk" mastectomy specimens to carcinogens and fatty acids as secondary modulators

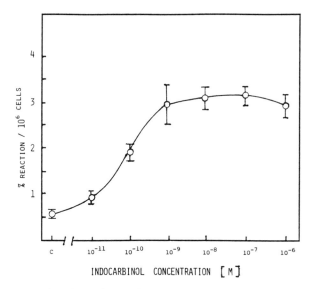

Fig. 1. Concentration-dependent effect of 13C on 2-hydroxylation of estradiol in MCF-7 cells. Tritium release was measured using 10^{-6}-10^{-11} M 13C. Values are % reaction per 10^6 cells.

Table 1. Responses in TDLU-HR and TDLU-LR.

Treatment	ras P21 GTP ASU mean ± SD		16α-hydroxylation % mean ± SD	
	TDLU-HR	TDLU-LR	TDLU-HR	TDLU-LR
Me$_2$SO	26.2	16.1	0.077	0.059
BP	91.9	25.9	0.239	0.082

Table 2. Effects of BP and fatty acids on biomarker levels.

Treatment	ras P21 GTP ASU mean ± SD	16α-hydroxylation % mean ± SD
Me$_2$SO	24.7 ± 1.1	0.15 ± 0.03
BP	88.4 ± 0.7	0.32 ± 0.02
LNA + BP	95.9 ± 0.7	0.57 ± 0.02
ARA + BP	111.2 ± 1.2	0.65 ± 0.05
EPA + BP	22.8 ± 1.5	0.25 ± 0.01

Table 3. Effect of BP on 2- and 16α-hydroxylation of estradiol.

Treatment	Estradiol Metabolism (%, mean ± SD)		Ratio C-16α
	C2/C16α	C-2	
Me$_2$SO	0.28 ± 0.003	0.039 ± 0.004	1:0.13
BP	0.18 ± 0.022	0.552 ± 0.059	1:3.06
	$p < 0.057$	$p < 0.00001$	

of cancer risk. Previous studies from our laboratory (4) have established an association between the levels of *ras* P21 expression and 16α-hydroxylation in various situations. Both parameters have also been associated with the progression of breast cancer (5). Therefore, these markers were selected for further study on the responsiveness of TDLU-HR and TDLU-LR to treatment with these agents. As shown in Table 1, TDLU-HR show higher levels of both parameters relative to TDLU-LR. TDLU-HR are also hyperresponsive to treatment with carcinogens relative to TDLU-LR. These results suggest that "normal" tissue in a breast containing a tumor is truely normal in its biochemical behavior.

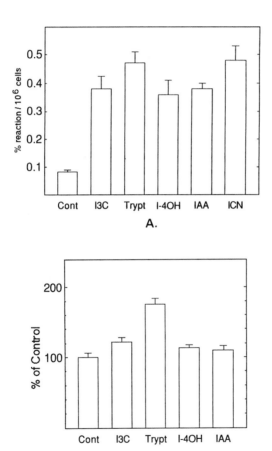

Fig. 2. a,b Effect of indoles on estradiol 2- and 16α-hydroxylation in MCF-7 cells. Values are triplicate detns. Cells were treated with the compounds for 5 days followed by a 2-day tracer incubation. The bars represent the % reaction. $p < 0.01$ for C-2. Only tryptophol showed a difference in reaction at C-16α-hydroxylation.

Secondary modulation with fatty acids also showed a specific pattern in both parameters when added togther with BP, while W-3 fatty acids decreased both biomarkers. This direct response in breast tissue is in agreement with laboratory and epidemiological data on the effects of both classes of fatty acids on breast cancer risk. Parallel responses were also observed when fatty acids alone were used (Figure 2). Additional studies from this laboratory have shown that transfection with oncogenes (ras, myc) and viruses (MMTV, HPV-16) also results in increased 16α-hydroxylation of estradiol.

The results suggest that dietary agents may have direct effects on target tissues in addition to any indirect responses arising from changes in the body milieu.

References

1. Telang NT, Axelrod DM, Wing GY, Bradlow HL, Osborne MP (1991) Biotransformation of estradiol by explant cultures of human mammary tissue. Steroids 56:37-43.

2. Telang NT, Bradlow HL, Kurihara H, and Osborne MP (1991) *In Vitro* Transformation of estradiol by explant cultures of murine mammary tissues. Breast Cancer Res and Treatment 13:173-181.

3. Telang NT, Basu A, Kukrihara H, Osborne MP, & Modak MJ (1988) Modulation in the expression of murine mammary tumor virus, *ras* protooncogene and of alveolar hyperplasia by fatty acids in mouse mammary explant cultures. Anticancer Res 8:971-976.

4. Telang NT, Narayanan R, Bradlow HL, & Osborne MP (1991) Coordinated expression of intermediate biomarkers for tumorigenic transformation in *ras*-transfected mouse mammary epithelial cells. Breast Cancer Res and Treatment (in press).

5. Schneider J, Kinne D, Fracchia A, Pierce V, Anderson KE, Bradlow HL, & Fishman J (1982) Abnormal oxidative metabolism of estradiol in women with breast cancer. Proc Natl Acad Sci USA 79P:3047-3051.

Estrogen Metabolism in Subcellular Preparations and Tissue Cultures of Syrian Hamster Liver and Kidney

Robert W. Brueggemeier, Mustapha A. Beleh, Denise L. Donley, and Young C. Lin

Summary

Estrogen metabolism was evaluated in both kidney and liver tissues from Syrian hamsters, a potential experimental model for estrogen carcinogenesis. In initial velocity studies, apparent K_ms for estrogen 2- and 4-hydroxylases ranged from 2-10 μM for liver and renal microsomes. Primary kidney cell cultures and short-term kidney tissue cultures were also utilized to examine estrogen biotransformations in intact cell systems. Both estrogen 2- and 4-hydroxylase activities were detected in these cultures. Estriol, catechol estrogens, and polar metabolites were identified from microsomal incubations. Catechol estrogens were more abundant in liver microsomal incubations than in kidney microsomal incubations; the amounts of polar metabolites were larger from renal microsomes than from liver microsomes. Kidney microsomal preparations from DES-treated hamsters yielded higher quantities of polar metabolites and lower amounts of catechol estrogens than microsomes from untreated hamsters. Kidney cultures from hamsters metabolize estradiol to yield small quantities of estrone and significant amounts of polar metabolites, and small amounts of catechol estrogens were isolated. Thus, kidney cultures from Syrian hamsters are capable of metabolizing estrogens and converting any catechol estrogens formed into more polar metabolites.

Introduction

The unique *in vivo* model of estrogen carcinogenicity in the Syrian hamster may provide important insights into the molecular processes by which estrogens induce cancer development. The relative carcinogenicity of certain estrogens in the Syrian hamster kidney tumor model correlates better with the ability of the estrogens to form catechol estrogens than with the relative affinity for the estrogen receptor (1,2). However, recent data on the induction of hamster kidney tumors by 11ß-substituted estrogens (such as Moxestrol) do not correlate with the rate of estrogen metabolism by estrogen 2-hydroxylase (3,4). Thus, the role of estrogen metabolism in hormonal carcinogenesis in this model is yet to be elucidated. Also, the question of whether it is the formation of the catechol itself, its own action, or further metabolism of the 2-hydroxyestrogen via oxidative or peroxidative pathways remains unanswered. A major problem is that the methodology for determination of catechol estrogen formation in microsomal assays utilizes conditions of high protein and steroid concentrations, which are unlikely to occur *in vivo*. We have begun to examine these issues by comparing estrogen metabolism in liver and kidney microsomal incubations with estrogen metabolism in primary kidney cell cultures (5). These present studies expand the earlier investigations and also examine metabolism in freshly isolated kidney tissue slices.

Microsomal Studies

Initial velocity studies of the conversion of estradiol to 2-hydroxyestradiol, as determined by the ^3H_2O release assay with the substrate [2-^{3}H]-estradiol, have been performed on freshly prepared, washed microsomes from both hamster liver and renal tissues. Both tissues demonstrate similar apparent K_ms of estrogen 2-hydroxylase of 2.85 μM and 6.25 μM for liver and renal microsomes, respectively. Similar results were also obtained by HPLC isolation of the catechol estrogen product using the substrate [6,7-^{3}H]-estradiol. Additional metabolites observed by HPLC isolation include estrone, estriol, and polar metabolites.

Primary Kidney Cell Cultures

Primary cultures of normal and DES-treated hamster kidney cells were incubated with [6,7-^{3}H]-estradiol (10 μM) for 48 hours. The media was removed, extracted with ethyl acetate, and the organic soluble radioactivity analyzed by reverse-phase HPLC. In the primary kidney cultures from untreated hamsters, the metabolite estrone was observed, but no catechol estrogens were observed. In addition, significant amounts of more polar metabolites were observed (5-10% formation from estradiol). In the primary kidney cultures from DES-treated hamsters, again estrone was observed but no catechol estrogens. Interestingly, much larger amounts of more polar metabolites were observed (15-20% formation; double the levels from untreated cells).

Additional experiments were performed at lower concentrations (100 n*M*) of estradiol. Again, significant amounts of more polar metabolites were formed and those levels increased with increasing duration of treatment. At these lower concentrations of estradiol, estriol formation was observed and estriol levels remained constant with increasing duration of treatment. In contrast to the previous experiments with high concentrations of estradiol, small amounts of catechol estrogens were formed in cells from untreated and 3-month-treated animals.   The levels of catechol estrogens formed decreased in cells from 6-month-treated hamsters and disappeared completely at longer treatment periods.   These results indicate that estrogen metabolism can be quantified in primary cultures of kidney cells from untreated hamsters and differences in the extent of catechol estrogen formation are observed in cells from animals treated with DES.

Kidney Tissue Slices

Examination of estrogen metabolism in hamster kidney and liver tissue slices has been initiated.   Isolated kidneys are sliced longitudinally with a scalpel into 1- to 2-mm-thick sections.   In this manner, each slice retains the tissue architecture and consist of cortex, medulla, and tubules.   Isolated livers were also sliced into 1- to 2-mm-thick sections. $[6,7-{}^3H]$-Estradiol (100 nM - 1 μM, 5.0 μCi) were incubated for 3 hours with liver tissue slices.   The media were removed and extracted three times with equal volumes of ethyl acetate containing 1% ascorbic acid (to minimize catechol estrogen degradation).   The organic extracts were analyzed by separation of the estrogen metabolites on reverse-phase HPLC with a radioactivity flow monitor.   Initial studies of estradiol metabolism by the hamster liver and kidney slices demonstrate that the liver slices are capable of metabolizing estrogens and producing significant quantities of polar metabolites for subsequent structural elucidation.   In addition, the slices produce small quantities of methoxyestrogens and catechol estrogens under the conditions employed.   Thus, the liver and kidney slices from untreated hamsters exhibit both oxidative and secondary pathways of estrogen metabolism.

References
1. Li JJ, Li SA, Klicka JK, Parsons JA, Lam LKT (1983) Relative carcinogenic activity of various synthetic and natural estrogens in the Syrian hamster kidney. Cancer Res 43:5200-5204.
2. Li SA, Klicka JK, Li JJ (1985) Estrogen 2- and 4-hydroxylase activity, catechol estrogen formation, and implications for estrogen carcinogenesis in the hamster kidney. Cancer Res 45:181-185.
3. Liehr JG, Purdy RH, Baran JS, Nutting EF, Colton F, Randerath E, Randerath K (1987) Correlation of aromatic hydoxylation of 11ß-substituted estrogens with morphological transformation *in vitro* tumor induction by these hormones. Cancer Res 47:2583-2588.
4. Li JJ, Li SA (1990) Estrogen carcinogenesis in hamster tissues: a critical review. Endocrine Rev 11:525-531.

5. Brueggemeier RW, Tseng K, Katlic NE, Beleh MA, Lin YC (1990) Estrogen metabolism in primary kidney cell cultures from Syrian hamsters. J Steroid Biochem 36:325-331.

Hormonal Regulation of Plasminogen Activation in the Human Endometrium

Bertil G. Casslén

Summary

Plasminogen activation is a crucial step in proteolytic events that result in the degradation of extracellular matrix proteins during processes involving tissue proliferation (i.e., tumor growth and metastasis). Hormonal regulation of tissue proliferation can be studied in the endometrium where proliferation is stimulated by estradiol and arrested by progesterone. Plasminogen activator activity of the endometrium increased in the proliferative phase under influence of estradiol and decreased after ovulation in response to progesterone. We found that the decreased plasminogen activator activity was the result of decreased production of urokinase plasminogen activator and increased production of plasminogen activator inhibitor 1. These changes combined to shift the activator/inhibitor balance to a reduced activator activity, which is relevant to the reduced need for plasminogen activation once proliferation is arrested.

Introduction

Plasminogen activation is intimately connected with cell proliferation. Plasmin is a broad-spectrum protease that is actively involved in pericellular proteolysis during biological processes like tissue invasion and remodeling, cell migration, and tumor growth. Degradation of the extracellular matrix is a constant feature of these processes. Plasmin activates latent collagenases, which subsequently degrade the collagen matrix. Also, plasmin directly degrades certain matrix proteins like laminin and fibronectin. Activation of the zymogen plasminogen is stimulated by specific proteases, plasminogen activators (PA). Urokinase PA (u-PA) is the activator that appears to be specifically involved in cell proliferation and tissue growth. Activation of plasminogen takes place on cell surfaces where plasminogen and uPA bind to specific receptors (1). Production of PAs is a feature common to all growing tissues and activation of the u-PA gene is an early event in the mitogenic response of stimulated cells (2). Functionally active u-PA bound to its receptor is the crucial factor that initiates plasminogen activation and thereby degradation of extracellular matrix by

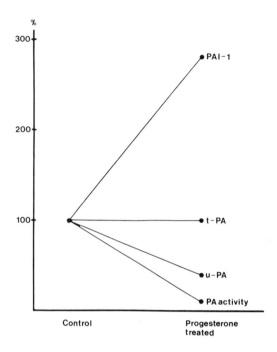

Fig. 1. Schematic presentation of the effects of progesterone (100 nmol/L) on the components of the plasminogen activating system in endometrial stromal cell cultures. Results are based on the mean values in culture medium after three days progesterone stimulation and are expressed as percent of the release in nonstimulated cultures. Progesterone shifted the activator/inhibitor balance towards lower PA activity. This resulted from decreased u-PA production and increased PAI-1 production.

tumor cells (3,4). Tissue PA (t-PA), the other known activator in humans, binds to fibrin and is mainly concerned with maintaining fluidity of the extracellular compartment. Both PAs are regulated by specific inhibitors (PAI). PAI-1 is released from endothelial cells and a number of other cell types and is regularly associated with the extracellular matrix. PAI-2 is produced by macrophages and the placenta.

Endometrial tissue proliferates promptly in response to estradiol during the proliferative phase of the menstrual cycle. Proliferation involves both the stroma and the epithelium. Progesterone, apart from differentiating the endometrium into the secretory state, abruptly turns off proliferation. This occurs also in the presence of estradiol. Endometrial tissue may thus serve as a model for hormonal regulation of cell functions associated with proliferation.

Endometrial tissue samples, obtained in the proliferative phase, release more PA activity in culture than those obtained in the luteal phase (5). Correspondingly, the PA activity of endometrial secretion increases during the proliferative phase *in vivo* to a maximum at midcycle and was then lower in the luteal phase (6,7). PA activity of the endometrium is secondary to both u-PA and t-PA (5,8). The release of u-PA was higher in the proliferative phase than in the luteal phase, whereas the release of t-PA did not vary over the menstrual cycle. Also, the release of u-PA from endometrial tissue in culture is depressed by progesterone, whereas the release of t-PA is not affected (9). PA activity results from the balance between PAs and PAIs. The present study was undertaken to study the hormonal regulation of PAs and PAIs, and their origin in glandular epithelial vs. stromal cells.

Material and Methods

Endometrial tissue was obtained preoperatively from uteri with nonendometrial pathology, digested with collagenase and the stromal and epithelial cells separated and cultured as described (10). u-PA was assayed in a radioimmunoassay (11). t-PA and PAI-1 were assayed in commercial ELISA kits [Immunolys, Biopool, Umeσ, Sweden]. u-PA receptors were assayed in endometrial membranes using 125_I labeled u-PA [Casslén, Gustavsson, unpublished]. Endogenously bound u-PA was removed by a brief acid treatment, allowing the total number of receptors to be measured. The occupied fraction was calculated as the difference between the total and the free fractions.

Results

Stromal as well as epithelial cell cultures released both u-PA and t-PA. Estradiol did not influence the release of the PAs in either cell type. On the other hand progesterone significantly reduced the u-PA production in stromal cells, but not in epithelial cells. The release of t-PA was not affected by progesterone stimulation. The release of PAI-1 was much higher in stromal than in epithelial cells, and it was further increased by progesterone in the stromal cells, but not in the epithelial cells. The number of u-PA binding sites was higher in membranes prepared from luteal phase endometria than in those from the proliferative phase. This was true for the total number as well as the free and occupied fractions.

Conclusions

Plasminogen activation has a key role in tissue proliferation. Endometrial tissue proliferates readily in response to estradiol *in vivo* and increasing amounts of PAs are released from the endometrial tissue during this phase. Soon after ovulation and in response to progesterone, PA activity decreases and the mitotic activity disappears in both the stroma and the epithelium. In this study we found that the reduced PA activity was due to reduced release of u-PA and increased release of PAI-1 from the endometrial stromal cells. This shifted the balance towards a lower PA activity. Secretion of t-PA was not affected by progesterone treatment. In contrast to the response in stromal cells, the release of u-PA and PAI-1 in epithelial cells was not altered by progesterone, since proliferation is arrested and mitotic activity disappears concomitantly in the epithelium and stroma *in vivo*. A similar response would have been expected in epithelial and stromal cells. *In vivo*, however, morphological differentiation of the endometrial epithelium is induced by the stroma (12). Thus, proliferation-related cell functions in the uterine epithelium may similarly be regulated by the stroma *in vivo*, where the epithelium occurs in functional relation to the stroma.

From the *in vivo* effects of estradiol on endometrial proliferation, it might be expected that estradiol would increase the release of u-PA from endometrial cells in culture. We were, however, unable to show such an increase. This may relate to the fact that it has not been convincingly shown that estradiol is mitogenic to endometrial cells *in vitro*. The increased receptor-binding of u-PA during the secretory phase may, at least, partly, explain the decresed release of u-PA, and also indicate a changed metabolism of u-PA during this phase. Alternatively, the finding suggests a function for membrane-bound u-PA during differentiation of the endometrium into its secretory state.

Acknowledgment

This study was supported by grants from the Swedish Cancer Foundation (2693-B90-02XA).

References

1. Stephens RW, Pöllänen J, Tapiovaara H, Leung K-C, Sim P-S, Salonen E-M, Rönne E, Behrendt N, Danö K, Vaheri A (1989) Activation of prourokinase and plasminogen on human sarcoma cells: A proteolytic system with surface-bound reactants. Cell Biol 108:1987-1995.
2. Grimaldi G, Di Fiore P, Locatelli EK, Falco J, Blasi F (1986) Modulation of urokinase plasminogen activator gene expression during the transition from quiescent to proliferative state in normal mouse cells. The EMBO Journal 5:855-861.
3. Ossowski L (1988) *in vivo* invasions of modified chorioallantoic membrane by tumor cells: the role of cell surfacebound urokinase. J Cell Biol 107:2437-2445.
4. Baker MS, Bleakley P, Woodrow GC, Doe WF (1990) Inhibition of cancer cell urokinase plasminogen activator by its specific inhibitor PAI-2 and subsequent effects on extracellular matrix degradation. Cancer Res 50:4676-4684.
5. Casslén B, Åstedt B (1983) Occurrence of both urokinase and tissue plasminogen activator in the human endometrium. Contraception 28:553-564.
6. Casslén B, Åstedt B (1981) Fibrinolytic activity of human uterine fluid. Acta Obstet Gynecol Scand 60:55-58.

7. Casslén B, Ohlsson K (1981) Cyclic variation of plasminogen activation in human uterine fluid and influence of an intrauterine device. Acta Obstet Gynecol Scand 60:97-101.
8. Casslén B, Thorell J, Åstedt B (1981) Effect of IUD on urokinase-like immunoreactivity and plasminogen activators in human uterine fluid. Contraception 23:435-445.
9. Casslén B, Andersson A, Nilsson IM, Åstedt B (1986) Hormonal regulation of the release of plasminogen activators and of a specific activator inhibitor from endometrial tissue in culture. Proc Soc Exptl Biol Med 182:419-424.
10. Casslén B, Siler-Khodr TM, Harper MJK (1990) Progesterone regulation of prolactin release from human endometrial stromal cells in culture: Potential bioassay for progestational activity. Acta Endocrinol 122:137-44.
11. Åstedt B, Holmberg L, Lecander I, Thorell J (1981) Radioimmunoassay of urokinase for quantification of plasminogen activators released in ovarian tumour cultures. Europ J Cancer 17:239-44.
12. Cunha GR (1976) Stromal induction and specification of morphogenesis and cytodifferentiation of the epithelia of the müllerian ducts and urogenital sinus during development of the uterus and vagina in mice. J Exp Zool 196:361-370.

Your Research—Our Lives

Pat Cody

Summary

DES Action is a consumer group representing those exposed *in utero* to diethylstilbestrol and their mothers. We work to educate the public and health-care providers about DES, to provide medical information and referrals, to monitor research, and to act as advocates for the DES-exposed. DES Action has 30 chapters in 22 states in the United States as well as foreign affiliates in Australia, Canada, England, France, Ireland, and the Netherlands. Research reports on such major concerns as fertility and pregnancy and risks for breast cancer make possible our special publications on these topics. As the DES-exposed cohort ages, there remain some major unanswered questions: effects on the children of DES daughters and sons? Extent of immune system impairment? Effects on the endocrine system? Research into these questions will shed light on anecdotally observed health effects from DES exposure.

DES Action began in 1975 when some DES mothers and DES daughters met to discuss their common concerns about appropriate care for the DES-exposed and the need for public and professional education, for research, and for physician referrals. Sixteen years later, we have the same concerns.

We have, of course, made progress. There has been a considerable amount of research at both laboratory and clinical levels on DES daughters, so that we have the kind of knowledge that guides our health-care decisions. We know that about 1 out of 1,000 daughters will develop clear-cell adenocarcinoma of the vagina/cervix. One out of two daughters is at risk for a variety of reproductive problems. Structural malformations and abnormalities cause infertility for some daughters: scanty cervical mucus, changes in endometrial tissue, blocked tubes, and anovulation. Daughters who achieve pregnancy have greater risks for ectopic pregnancy, miscarriage because of a T-shaped uterus, or other changes, and premature delivery because of incompetent cervix or small uterus. Such premature deliveries sometimes extend the DES trauma to the third generation in that birth injuries are sustained because of the structural changes DES created in the uterus of the DES daughter.

Unfortunately there are serious gaps in the research. There have been very few studies on the women given DES during pregnancy, and these studies have been limited to risks for cancer of the reproductive organ, in particular, breast cancer. A report by E.R. Greenberg et al. (1), describes a significant increase in risk for breast cancer for DES mothers.

Studies on DES sons have been sparse, and there has not been a single study large enough (1,000 DES-exposed and 1,000 controls) to provide data that can give good risk assessments. The largest study (2) of 308 sons from the Dieckmann cohort concerned only the reproductive system. It showed increased risks for epididymal cysts and/or hypoplastic testes, severe pathological changes in spermatozoa, and for cryptorchidism.

We have always believed it does not make biological sense that exposure *in utero* to this powerful nonsteroidal synthetic estrogen would affect only one body system, the reproductive system. A monograph by Blair (1981) described the results of her experiment with DES and neonatal mice (3). She concluded that "The effect of DES upon the developing immune system during the perinatal period is significant. There are immediate effects which are dramatic in the thymus. Even after the thymus and peripheral lymphoid organs return to normal weight and histologic appearance, both B cell and T cell responses are abnormal. These impairments can be found even in 17-month old animals, and indeed may become more severe as the animals age."

In order to stimulate interest in doing a similar study on DES-exposed people, DES Action asked readers of its newsletter as well as other DES-exposed to fill out a detailed health history questionnaire. The results of this study (4) stated, "Conditions that suggest possibly impaired immune function—that is, respiratory tract infections, asthma, arthritis, and lupus—were reported more frequently among the persons with DES exposure. Conditions that may involve altered endocrine function were also more frequent among such persons."

Since participants in the above inquiry were self-selected, we realized that a more rigorous study was needed. The directors of the DESAD project worked with Dr. Blair to develop their 1986 questionnaire (5). The authors concluded that "The information presented in this preliminary communication also supports the concept that human exposure before birth to DES may subsequently affect the adult immune system."

This DESAD report refers only to DES daughters. The Wingard and Turiel study covered mothers, daughters, and sons and showed impaired immune function in all three populations. We need studies of the mother and the son cohorts on immune impairment. We need studies in all groups of endocrine system effects; of the children of DES sons and daughters, to learn if there are risks for a "third-generation" effect; that is, of genetic damage, particularly as it would apply to a risk for cancer. We need studies on the long-term health of clear-cell cancer survivors, on the risks for recurrences, and on successful treatment methods for recurrence. Our DES Cancer Network can assist by providing access to members who had clear-cell cancer.

There is more than scientific curiosity in our queries. We represent a large DES exposed population, both in the United States and in other countries. DES was administered to pregnant women in the U.S. beginning in 1938, the year it was first synthesized by Sir Charles Dodds. White, one of the principal physicians at the Joslin Diabetes Center in Boston, testified in 1979: "When stilbestrol became available in 1938, I began using it for the treatment of pregnant diabetics. On the basis of my clinical experience, I devised a dosage schedule commencing early in pregnancy and continuing until delivery."

Experimental use of DES during pregnancy occurred from 1938 on, but it was not until publication of the Smith report (6) that extensive prescription began. The report by Dieckmann et al. (7) concluded that there was no therapeutic value to such prescription, but five years later did little to stem the enthusiasm with which DES was prescribed. The National Cancer Institute in its request for proposal for the DESAD project in December 1973 stated that ".....among 62 million births during the potential exposure time (1943-1959), there would be 31 million females, of whom 2.8 million have been exposed to estrogen *in utero*, and 1.9 million to synthetic estrogens." If there were 1.9 million females, there would also be 1.9 million males during those years, for a total of 3.8 million children. For the period 1960-1970, the Boston Collaborative Drug Surveillance Program (Boston University Medical Center) reported that 100,000 DES prescriptions were written each year for pregnant women, a total of one million during the last decade of approved use, when use was reported to decline.

Accordingly, for the years 1943-1970, we estimate there were a total of at least 4.8 million children plus the same number of mothers, for a total of 9.6 million DES-exposed in the U.S. The FDA warning (DES has never been banned) did not appear until November 1971, so use continued through that year. Indeed, many obstetricians did not get the message, because a prescription audit for 1974 showed 11,000 prescriptions written that year for DES for pregnant women (8). Use of DES by pregnant women in other countries continued until 1975 in the Netherlands, 1977 in France, 1983 in Hungary, for example. DES was used during pregnancy in every country where U.S. drug companies had markets. At present we have DES Action groups in Australia, Canada, England, France, Ireland, and the Netherlands, and the European Parliament is currently conducting a study on DES exposure in the 12 European Economic Community nations in order to plan a program for public and professional education.

References

1. Greenberg ER et al (1984) Breast Cancer in Mothers Given Diethylstilbestrol in Pregnancy. N Engl J Med 311:1393-1398.
2. Gill WB et al (1979 Association of Diethylstilbestrol Exposure *in Utero* with Cryptochidism, Testicular Hypoplasia and Semen Abnormalities. J of Urology 122:36-39.
3. Blair PB (1981) Immunologic Consequences of Early Exposure of Experimental Rodents to DES. Editors Herbst AL and Bern HA in Developmental Effects of Diethylstilbestrol in Pregnancy, Thieme and Stratton, 167-178.

4. Wigard DL and Turiel J (1988) Long-term Effects of Exposure to Diethylstilbestrol. Western J Med 149:551-554.
5. Noller KL et al (1988) Increased occurrence of autoimmune disease among women exposed *in utero* to diethylstilbestrol. Fertility and Sterility 49:1080-1082.
6. Smith OW (1948) Diethylstilbestrol in the prevention and treatment of complications of pregnancy. Am J Ob Gyn 56:821-833.
7. Dieckmann WJ et al (1953) Does the administration of diethylstilbestrol during pregnancy have therapeutic value? Am J Ob Gyn 66:1062-1080.
8. The Wall St. Journal, Dec. 23, 1975.

Prostaglandin H Synthase Peroxidase Catalyzed Metabolism of Estrogens in Syrian Hamster and Rabbit Kidney

Gisela H. Degen

Summary

Since prostaglandin H synthase (PHS) peroxidase can catalyze metabolic activation of both stilbene and steroid estrogens *in vitro*, it is of relevance to study this enzymatic activity in a target tissue for their carcinogenic action. Microsomal preparations from male Syrian golden hamster kidney supplemented with arachidonic acid (ARA) convert radiolabeled diethylstilbestrol (DES) to the oxidative metabolite Z, Z-dienestrol (Z,Z-DIES) and to protein-bound product(s). PHS-mediated (ARA-dependent) oxidation of DES can be clearly demonstrated in incubations with microsomes from hamster medulla/papilla, but is negligible with those from cortex. This intraorgan distribution of PHS in hamster kidney resembles that observed for rabbit kidney. The data suggest that PHS-peroxidase can contribute to the metabolic activation of carcinogenic estrogens in hamster kidney but its precise role remains to elucidated.

Introduction

Several synthetic and natural estrogens are known to induce kidney tumors in male Syrian hamsters. It seems this process also involves a nonhormonal mechanism and is modulated by compounds that could affect oxidative metabolism (1). Since it has been shown that not only monooxygenases (MFO), but also purified prostaglandin H synthase (PHS) peroxidase catalyze metabolic activation of both stilbene and steroid estrogens *in vitro* (2), its activity in renal tissue is of considerable interest.

Results

Microsomes from male Syrian golden hamster kidney supplemented with arachidonic acid (ARA) convert radiolabeled diethylstilbestrol-(DES) to the oxidative metabolite Z,Z-dienestrol (Z,Z-DIES) and to protein-bound products.

Peroxides in microsomal preparations apparently also support DES-activation by PHS-peroxidase (incomplete inhibition of ARA-dependent DES-oxidation by PHS-cyclooxygenase inhibitors; "background" oxidation by nonsupplemented but not by heat-inactivated microsomes).

Microsomes prepared from dissected kidneys showed that enzyme activities involved in estrogen metabolism are unevenly distributed within the target tissue: MFO-mediated (NADPH-dependent) oxidation of DES, which accounts for the majority of metabolism in total kidney is found in the cortex (3). Conversely, PHS-catalyzed (ARA-dependent) oxidation of DES can be clearly demonstrated in incubations with microsomes from hamster medulla/papilla, but is not significant with those from the cortex. This preferential localization has been corroborated by Western-immunoblot analysis for PHS-protein (4). Interestingly, in incubations with renal microsomes from hamsters pretreated *in vivo* with DES (for 3 months), both the PHS- and the MFO- mediated oxidation of DES were decreased rather than increased (5).

Conclusions

Monooxygenases and peroxidases may act in concert to generate reactive estrogen intermediates: catechol metabolites of steroid estrogens made by MFO require further oxidation. The data suggest that PHS-peroxidase can contribute to the metabolic activation of carcinogenic estrogens in hamster kidney, but its exact role has yet to be clarified.

References

1. Li, JJ, Li SA (1987) Estrogen carcinogenesis in Syrian hamster tissues role of metabolism. Fed Proc 46:1858-1863.
2. Freyberger A, Degen GH (1989) Covalent binding to proteins of reactive intermediates resulting from prostaglandin H synthase-catalyzed oxidation of stilbene and steroid estrogens. J Biochem Toxicol 4:95-103.
3. Degen GH, Blaich G, Metzler M (1990) Multiple pathways for the oxidative metabolism of estrogens in Syrian hamster and rabbit kidney. J Biochem Toxicol 5:91-97.
4. Fischer B (1989) Gewinnung eines gegen Prostaglandin-H-Synthase gerichteten polyklonalen Antiserums and PHS-Nachweis in unterschiedlichen Geweben verschiedener Spezies. Diploma-Thesis, University of Wuerzburg.
5. Blaich G et al. (unpublished data).

Peroxidative Metabolism of Diethylstilbestrol in Ram Seminal Vesicle Cell Cultures: An *In Vitro* Model for Studies of Estrogen-Induced Genotoxicity

Gisela H. Degen and Jurgen Foth

Summary

The metabolism of diethylstilbestrol (DES) is characterized in ram seminal vesicle (SEMV) cells in culture. These cells contain prostaglandin H synthase (PHS) peroxidase but lack detectable monooxygenase (MFO) activity. HPLC analysis reveals that DES is converted to the peroxidative metabolite Z,Z-dienestrol (Z,Z-DIES) and to sulfate conjugates, but not to hydrozylated DES-metabolites or to glucuronides. The rates of oxidative metabolism and of phase II metabolism are similar in growing SEMV cells and in almost confluent cultures. Compounds known to modulate PHS activity increased (arachidonic acid) or decreased (indomethacin) Z,Z-DIES formation. The results clearly indicate that SEMV cells catalyze PHS-dependent oxidation of DES in the absence of detectable monooxygenase activity. These features and recent data indicating that DES can induce micronuclei in these cells make them an attractive *in vitro* model for further investigations of the role of PHS in mediating estrogen-induced genotoxicity.

Introduction

Prostaglandin H synthase (PHS) has been found to metabolize stilbene estrogens such as diethylstilbestrol (DES) as well as steroid estrogens *in vitro* to reactive intermediates (1). The enzyme occurs in several target cells and tissues, and PHS-peroxidase-dependent oxidation has been suggested to play a role in the neoplastic and genotoxic effects of stilbene and steroid estrogens (2). However, it still remains uncertain whether metabolic activation is required for mediating their adverse effects. Recently we derived a cell line from ram seminal vesicles

Table 1. Conversion of DES in SEMV cell cultures.

Incubation[a] of	Growing	Confluent	Growing
Cells x 10^5 at 0 h	7.4	14.2	8.0
Cells x 10^5 at 24 h	14.8	14.3	13.9
with DES (μM)	2	2	20
Product analysis[b]—(pmol total formed in 24 h)			
Sulfate conjugates	417 ± 121	553 ± 9	3500 ± 610
Z,Z-DIES			
(free)	162 ± 1	237 ± 57	1520 ± 170
(sulfated)	42	55	350
in Control[c]	69 ± 6	148 ± 4	1180 ± 140
Net Production	135	144	690
Rates of Product Formation[d] (nmol/24 h x 10^6 cells)			
Sulfates	0.28-0.56	0.39	2.52-4.38
Z,Z-DIES	0.09-0.18	0.10	0.50-0.86

[a]SEMV cells incubated with ^{14}C-DES in medium for 24 h;
[b]Metabolite analysis was carried out as described (4).
[c]Amount of Z,Z-DIES arising from nonenzymatic oxidation determined in medium controls without cells.
[d]Calculated from product formation by the given cell numbers at the start and end of 24 h incubation.

(SEMV cells) (3) to conduct studies on the PHS-mediated metabolism of estrogens in intact cells with the goal of relating this to an endpoint for genotoxicity such as micronucleus formation inducible in this *in vitro* model. Radiolabeled estrogen (^{14}C-DES) has been used to assess the drug-metabolizing capability of SEMV cell cultures; the metabolite profile has been analyzed by means of reverse phase HPLC with on-line radioactivity detection in incubation extracts and after enzymatic hydrolysis of conjugate fraction (4).

Results

The pattern of DES metabolites produced by SEMV cell cultures is rather simple: DES was metabolized to its peroxidative metabolite Z,Z-dienestrol (Z,Z-DIES) and to sulfate conjugates. The conjugate fraction is cleaved completely by sulfatase (but not by β-glucuronidase) and contained parent compound (present as E- and Z-isomer) and about 10% Z,Z-DIES. Hydroxylated DES-metabolites, which are characteristic for MFO-dependent oxidation of DES, were not detectable in either the free or conjugated metabolite fraction. The amounts of Z,Z-DIES and of sulfate conjugates clearly increased with time of incubation (data not shown). Conjugates were detected after 4 h whereas SEMV-cell mediated DES-oxidation can be masked after short incubation periods by nonenzymatic "background" production of Z,Z-DIES; its amount was clearly above control values at 24 h (Table 1).

The extent of DES conversion in cultured SEMV cells incubated for 24 h (with radiolabeled estrogen at 2 μM) was comparable for growing SEMV cells and for almost confluent cultures (Table 1). Increasing the substrate concentration 10-fold (DES 20 μM) resulted in an increase for the rates of conjugation (by a factor of 8-9) and DES-oxidation (factor of 5-6).

A comparison of the rate of arachidonic acid turnover to prostaglandins (8-17 nmol/24 h and 10^6 cells) (2) on one hand and DES oxidation on the other (Table 1) reveals that DES is cooxidized despite the presence of competing endogenous cosubstrates of PHS. Compounds expected to modulate PHS-dependent co-oxidation of DES increased (arachidonic acid) or inhibited (indomethacin 5 μM) Z,Z-DIES formation by 60 and 50%, respectively (4).

Since this treatment was genotoxic for SEMV cells it could be used to manipulate the extent of DES peroxidation. The DES concentrations used to investigate its metabolism were not acutely toxic for SEMV cells, but induced micronuclei (5).

References

1. Freyberger A, Degen GH (1989) Covalent binding of reactive intermediates resulting from prostaglandin H synthase-catalyzed oxidation of stilbene and steroid estrogens. J Biochem Toxicol 4:95-103.
2. Degen GH (1990) Role of prostaglandin-H synthase in mediating genotoxic and carcinogenic effects of estrogens. Environmental Health Perspectives 88:217-223.
3. Freyberger A, Schnitzler R, Schiffmann D, Degen GH (1987) Prostaglandin-H-synthase competent cells derived from ram seminal vesicles: a tool for studying cooxidation of xenobiotics. Molecular Toxicology 1:503-512.
4. Foth J, Degen GH (1992) Prostaglandin H synthase dependent metabolism of diethylstilbestrol by ram vesicle cell cultures. Arch Toxicol (in press).
5. Foth J, Schnitzler R, Jager M, Koob M, Metzler M, Degen GH (unpublished data).

In Vivo Effects of Progesterone on Human Breast 17β-Dehydrogenase and Epithelial Cells Mitotic Activities

Bruno de Lignieres, Jacques Barrat, Sabine Fournier, Kahil Nahoul, Gustavo Linares, and Genevieve Contesso

Summary

Conflicting results have suggested that progesterone effects on breast epithelial cell proliferation could differ *in vitro* and *in vivo*. This difference could be explained by higher 17β-dehydrogenase reductive activity in heterogeneous breast tissue, including fat and stroma, stimulated by progestins *in vivo*. In the present study, normal breast tissue samples were obtained from areas adjacent to benign lesions after 11 to 13 days of topical application on breast skin of either placebo, estradiol, or progesterone. Mean progesterone concentration within breast tissue was significantly increased in the progesterone-treated group in comparison with the two other groups, but estradiol/estrone ratio was decreased, although not significantly. Mitotic activity in lobular epithelial cells was significantly lower in the progesterone treated group. Eleven to 13 days of *in vivo* progesterone stimulation, similar to normal luteal phase duration or recommended progestin sequential treatment, did not lead to an increased 17β-dehydrogenase reductive activity, but actually reduced both mitotic activity in normal lobular epithelial cells.

Introduction

Many critical clinical decisions are now based on insufficient and conflicting data (1) regarding progesterone influence on normal epithelial breast cells (1-4). It has been suggested that progestins may stimulate the reductive 17β-hydroxysteroid dehydrogenase activity, thus converting estrone to more active estradiol (5), instead of converting estradiol to estrone as previously described (2).

In the present study, we tried to induce *in vivo* high stable tissue concentrations of either progesterone or estradiol, at least 10 days before breast

Table 1.

Treatment group	P/E_2	E_2/E_1	Mitotic index
Placebo $(n=9)$	5.2	1.48	0.1
Progesterone $(n=10)$	124.3**	0.86	0.04*
Estradiol $(n=13)$	0.88**	12.01**	0.2

*$p < 0.05$
**$p < 0.01$

surgery. For each patient, actual plasma and tissue concentrations of progesterone, estradiol, and estrone at time of mitotic counting were available for the first time.

Methods

Breast tissue samples were taken during surgery in premenopausal women with various benign breast diseases. Surgery was scheduled between days 11 and 13 of their menstrual cycle, before presumed ovulation and endogenous production of progesterone. Each patient was treated 11 to 13 days before surgery by daily percutaneous application on the breast of either a placebo gel, a gel containing progesterone, or a gel containing estradiol. Treatments were assigned at random and the study conducted blindly. Normal glandular breast tissue samples were obtained from areas adjacent to benign lesions. These samples were separated into two fragments, one for intratissue evaluation of steroids (6), and one for mitotic counting by light microscopy in areas showing normal lobular organization. Areas of fibrosis or adjacent cysts were excluded. The results were expressed as the mean number of mitotic figures observed by the same investigator per lovular unit in at least three different areas of the sample, ignoring treatment and hormonal values.

Results

The mean estradiol concentration in breast tissue was significantly higher (3,409 pg/g) in the estrogen-treated group than in the placebo (365 pg/g) and progesterone (523 pg/g)-treated groups. The mean progesterone concentration in breast tissue was significantly higher (69.1 ng/g) in the progesterone-treated group than in the placebo- (1.95 ng/g) and the estradiol (3 ng/g)-treated group. Mean progesterone/estradiol ratio (P/E_2), estradiol/estrone ratio (E_2/E_1), and mitotic index in each group are indicated in Table 1.

Discussion

Sustained high concentrations of progesterone in human breast tissue for 11 to 13 days do not lead to an increase in conversion of estrone to estradiol or to higher mitotic index. In the present study, high concentrations of progesterone in breast tissue coincide with the lowest reductive 17β-hydroxysteroid dehydrogenase activity as well as the lowest mitotic index. This does not imply however, that a shorter time of exposure to progesterone will have induced similar results.

References

1. McCarty D (1989) Proliferative stimuli in the normal breast: estrogens or progestins ? Hum Pathol, 20:1137-1138.
2. Gompel A, Malet C, Spritzer P, Lalrdrie JP, Kuttenn F Mauvais-Jarvis P (1986) Progestin effects on cell proliferation and 17β-hydroxysteroid dehydrogenase activity in normal human breast cells in culture. J Clin Endocrinol Meta, 63:1174-1180.
3. Gambrell RD (1990) Estrogen therapy and breast cancer. Int J Fertil, 36:202-204.
4. Barrat J, Lignieres B de, Marpeau L, Larue L, Fournier S., Nahout K, Linares, G, Giorgi M, Contesso G (199) Effect in vivo de l'administration local de progesterone sur l'activite mitotique des galactophores humains. J Gynecol Obstet Biol Reprod, 19:269-274.
5. Coldham N, James V (1990) A possible mechanism for increased breast cell proliferation by progestins through increased reductive 17β-hydroxysteroid dehydrogenase activity. Int J Cancer, 45:174-178.
6. Boevr J de, Vermeugen C, van Malle G, Vanderkerckhove D (1983) Steroid concentrations in serum, glandular breast tissue and breast cyst fluid of control and progesterone treated patients. In "Endocrinology of Cystic Breast Disease" Angeli A. (ed), Raven press, New York, p. 93-99.

DNA Adduct Profiles in Hamster Kidney Following Chronic Exposure to Various Carcinogenic and Noncarcinogenic Estrogens

Richard P. DiAugustine, Michael Walker, Sara Antonia Li, and Jonathan J. Li

Summary

The generation of specific estrogen-induced DNA adduct modifications in the hamster kidney following chronic exposure has been reported. Moreover, these covalent DNA alterations produced by estrogens have been suggested to play a critical role in estrogen-induced renal tumorigenesis in this species. Employing the P-1 nuclease postlabeling methods, we have studied the generation of DNA adduct modifications by various strongly carcinogenic (Ethinylestradiol, EE) and noncarcinogenic (17α-estradiol, β-dienestrol, indanestrol) estrogens and compared these data to untreated or cholesterol-treated castrated male hamsters at 5.0 and 7.0 months. No significant differences were found between DNA adduct profiles ($\sim$ 10 spots) in these control groups and those generated from any of the estrogenic compounds tested, whether carcinogenic or not. These data coupled with the very poor metabolism of Moxestrol (11β-methoxy EE) seen in the hamster kidney weaken the view for a significant role for renal DNA adduct alterations, which appears evidently indigenous, in the estrogen-induced neoplastic transformation of the hamster kidney.

Introduction

Estrogens are considered to have a causative role in tumor formation in a number of mammalian species. Chronic administration of estrogens induces a high incidence of renal tumors in male Syrian hamsters. This experimental model has been studied intensely to understand the biochemical basis for hormone-induced neoplasia (1). One concept holds that renal tumorigenesis occurs as a result of the genotoxic effects of estrogens or their metabolites (2). In one series of studies, it was shown that various carcinogenic estrogens modify the hamster kidney covalent DNA adduct profile as determined by ^{32}P-postlabeling (3-5). In the present study we examine structurally diverse estrogens, possessing strong-, weak-, or nontumorigenic activities, for their capacity to influence renal DNA adducts. The data are evaluated against the tumorigenic, hormonal, and catechol-forming properties of the different estrogens.

Methods

Hormone pellets (20 mg) were implanted s.c. in the adult male castrated Syrian golden hamsters (90-100 g) as described previously (6). New pellets were implanted every 2.5 months. Control animals received cholesterol or no pellets.

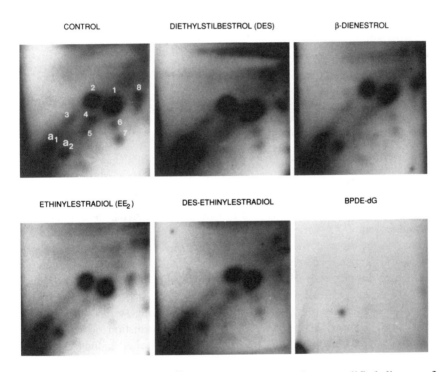

Fig. 1. TLC adduct maps of ^{32}P-postlabeled (P1-nuclease-modified digests of DNA. The DNA was obtained from kidneys of castrated male Syrian hamsters treated continuously for 5 months with cholesterol (control) or various estrogens as indicated. The major DNA adducts have been designated a_1, a_2, and 1-8. Postlabeling of 7R, 8S, 9S-trihydroxy-10R-(N^2-deoxyguanosyl-3^1-phosphate) 7,8,9,10-tetrahydrobenzo[a]pyrene (BDPE-dg standard, Midwest Research Institute, Kansas City, MO) yielded a single adduct as shown in the lower right panel. The solvents used were (D1) 1.0 M sodium phosphate, pH 6.5; (D3) 4.0 M lithium formate, 7.0 M urea, pH 3.6; (D4) 1.2 M lithium chloride, 0.5 M.

Table 1. Estrogenic and tumorigenic activity of certain steroidal and stilbene estrogens in the hamster kidney.[1]

Estrogens	Competitive Binding (%)[2,4]	Induction Prog. Receptor[3,4]	Number of Animals With Tumors/n	Percent of Tumor Incidence
17β-Estradiol	90 ± 1	49 ± 6	10/10	100
DES	90 ± 1	52 ± 3	10/10	100
Moxestrol	85 ± 2	60 ± 2	10/10	100
Estriol	84 ± 2	35 ± 3	4/7	57
Ethinylestradiol (EE)	90 ± 1	56 ± 3	2/20	10
17α-Estradiol	84 ± 3	6 ± 1	0/8	0
βDienestrol	8 ± 1	ND[5]	0/10	0
Indanestrol	78 ± 4	29 ± 5	0/8	0
EE + DES	90 ± 2	54 ± 3	0/10	0

[1]Duration of estrogen treatments was 9.0-9.5 months. Pellets were implanted every 2.5 months.
[2]Competitive binding for ER was carried out in hamster renal tumor cytosol at 100-fold excess using 5 nM [^{3}H]-estradiol.
[3]Data expressed as fmol/mg cytosol protein.
[4]Values represent mean ± SEM.
[5]ND, not detectable.

After 5 and 7 months of treatment kidneys were removed, decapsulated, and stored frozen. DNA was isolated and digested as previously described (7). An aliquot of the digest corresponding to approximately 0.5 μg DNA was analyzed by HPLC to quantify deoxyguanosine and monitor digestion. DNA adducts were determined by nuclease P1-modified ^{32}P-postlabeling analysis (8). The solvents for TLC maps (PEI-cellulose) are given in the legend of Figure 1. Estrogen-receptor competition binding and quantitation of progesterone receptor were performed as previously described (9, 10). The formation of catechols was assessed by HPLC using [^{14}C]-estrogen substrata after kidney microsomal incubations.

Results and Conclusion

As shown by the TLC maps in Figure 1, multiple DNA adducts were observed by ^{32}P-postlabeling digests of DNA from kidneys of control and estrogen-treated hamsters. Chronic treatment with either strongly carcinogenic (17β-estradiol, DES), weakly carcinogenic (ethinylestradiol), or noncarcinogenic (β-dienestrol, 17α-estradiol, indanestrol) estrogens did not appear to alter the covalent DNA adduct profiles seen in untreated hamster kidneys. Moreover, DNA profile were

Table 2. Catechol estrogen formation of various steroidal and stilbene estrogens in liver and kidney microsomes of castrated Syrian hamsters.

	Catechol estrogen formation (pmoles catechol formed/min/mg protein)	
Radiolabeled Estrogens	Liver	Kidney
[4-^{14}C]-Estrone	228 ± 12	4.3 ± 0.30
[4-^{14}C]-17β-Estradiol	504 ± 31	1.4 ± 0.20
[4-^{14}C]-Ethinylestradiol	293 ± 29	0.1 ± 0.05
[^{3}H]-Moxestrol	241 ± 35	0.02 ± 0.01
[2-^{14}C]-Diethylstilbestrol	326 ± 14	2.9 ± 0.30

essentially the same in all hormone-treated groups regardless of the type of estrogen used. Receptor binding and tumorigenic properties of the various estrogens evaluated are compared in Table 1. The TLC solvents used for the adduct maps were designed to display major adducts, and it is expected that under these conditions some minor adducts were not visualized. The findings confirm that kidneys of untreated hamsters accumulate "indigenous" covalent DNA adducts previously reported (12). In light of these data, the significance of estrogen-induced DNA (lipophilic) adducts in hormonal carcinogenesis is doubtful.

It is also notable that we could not correlate tumorigenicity with the capacity of the estrogen to form reactive catechol intermediates. As shown in Table 2, kidney microsomes are much less active than hamster liver microsomes in converting the labeled estrogens to corresponding catechols. The potent tumorigenic estrogen Moxestrol (11p-methoxyl ethinylestradiol) in particular is very poorly metabolized to catechols *in vitro* by kidney microsomes. Therefore, it is unlikely that the tumorigenic potency of estrogens derives from their capacity to form reactive metabolites.

References

1.   Li JJ, Li SA (1990) Estrogen carcinogenesis in hamster tissues; a critical review. Endocrine Rev 11:524-531.
2.   Li JJ, Li SA (1987) Estrogen carcinogenesis in Syrian hamster tissues: role of metabolism. Fed Proc. 16:1858-1853.

3.   Liehr JG, Randerath K, Randerath E (1985) Target organ-specific covalent DNA damage preceding diethylstilbestrol-induced carcinogenesis. Carcinogenesis (Lond.) 6:1067-1069.

4.   Liehr JG, Avitts TA, Randerath E, Randerath D (1986) Estrogen-induced endogenous DNA adduction: possible mechanism of hormonal cancer. Proc. Natl. Acad. Sci. USA 83:5301-5305.

5.   Liehr JG, Hall ER, Avitts TA, Randerath E, Randerath K (1987) Localization of estrogen-induced DNA adducts and cytochrome P-450 activity at the site of renal carcinogenesis in the hamster kidney. Cancer Res. 47:2156-2169.

6.   Li JJ, Kirkman H, Hunter RL (1969) Sex difference and gonadal hormone influence on Syrian hamster kidney esterase isoenzymes. J Histochem Cytochem 17:386-393.

7.   Jahnke GD, Thompson CL, Walker MP, Gallagher JE, Lucier GW, DiAugustine RP (1990 Multiple DNA adducts in lymphocytes of smokers and nonsmokers determined by ^{32}P-postlabeling analysis. Carcinogenesis (Lond.) 11:205-211.

8.   Reddy MV, Randerath K (1986) Nuclease P1-mediated enhancement of sensitivity of ^{32}P-postlabeling test for structurally diverse DNA adducts. Carcinogenesis (Lond.) 7:1543-1551.

9.   Li JJ, Talley DJ, Li SA, Villee CA (1974) An estrogen binding protein in the renal cytosol of the intact, castrated, and estrogenized golden hamster. Endocrinology 95:1134-1141.

10.   Li JJ, LI SA (1981) Estrogen-induced progesterone receptor in the Syrian hamster kidney II. Modulation by synthetic progestins. Endocrinology 108.

11.   Li JJ, DiAugustine RD, Walker MP, Haaf H, Li SA (1993) DNA Adduct modifications in hamster kidney following chronic treatment to various carcinogenic and noncarcinogenic estrogens. Carcinogenesis, in press.

12.   Randerath, K., Liehr, JG, Gladek A, Randerath E (1989) Age-dependent covalent DNA alterations (I-compounds) in rodent tissues: species, tissue and sex specificities. Mutation Res 219:121-133.

Hormone-Dependent Activation of c-Ki-ras in N-Methyl-N-Nitrosourea (MNU)-Induced Mouse Mammary Tumors

Raphael C. Guzman, Rebecca C. Osborn, Shigeki Miyamoto, Ramasamy Sakthivel, Soo-In Hwang, and Satyabrata Nandi

Summary

Mouse mammary epithelial cells (MMEC) cultured in the presence of mammogenic hormones (progesterone and prolactin), treated with MNU, and transplanted to syngeneic mice developed a high frequency of hyperplastic alveolar nodules (HAN) and carcinomas. The majority of these transformants had activated c-Ki-ras with a specific point mutation in the twelfth codon (G35—A35). In contrast, MMEC cultured with EGF developed a low frequency of ductal hyperplasias. MMEC cultured with lithium developed a high frequency of HAN and carcinomas, but no c-Ki-ras has been detected. To determine whether these findings parallel mammary carcinogenesis in vivo, mice were pituitary isografted to increase their levels of progesterone and prolactin and injected with MNU. Greater than 90% of the treated mice developed mammary carcinomas and the majority of these cancers had an identical phenotype to those induced in vitro in the presence of progesterone and prolactin. The majority (75%) of the cancers induced in vivo also had the identical point mutation in the c-Ki-ras protooncogene to those found in the in vitro studies. These studies suggest that the hormonal milieu at the time of carcinogen exposure affects not only the incidence and phenotype of the mammary lesions, but also the molecular events associated with mammary carcinogenesis.

Introduction

Ovarian and pituitary hormones play an essential role in mouse mammary carcinogenesis, being required for the proliferation and differentiation of the mammary epithelial cells that are at risk to the carcinogenic insult. However, the role of hormones in determining the phenotype of the mammary cancers and the mechanisms underlying the molecular events associated with mammary carcinogenesis are poorly understood.

In order to attempt to achieve an understanding of the role of hormones in mouse mammary carcinogenesis, we have developed a serum-free culture system in which mouse mammary epithelial cells (MMEC) can be grown, be induced to differentiate, and be neoplastically transformed with chemical carcinogens. In this culture system MMEC grow inside a three-dimensional collagen matrix. The MMEC can be grown with a variety of mitogens including mammogenic hormones, growth factors, lipid metabolites, and lithium ions. We have used this culture system to transform MMEC to both preneoplastic and neoplastic states with either the direct acting alkylating chemical carcinogen MNU or the polycyclic hydrocarbon 7,12 dimethylbenz(a)anthracene, which must be metabolized to its proximate carcinogenic form (1,2).

Transformation is assayed in this system by transplanting the carcinogen treated cells from cultures to the parenchyma-free mammary fat pads of syngeneic mice. Resultant outgrowths are scored as to the morphological development of preneoplastic or neoplastic lesions.

We have observed that the types of mammary lesions induced in this *in vitro* transformation system are greatly influenced by the mitogens present around the time of MNU carcinogen treatment. When MMEC are grown with either EGF or *b*-FGF predominately ductal hyperplasias are induced. However, if MMEC are grown with the mammogenic hormones progesterone and prolactin (P+Prl) or lithium, then predominately hyperplastic alveolar nodules and carcinomas are induced. Additionally, the majority of the carcinomas induced in MMEC cultured in P+Prl are carcinomas with extensive squamous metaplasia.

When activation of protooncogenes was examined in these different types of lesions, we observed the activation of c-Ki-*ras* in the majority of the hyperplastic nodules and carcinomas that were induced in the presence P+Prl, but did not detect this gene mutation in mammary lesions induced with other mitogens (3). In order to determine the biological relevance of the *in vitro* transformation studies to mouse mammary carcinogenesis *in vivo*, we report here parallel *in vivo* studies. Five-week-old female BALB/C mice were assigned to four different experimental groups: A. untreated; B. pituitary isografted at 5 weeks of age; C. pituitary isografted at 5 weeks of age and treated I.V. with 50μg/g MNU; D. treated with MNU. Pituitary isografts were used to produce high levels of P+Prl to simulate our *in vitro* studies. We examined whether the carcinomas induced would have similar morphologies to those induced *in vitro* and whether the same point mutation would be found in c-Ki-*ras*.

Results

Mammary carcinomas occurred only in mice that received a pituitary isograft and MNU treatment (Group C). After 7 months of treatment, 90% of the mice developed carcinomas. The histopathology of 20 carcinomas was examined and of these, 75% were carcinomas with squamous metaplasia. The DNA of 12 carcinomas was amplified using polymerase chain reaction followed by hybridization to allele-specific oligonucleotides of either the wild-type c-Ki-*ras*

(G35) or the mutated c-Ki-*ras* (A35). A specific point mutation (G35—A35) in the c-Ki-*ras* protooncogene was observed in 75% of the carcinomas.

Discussion

We have demonstrated that MNU is a potent mammary carcinogen in mice and have confirmed that elevated levels of mammogenic hormones are essential for mouse mammary carcinogenesis (4). The majority of the carcinomas had an identical morphology and the identical point mutation to that of carcinomas induced in the presence of P+Prl *in vitro*. The present study strengthens the biological significance of our *in vitro* transformation system and provides additional evidence for our hypothesis that the mitogens present around the time of carcinogen treatment greatly influence the phenotype and the molecular events in mammary carcinogenesis. These parallel studies using the *in vivo* and *in vitro* systems may help to dissect out the role of hormones in mammary carcinogenesis under physiological as well as defined experimental conditions.

Acknowledgment

This work was supported by Grant CA05388-31A1 from the National Cancer Institute.

References

1. Guzman RC, Osborn RC, Bartley JC, Imagawa W, Asch BB, Nandi S (1987) *In vitro* transformation of mouse mammary epithelial cells grown serum-free inside collagen gels Cancer Res 47:275-280.
2. Miyamoto S, Guzman RC, Osborn RC, Nandi S (1988) Neoplastic transformation of mouse mammary epithelial cells by *in vitro* exposure to *N*-methyl-*N*-nitrosurea. Proc Natl Acad Sci USA 85:477-481.
3. Miyamoto S, Sukumar S, Guzman RC, Osborn RC, Nandi S (1990) Transforming *c-Ki-ras* mutation is a preneoplastic event in mouse mammary carcinogenesis induced in vitro by *N*-methyl-*N*-nitrosourea 10:1593-1599.
4. Medina D (1988) The preneoplastic state in mouse mammary tumorigenesis. Carcinogenesis 9:1113-1119.

Growth Hormone Regulation of the c-*myc* Gene During Sex-Differentiated Rat Liver Carcinogenesis

Inger Porsch-Hällström, Jan-Åke Gustafsson, and Agneta Blanck

Summary

The expression of the c-*myc* gene was analyzed at different stages of rat liver carcinogenesis in the resistant hepatocyte model (RH-model). During promotion of diethylnitrosamine (DEN)-initiated Wistar rats with 2-acetylaminofluorene (2-AAF) and partial hepatectomy (PH), the hepatic c-*myc* expression was increased in males, but not in females, from one day after PH. Continuous growth hormone (GH) infusion decreased the expression to the level in females. A higher c-*myc* mRNA level compared with the respective surrounding livers was observed in nodules from males isolated 6 weeks. This elevated c-*myc* RNA level was also seen in 8 and >11 months after DEN treatment and in hepatomas, while in females an increased expression was noted only in >11 month nodules and hepatomas. GH infusion to nodule bearing males decreased c-*myc* mRNA levels in surrounding livers, and in nodules 8 but not 11 months after DEN.

Introduction

Growth of enzyme-altered foci in the RH-model is sex differentiated ($\male > \female$) and males have a markedly shorter latency period for tumor development than females (1,2). This dimorphism is due to the sex-differentiated secretion pattern of GH from the pituitary, and "feminization" of the secretory pattern by continuous GH administration to males during promotion results in a decrease focal growth to the female level (1). In search for mediators of this response on the cellular level we observed that during the period when the sex differences in growth rate are first manifested, the expression of the c-*myc* gene was increased several fold in males, but not in females or in noninitiated males (3). The c-*myc* gene is shown to be involved in the regulation of cell proliferation and differentiation and has been implicated in the etiology of several malignancies (4), including overexpression and amplification of the gene in liver tumors in man and experimental animals (5-7).

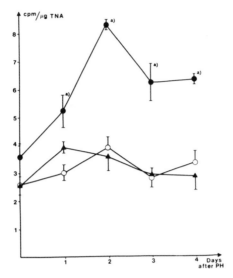

Fig. 1. Expression of the c-*myc* gene in male (●), female (○) and GH-treated male (▲) Wistar rats during promotion in the RH-model. Mean ± SEM of four animals per point.

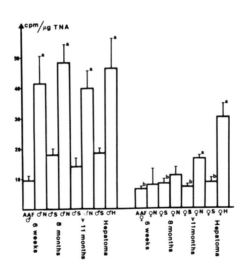

Fig. 2. Expression of the c-*myc* gene in male and female hepatomas, in individual nodules 8 and 11 months after DEN initiation compared with respective surrounding tissue, and in pooled nodules 6 weeks after DEN compared with uninitiated 2-AAF-treated animals, as no nodule-free surrounding can be collected at this time. Mean ± SEM of 3 to 6 points.

Table 1. Effects of growth hormone on the expression of the c-*myc* gene in nodules and surrounding livers in male rats 8 and 11 months after initiation in the RH-model.

Time after initiation	RH	c-*myc* expression (cpm/μg TNA)[a]	
		Surrounding	Nodules
8 months	-	18.0 ± 2.0	48.3 ± 7.9
	+	11.6 ± 1.1	15.9 ± 1.8
11 months	-	18.6 ± 1.7	56.3 ± 13.4
	+	11.6 ± 0.8	42.5 ± 5.0

[a]Data expressed as the mean $\pm$ SEM.

Results

The expression of the c-*myc* gene, analyzed by hybridization of RNA in samples of total nucleic acids (TNA) to ^{35}UTP-labeled complementary *myc* RNA in solution (3), increased in males, but not in females, from 1 day after PH in the RH-model. Continuous GH infusion to males during promotion down-regulated the expression to the female level (Fig. 1). The expression of the gene was increased when compared with the respective surrounding liver in male nodules isolated 6 weeks and 8 and >11 months after DEN initiation and in hepatomas, while in females an elevated expression could only be observed in >11 month nodules and in tumors (Fig. 2). Continuous infusion of GH to nodule-bearing males for 1 week before sacrifice feminized c-*myc* expression in the surrounding tissue, and downregulated nodular c-*myc* 8 but not 11 months after initiation (Table 1).

Conclusions

The results show a GH-dependent sex difference in the expression of the c-*myc* gene during promotion and parts of progression in the RH model. These findings might reflect a role for the c-*myc* gene in liver carcinogenesis, of possible importance for the occurrence of sex differences in hepatocarcinogenesis.

References

1. Blanck A, Hansson T, Eriksson LC, Gustafsson J-Å (1987) Growth hormone modifies the growth rate of enzyme altered hepatic foci in male rats treated according to the resistant hepatocyte model. Carcinogenesis 8:1585-1589.

2. Blanck A, Hansson T, Gustafsson J-Å, Eriksson LC (1986) Pituitary grafts modify sex differences in liver tumor formation in the rat following initiation with diethylnitrosamine and different promotion regimens. Carcinogenesis 7:981-985.

3. Porsch Hällström I, Gustafsson J-Å, Blanck A (1989) Effects of growth hormone on the expression of c-*myc* and c-*fos* during early stages of sex-differentiated rat liver carcinogenesis in the resistant hepatocyte model. Carcinogenesis 10:2339-2343.*

4. Cole MD (1986) The *myc* oncogene: its role in transformation and differentiation. Ann Rev Genet 20:361-384.

5. Gu JR (1988) Molecular aspects of human hepatic carcinogenesis. Carcinogenesis 9:697-703.

6. Makino R, Hayashi K, Sato S, Sugimura T (1984) Expression of the c-Ha-*ras* and c-*myc* genes in rat liver tumors. Biochem Biophys Res Commun 119:1096-1102.

7. Nagy P, Evarts RP, Marsden E, Roach J, Thorgeirsson SS (1988) Cellular distribution of c-*myc* transcripts during chemical hepatocarcinogenesis. Cancer Res 48:5522-5527.

*Some of the data have previously been published (Ref. 3) and are used with the permission of Oxford University Press.

Fetal Stromal Cells Produce a TGF that Elicits Hyperplasia in Adult Mammary Epithelium

Howard L. Hosick, Tracy G. Ram, Sylvia A. Oliver, Vasundara Venkateswaran, and Takuya Kanazawa

Summary

Fetal salivary mesenchyme (SM) transplanted into adult mouse mammary gland stimulates intense local epithelial hyperplasia and these areas are particularly vulnerable to transformation. We have developed a culture model that successfully duplicates *in vitro* the essential features of this system. SM cells increase the growth rate of mammary epithelium in collagen gels and provoke colony formation of NRK clone 49 and mammary epithelial cells in soft agarose (up to 51 % colony-forming efficiency). A molecule in SM cell-line conditioned medium competes for EGF receptors; it can be removed from conditioned medium by immunoprecipitation with anti-EGF antibodies. EGF antibodies also remove the growth-stimulatory activity. SDS-PAGE of radiolabeled immuno-precipitates resulted in a single band with an apparent MW of 15 Kd. Thus, the stimulatory molecule is considerably larger than either EGF or TGF-α. Further characterization of the TGF is in progress. Similar studies are also underway with adult mammary stromal cells. (Supported by NIH grant CA-46885.)

Introduction

When fetal salivary mesenchyme (SM) is transplanted into adult mouse mammary glands, the local epithelium responds by proliferating intensely to form ductal alveolar nodules (DANs) (1). When DAN-bearing mice (either intact or ovariectomized) are injected with dimethyl benz(a)anthracene or infected with mouse mammary tumor virus, the incidence of adenocarcinomas is much greater within DANs than in adjacent gland areas (2). These observations implicate stroma-induced changes in epithelial characteristics during mammary tumorigenesis *in vivo*. We have utilized tissue-culture procedures to determine

Table 1. Colony formation by normal mammary epithelial cells in soft agarose in response to fetal mesenchyme cells.

Stromal Cell Type	% Colony Formation (after two weeks)
None (10% serum)	0.0
Fetal salivary mesenchyme	13.8 ± 1.8
Fetal mammary fat pad	7.8 ± 1.1

if SM cells produce growth factor(s) that could account for the hyperplastic response of adjacent epithelium *in vivo*. We have begun to characterize one such molecule.

Results

SM cell lines were established. Conditioned medium from these lines stimulated sprouting and proliferation of mammary epithelial organoids suspended within collagen gels (3). A molecule in conditioned medium competed for EGF-receptor sites on mammary epithelial cell membranes. Therefore, we tested further the properties of the EGF-related molecule in conditioned medium.

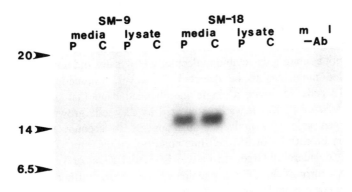

Fig. 1. SDA-PAGE of anti-EGF immunoprecipitated samples collected from [^{35}S]-methionine/cysteine-labeled cultures grown on plastic (P) or collagen gel (C) substrata. Labeled medium and cell lysates were immunoprecipitated with rabbit anti-mouse EGF antiserum and electrophoresed in 18% polyacrylamide gels under reducing conditons. Analyses of early (SN-9) and later passage (SM-18) cells are shown. Other methods as in Ram et al. (3).

Table 2. Colony formation by NRK cells in soft agarose in response to adult mammary fibroblasts.

Source of Conditioned Medium	% Colony Formation (± sem)	Colony Diameter Range (μm)
None (defined medium only)	0.0	
Virgin gland fibroblasts	1.6 ± 1.8	18 (10-30)
Pregnant gland fibroblasts	8.9 ± 1.0	20 (10-30)

By definition, transforming growth factors stimulate the anchorage-independent growth of NRK clone 49 cells (4). Conditioned medium stimulated up to 50% of NRK cells to form colonies in soft agarose. We also tested for the ability of mammary epithelial cells to grow in suspension in soft agarose in response to fetal mesenchyme [Table 1; (5)]. SM provoked a significant response in mammary epithelial cells as well, as did another fetal mesenchyme (from mammary fat pad precursor) that induces hyperplasia in adult mammary glands *in vivo* (2). SM cell-line conditioned medium treated with anti-EGF antibodies lost most of its ability to stimulate growth of mammary cells in collagen gels and NRK cells in soft agarose. The substance(s) that competes for EGF receptor sites was also completely removed (3). Immunoprecipitates were prepared from [^{35}S]-methione/cysteine-labeled cultures of SM cells and their conditioned medium, and analyzed by SDS-PAGE (Fig. 1). Very early-passage cells did not contain a detectable molecule. Cell lysates did not contain enough radiolabeled molecules to be detected. However, immunoprecipitates from passage 18 cells contained a single radiolabeled band that migrated with an apparent MW of 15 Kd. It was synthesized by SM cells grown on both plastic and collagen gel. This molecule thus appears to account for the growth-stimulatory bioactivity of SM cell-line conditioned medium. This EGF-related protein is considerably larger than either EGF (6.1 KDa) or TGF-α (5.7 KDa). It may be a form of the TGF-α precursor protein (6). Further characterization of this molecule is underway.

We have begun tests to determine if mammary stromal cells also produce TGFs under specific conditions. In one such experiment shown in Table 2, fibroblastoid cells were isolated from mammary glands of virgin and pregnant mice. Conditioned medium was isolated from these cells and added to cultures of NRK cells in soft agarose. Both cell populations stimulated some colony formation, but medium from cells of pregnant animals was about five times more potent. We conclude from these experiments: (1) stromal cells of the adult mouse gland can produce one or more potent TGFs in culture, and (2) production of this TGF(s) coincides with intense growth of adjacent epithelium *in vivo*.

Discussion

We have devised culture procedures in which mammary epithelial cell responsiveness to stromal cells mimics that observed *in vivo*. Using this system, we have demonstrated that fetal mesenchyme tissue that provokes hyperplasia and preneoplasia *in vivo* produces transforming growth factor(s) that are likely to mediate its effects on epithelium. Preliminary results now indicate that certain populations of mammary stromal cells produce functionally analogous factors. We believe that these observations provide solid evidence about how stroma can contribute actively to early tumorigenic events.

References

1. Sakakura T, Sakagami Y, Nishizuka Y (1979) Persistence of responsiveness of adult mouse mammary gland to induction by embryonic mesenchyme. Devel Biol 72:201-210.
2. Sakakura T, Sakagami Y, Nishizuka Y (1981) Accelerated mammary cancer development by fetal salivary mesenchyme isografted to adult mouse mammary epithelium. J Natl Cancer Inst 66:953-959.
3. Ram TG, Venkateswaran V, Oliver SO, et al (1991) Transforming growth factor related to epidermal growth factor is expressed by fetal mouse salivary mesenchyme cells in culture. Biochem Biophys Res Comm 175:37-43.
4. DeLarco JE, Todaro J (1970) Growth factors from murine sarcoma virus-transformed cells. Proc Natl Acad Sci USA 75:4001-4005.
5. Kanazawa T and Hosick H (1991) Stimulation of anchorage dependent and anchorage independent growth of primary mammary epithelial cells by fetal salivary mesenchyme cells. Proc Am Assoc Can Res 32:43.
6. Ignotz RA, Kelly B, Davis RJ, et al (1986) Biologically active precursor for transforming growth factor type α, released by retrovirally transformed cells. Proc Natl Acad Sci USA 83:6307-6311.

Induction of Catechol Estrogen Formation by Indole-3-Carbinol

Peter H. Jellinck, Jon J. Michnovicz, and H. Leon Bradlow

Summary

Dietary indoles in cruciferous vegetables induce cytochrome P-450 isozymes and have prevented tumors in various animal models. Because estradiol (E_2) metabolism is also cytochrome. P-450-mediated and linked to breast cancer risk, indoles may similarly reduce the incidence of estrogen-responsive tumors in humans. We have examined the effect of one of these, indoles-3-carbinol (IC) in female Sprague-Dawley rats for induction of hepatic estradiol 2-hydroxylase and also on estradiol-2-hydroxylation in male volunteers given IC (500 mg daily for 1 wk). In both cases, it produced a large increase in the conversion of E_2 to its less active 2-hydroxylated metabolite and therefore has the potential to provide a new chemopreventive approach to estrogen-dependent diseases in humans. The dimer of IC, to which it is converted in the stomach, was effective at much lower doses and was more active when injected into rats i.p. Evidence is provided that the induced isozyme is cytochrome P-450IA2.

Introduction

A wealth of animal and human data have provided evidence that estrogens play a role in the initiation and/or maintenance of mammary tumors. The metabolism of estradiol (E_2), which is primarily oxidative, yields estrone (E_1) and consists of two alternative hydroxylative pathways: hydroxylation at the C-2/4 and at the 16α positions. The products of these competing reactions have markedly different biological properties. The 16α-hydroxyestrogens-estriol and 16α-hydroxyestrone (16α-OHE)-demonstrate uterotrophic activity comparable to that of the parent compound while the ring A hydroxylated products—the catechol estrogens—are rapidly inactivated but may have a role in neuroendocrine events. In earlier studies (1,2), it was shown that 16α-hydroxylation of estrogens was increased by 50% in women with breast and endometrial cancer and this reaction was also elevated in strains of mice with high incidence of tumors and low in strains with low cancer incidence. This risk was ascribed to the unique property of 16α-OHE, to form covalent adducts with amino groups on biological macromolecules. Thus, shifting estrogen metabolism away from the formation of this product towards that of catechol estrogens should decrease cancer incidence, and this has been found to be true for endometrial cancer in female smokers in whom the 2-hydroxylation of E_2 is elevated by 50-70% (3).

Epidemiological research suggests that increased consumption of cruciferous vegetables (e.g., broccoli, cabbage, and brussels sprouts) reduced cancer incidence (4) and this effect has been ascribed to the ability of compounds such as indole-3-carbinol (IC) in such vegetables to induce specific cyt. P-450s (5). For this reason we have tested IC and its dimer (diIC), to which IC is converted in the stomach, for their effect on the induction of estradiol 2-hydroxylase in female rat liver microsomes. We have also looked for an effect on the 2-hydroxylation of E_2 in humans and provide some evidence that the induced isozyme is cytochrome P-450IA2.

Results

1. Dietary indole-3-carbinol (IC), present in cruciferous vegetables, increased the rate of 2-hydroxylation of estradiol in both humans and rats. 2. The dimer of IC was more active than IC and was still effective when administered intraperitoneally, unlike the parent compound. 3. In the rat, the increase in estrogen metabolism by IC could be prevented by prior treatment with ethionine. 4. The change in metabolic pattern of ^{14}C-androstenedione induced in female rats by IC or diIC was the same as that produced by isosafrole, a known inducer of cyt. P-450IA2.

Conclusions

The results indicate that IC is a potent inducer of the 2-hydroxylation of E_2 in both humans and rats when administered orally and are consistent with previous reports on the inducing properties of dietary indoles in cruciferous vegetables (5). This hydroxylation of E_2 has been observed in several tissues (6) and may occur in an estrogen-responsive tissue such as the breast. We have also found recently that IC administered in a semisynthetic diet to female C3H mice significantly reduced the incidence of spontaneous mammary tumors.

Dietary IC, on exposure to low pH, undergoes dimerization to DiIC and also polymerization (5,7). The conversion of orally administered IC to diIC in the stomach is supported by our findings that the dimer was effective at much lower doses and was more active when injected into rats i.p. It has been proposed (8, 9) that the products of IC are able to bind to the aryl hydrocarbon receptor, thereby inducing P-4501 isozymes. Our present findings indicate that the primary isozyme induced is P-450IA2 because liver microsomes from IC- or diIC-treated rats gave the same metabolic pattern with ^{14}C-androstenedione as did microsomes from animals treated with isosafrole (induces cyt. P-450IA2), but not MC (induces cyt. P-450IA1) (10). This isozyme has also been shown to be involved in the conversion of E_2 to it 2- and 4-hydroxylated derivatives (11), and we hope to confirm these results by immunochemical analysis.

The relative flux of estrogens through the competing C-2 and C-16α pathways is linked to risk for estrogen-dependent tumors in humans (3,8,12). The present study indicates that a readily available dietary indole (IC) can enhance estradiol metabolism and increase its 2-hydroxylation. This modulation may presage new therapeutic strategies directed at reducing the risk for estrogen-dependent diseases such as breast cancer.

Acknowledgments

This work was supported by grants MT 7688 from the Medical Research Council of Canada (P.H.J.), CA 39734, CA 44458, and CTR 2016 (H.L.B. and J.J.M.).

References

1. Fishman J, Schneider J, Hershcopf RJ, and Bradlow HL (1984) Increased estrogen-16α-hydroxylase activity in women with breast and endometrial cancer. J Steroid Biochem 20:1077-1081.
2. Bradlow HL, Hershcopf RJ, Martucci CP, and Fishman J (1985) Estradiol 16α-hydroxylation in the mouse correlates with mammary tumor incidence and presence of murine mammary tumor virus: A possible model for the hormonal etiology of breast cancer. Proc Natl Acad Sci U.S.A. 82:6295-6299.
3. Lesko SM, Rosenberg L, Kaufman DW et al (1985) Cigarette smoking and the risk of endometrial cancer. N Engl J Med 313:593-596.
4. Young TB and Wolf DA (1988) Case-control study of proximal and distal colon cancer and diet in Wisconsin. Int J Cancer 42:167-175.
5. Bradfield CA and Bjeldanes LF (1987) Structure-activity relationships of dietary indoles: A proposed mechanism of action as modifiers of xenobiotic metabolism. J Toxicol Environ Health 21:311-323.
6. Jellinck PH, Hahn EF, Norton BI, and Fishman J (1984) Catechol estrogen formation and metabolism in brain tissue: Comparison of tritium release from different positions in ring A of the steroid. Endocrinology 115:1850-1856.
7. Leete E and Marion L (1953) The hydrogenolysis of 3-hydroxymethylindole and other indole derivatives with lithium aluminum hydride. Can J Chem 31:775-784.
8. Gillner M, Bergman J, Cambillau C et al (1985) Interactions of indoles with specific binding sites for 2,3,7,8-Tetrachlorodibenzo-p-dioxin in rat liver. Mol Pharmacol 28:357-363.
9. Michnovicz JJ and Bradlow HL (1990) Induction of estradiol metabolism by dietary indole-3-carbinol in humans. J Natl Cancer Inst 81:947-949.

10. Waxman D (1988) Interactions of hepatic cytochromes P-450 with steroid hormones. Regioselectivity and stereospecificity of steroid metabolism and hormone regulation of rat P-450 enzyme expression. Biochem Pharmacol 37:71-84.

11. Ghazi A, Dannan DJ, Porubek SD et al (1986) 17 β-estradiol 2- and 4-hydroxylation catalyzed by rat hepatic cytochrome P-450: Roles of individual forms, inductive effects, developmental patterns, and alterations by gonadectomy and hormone replacement. Endocrinology 118:1952-1960.

12. Schneider J, Bradlow HL, Strain G et al (1983) Effects of obesity on estradiol metabolism: decreased formation of nonuterotropic metabolites. J Clin Endocrinol Metab 6:973-978.

Cytochrome P-450 Mediated Activation and Irreversible Binding of Tamoxifen to Rat and Human Liver Proteins

David Kupfer and Chitra Mani

Summary

Tamoxifen (TXF), an antiestrogen, widely used for treatment of human breast cancer, elicits in rare cases endometrial cancer. In rats, TXF induces hepatocellular carcinoma. Neither the mechanism of TXF anticancer activity nor its carcinogenicity are fully understood. It has been suggested that TXF metabolites contribute to its antiestrogenic-anticancer activities. Rat liver microsomes metabolize TXF to the N-oxide, N-desmethyl, and 4-hydroxy and to a putative TXF epoxide. Our study demonstrates a novel route of TXF metabolism. Incubation of TXF with rat or human liver microsomes yields a reactive intermediate (txf*) that binds irreversibly to proteins. This reaction is catalyzed by cytochrome P-450 monooxygenases. Additionally, it appears that the microsomal flavin-containing monooxygenase (FMO) is also involved in TXF binding. A speculation that the therapeutic and/or carcinogenic activity of TXF may involve some form of txf* is presented.

Introduction

Tamoxifen (TXF) (Fig. 1), a therapeutic agent for breast cancer, is a triphenylethylene antiestrogen. The antiestrogenic activity of TXF was the prime factor in its development as a therapeutic agent (1). Several studies suggested that the antiestrogenic activity of TXF involves binding of TXF or its metabolite(s) to the estrogen receptor (ER), at the estrogen binding site and/or at the antiestrogen binding site (2,3). However, despite numerous studies, the mechanism of the estrogenic/antiestrogenic action of TXF is still not fully understood. It has been proposed that TXF might be used in postoperative long-term breast cancer therapy and prophylactically in women at high risk for breast cancer. However, of some concern are the observations that TXF has evoked, in rare cases, endometriosis and increased incidence of endometrial cancer (4). Also, TXF induces ovarian and hepatocellular carcinoma in laboratory animals. The mechanism of the carcinogenic effects of TXF is not known. The current study demonstrates that TXF undergoes metabolic activation and irreversible binding to proteins and examines the nature of the enzymes catalyzing that reaction.

Results and Discussion

Incubation of [^{14}C]-tamoxifen with liver microsomes from untreated rats or from phenobarbital-treated rats (PB-microsomes), in the presence of NADPH, yielded radiolabeled microsomal proteins (Table 1). There was a much higher binding of TXF in PB-microsomes, suggesting that induced enzymes catalyzed the formation of the reactive intermediate (txf*) or that PB increased the number of txf*-binding sites in the microsomal proteins. Each set of microsomes represents a pooled sample from livers of 4-8 male or female rats.

The binding of TXF to proteins appears to be covalent. Washings with solvents of various polarities did not dissociate the radioactivity and SDS-PAGE of the adduct revealed a narrow radioactive band at approximately Mr = 54 KD. This suggests that the binding at 54 KD might be to a P-450. TXF binding is catalyzed by cytochrome P-450 monooxygenase: carbon monoxide and inhibitors of cytochrome P-450 monooxygenases markedly diminish binding (Table 2).

Control male and female liver microsomes exhibit low binding of TXF, suggesting that constituitive sex-specific P-450s do not contribute to activation of TXF. The findings that PB-treatment markedly increased the rate of binding of TXF, suggests that P-450b/e (IIB1/IIB2) and/or P-450p (IIIA1), are involved in generating the reactive intermediate. However, the possibility that PB treatment increased the number of txf*-binding sites, has not been ruled out.

Heating the microsomes at 50° for 90 seconds, known to inactivate liver flavin-containing monooxygenase (FMO) but not cytochrome P-450, markedly diminished binding of TXF (Table 3). Incubations at pH 8.6, optimal for FMO, produced greater binding than incubations at pH 7.4. Additionally, alternate substrates of FMO significantly inhibited TXF binding. This suggested that FMO, is also involved in catalysis of the irreversible binding of TXF.

Human liver microsomes exhibit lower binding than liver from control rats, 0.12 vs. 0.38 nmol/60min/mg protein. Whether the low activity in human is due to low rate of txf* formation, or due to high rate of txf* inactivation or due to low concentration of txf* binding sites is not known.

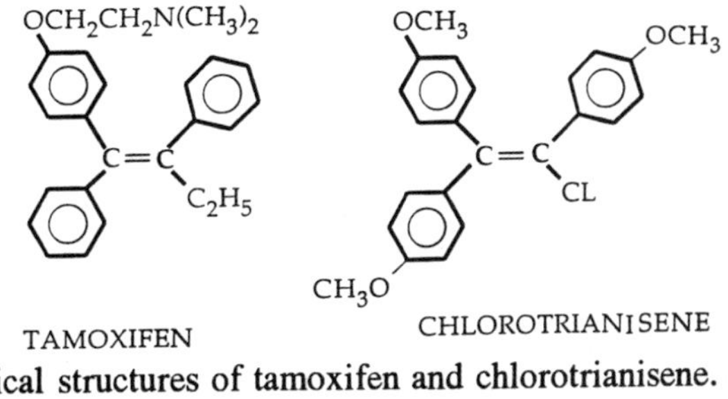

Fig. 1. Chemical structures of tamoxifen and chlorotrianisene.

Table 1. The effect of (PB) and (MC) treatment of rats on binding of tamoxifen (equivalents) to liver proteins.

Treatment	Incubation		Tamoxifen Bound
	Sex	(min)	(nmol/mg protein)
Control	M	60	0.38
PB	M	60	2.24
Control	M	60	0.40
MC	M	60	0.37
Control	F	30	0.31
	F	60	0.60
PB	F	30	1.14
	F	60	2.26
PB	M	60	2.59

Table 2. The influence of various gas mixtures and inhibitors of P-450 on binding of tamoxifen equivalents to male PB-microsomal proteins.

Atmosphere/Additions	Binding of Tamoxifen (nmol/60 min/mg protein)	
Oxygen	1.62	
$N_2:O_2(4:1)$	1.96	(100%)
$CO:O_2(4:1)$	0.19	(10%)
	1.98	(100%)
SKF525A, 0.5 mM	0.13	(7%)
Metyrapone, 0.5 mM	0.15	(8%)
	2.14	(100%)
Benzylimidazole, 0.01 mM	1.09	(51%)
Benzylimidazole, 0.10 mM	0.30	(14%)

We observed that FMO catalyzes the N-oxidation of TXF and that inhibition of FMO is accompanied by decrease in TXF binding. Also, radiolabeled TXF N-oxide can undergo irreversible binding, without significant accumulation of TXF. Additionally, we found that demethylation is not essential for binding, hence, nitrone is apparently not involved. Rat liver microsomes yield a putative tamoxifen epoxide (5). Hence, it is conceivable that txf* is a metabolite of TXF-N-oxide, possibly the N-oxide-epoxide.

Table 3. Effects of pH and heat treatment of male PB-microsomes and of FMO-alternate substrates on the binding of tamoxifen (equivalents) to microsomal proteins.

Experimental Conditions		Tamoxifen Bound (nmol/60min/mg protein)	
Control,	(pH 7.4)	1.53	(100%)
	(pH 8.6)	2.19	(143%)
Control		2.11	(100%)
	50°, 90 seconds	1.05	(50%)
Control		2.14	(100%)
	methimazole, 0.2 mM	0.72	(34%)
Control		2.17	(100%)
	chlorpromazine, 10 μM	1.30	(60%)

Conclusion

Earlier studies demonstrated that tamoxifen treatment of rats yields a modified uterine estrogen receptor (ER) and eliminates its affinity for estradiol (6). Also, we observed that metabolic activation of chlorotrianisene (TACE) (7), an antiestrogenic triphenylethylene, is accompanied by a decrease in estradiol binding to ER (8). It is tempting to speculate that the antiestrogenic/anticancer and carcinogenic activity of TXF involves the binding of txf* to the ER and to other macromolecules.

Acknowledgment

This work was supported by an NIH grant ES00834.

References

1. Jordan VC (1988) The development of tamoxifen for breast cancer therapy: a tribute to the late Arthur L. Walpole. Breast Cancer Res. and Treatment 11:197-209.
2. Sutherland RL, Murphy LC, Foo MS, Green MD, Whybourne AM, Krozowski ZS (1980) High-affinity anti-oestrogen binding site distinct from the oestrogen receptor. Nature 288:273-275.
3. Katzenellenbogen BS, Miller MA, Eckert RL, Sudo K (1983) Antiestrogen pharmacology and mechanism of action. J. Steroid Biochem. 19:59-68.

4. Killackey MA, Hakes TB, Pierce VK (1985) Endometrial adenocarcinoma in breast cancer patients receiving antiestrogens. Cancer Treatment Reports 69:237-238.

5. Reunitz PC, Bagley JR, Pape CW (1984) Some chemical and biochemical aspects of liver microsomal metabolism of tamoxifen. Drug Metab. Dispos. 12:478-483.

6. Nakao M, Sato B, Koga M, Noma K, Kishimoto S, Matsumoto K. (1985) Identification of immunoassayable estrogen receptor lacking hormone binding ability in tamoxifen-treated rat uterus. Biochem. Biophys. Res. Comm. 132:336-342.

7. Juedes MJ, Kupfer D. (1990) Role of P-450c in the formation of a reactive intermediate of chlorotrianisene (TACE) by hepatic microsomes from methylcholanthrane treated rats. Drug. Metabol. Dispos. 18:131-137.

8. Kupfer D, Bulger WH (1990) Inactivation of the uterine estrogen receptor binding of estradiol during P-450 catalyzed metabolism of chlorotrianisene (TACE). FEBS Letters 261:59-62.

Neonatal Diethylstilbestrol Prevents Spontaneously Developing Mammary Tumors

Coral A. Lamartiniere and Michael B. Holland

Summary

Our laboratory has been investigating the effects of perinatal exposure to hormonally active chemicals for predisposing adults to biochemical insult. In experiment I, female Sprague-Dawley rats were treated with diethylstilbestrol (DES) on days 2, 4, and 6 post-partum, followed by aflatoxin B_1 (AFB_1) during puberty and with phenobarbital (PB) in the drinking water from 6 through 16 months of age. Controls received propylene glycol (PG) or no treatment (NT) neonatally followed by similar AFB_1 and PB treatment. Incidences of gross mammary lesions were 67% and 8% in control and DES treated female rats, respectively. In experiment II female rats treated neonatally with PG or DES only have gross mammary lesion incidences of 79% and 13%, respectively, at 14 months of age. The results of experiment II suggest that the formation of tumors in experiment I is not due to the AFB_1 treatment, but is a consequence of spontaneous development. In experiment III, 6-month-old rats having received no PG treatment or DES neonatally followed by 50 mg dimethylbenzanthracene (DMBA) on day 50 had mammary tumor incidences of 100, 100, and 90%, respectively. The latency of tumor development was, however, greater in DES-treated females than in the NT and PG females. Our results reveal that neonatal exposure to the nonsteroidal estrogen, DES, exerts a chemopreventive effect on spontaneously developing but not on chemically induced mammary tumors. This may occur via altered imprinting mechanisms on the hypothalamic-pituitary axis or as a consequence of direct action on the differentiation of the mammary.

Introduction

Developmental modifications during an early period of differentiation can be expressed in later life as beneficial or adverse effects. In humans and rodents, the perinatal period of development is recognized as a time during which critical imprinting events are still taking place in the brain (1). Exposure to DES and other hormonally active chemicals during this critical period of development has been shown to alter the ontogeny of endocrine secretion, brain morphology, sexual behavior, hepatic metabolism, and susceptibility to carcinogenesis. Another tissue that is known to undergo critical differentiation is the mammary gland. At birth and during the first week postpartum in the rat, the mammary gland is composed of a single primary or main lactiferous duct that branches into secondary ducts, to alveolar buds, and finally into lobules. Pregnancy has been reported to promote differentiation of the mammary gland and lower the susceptibility of normal epithelial cells to carcinogenic stimuli (2).

Work in our laboratory has been concerned with investigating predisposition for biochemical insult as a consequence of neonatal exposure of rats to hormonally active xenobiotics. We have been studying activation/detoxication enzymology, formation, and persistence of AFB_1-DNA adducts and hepatocarcinogenesis in rats exposed neonatally to DES and to AFB_1 postpubertally. This report is concerned with the chemopreventive effect of neonatal DES treatment against spontaneously developing mammary tumors.

Results

Experiment I. Offspring of birth-dated Sprague-Dawley CD rats (Charles River Breeding Laboratories, Raleigh, NC) were used. Neonatal rats received subcutaneous injections of 1.45 μmol of DES (390 μg) in 0.02 ml PG on days 2, 4, and 6 after parturition or PG or no treatment during the neonatal period. From days 34-43 postpartum, all rats received 40 μg AFB_1 daily via intragastric intubation. At 6 months of age, all animals were treated with 0.05% PB until they were necropsied at 16 months of age.

Female rats not treated neonatally but receiving AFB_1 postpubertally and PB during adulthood (NT-AFB_1-PB females) had mammary tumor incidences of 56% (10/18) and averaged 2.2 tumors/animal (37/17). Animals treated neonatally with PG, postpubertally with AFB_1 and in adulthood with PB (PG-AFB_1-PB females) had tumor incidences of (75%) 18/24. The PG-AFB_1-PB females averaged 3.4 tumors/animal (82/24). Surprisingly, females exposed to DES neonatally, postpubertally to AFB_1, and in adulthood to PB (DES-AFB_1-PB females) had the lowest incidence of tumors (8%) 3/37 and averaged 0.2 tumors/animal (9/37, $p < 0.001$ compared to NT-AFB_1-PB and PG-AFB_1-PB females; Fisher Exact Test).

Experiment II. Female rats were treated only with PG or DES neonatally as in Experiment I. At 14 months of age, we have data on palpable tumors only. The PG-females have 79% incidence (11/14) of gross mammary lesions. The DES-females have gross mammary lesion incidences of 13% (2/15 $p < 0.001$ compared to PG-females). These animals will be necropsied at a later date.

Experiment III. Female rats were treated neonatally with DES, PG, or received no treatment. At 50 days of age, they received 50 mg of DMBA or sesame oil (SO) intragastrically. Female rats receiving no treatment or PG neonatally plus DMBA were the first to have palpable tumors (49-63 day tumor latency). DES-DMBA treated females had a longer latency period (165-195 days) for the formation of palpable tumors as compared to the other DMBA groups. Animals were killed and necropsied at 230 days of age. Animals not receiving DMBA had 17% incidence of gross mammary tumors 67% (4/24) and low number of tumors/animal (0.2;5/24). All female rats receiving no treatment or PG neonatally and receiving DMBA at 50 days of age developed tumors; the average number of tumors/animal was 5.8 (23/4) and 4.4 (35/8), respectively. Female rats treated neonatally with DES and postpubertally with DMBA had 90% (9/10) incidence of mammary tumors and the average number of tumors/animal was 3.5 (35/10). The average number of tumors/animal for NT-DMBA and PG-DMBA treatment groups was 5.8 (23/4) and 4.4 (35/8), respectively.

Discussion

Experiment I was designed to investigate predisposition for hepatocarcinogenesis as a consequence of neonatal exposure to the hormonally active xenobiotic, DES. The procarcinogen, AFB_1, is well documented to be a hepatocarcinogen, but not a mammary carcinogen. Since the original intent of the study was directed towards liver tumorigenesis, PB was used as a promotor. At necropsy (16 months) we were surprised to find a high incidence 67% (28/42 of mammary tumors in control female rats (PG-AFB_1-PB and NT-AFB_1-PB females) and a low incidence in DES-AFB_1-PB female rats 8% (3/37 $p <$ 0.001).

Since there were no reports of AFB_1 being a mammary carcinogen and Prejean et al. (3) had reported a high incidence of spontaneous tumors in Sprague-Dawley rats we set up Experiment II. The aim was to confirm their results and to see whether neonatal exposure to DES would prevent or retard the development of spontaneously developing mammary tumors as opposed to AFB_1 being responsible for the observed mammary tumors in Experiment I. The results available to date (14-month-old female rats) indicate that control female Sprague-Dawley rats do develop a high incidence of spontaneous mammary tumors. Apparently AFB_1 treatment was not necessary for the development of mammary tumors in Experiment I. Furthermore, neonatal DES treatment is either preventing, or at the very least, increasing the latency period for development of spontaneous mammary tumors.

Experiment III was designed to determine if neonatal DES treatment could increase the latency or prevent the development of chemically induced mammary cancer. Since DMBA is a procarcinogen it must be metabolized prior to being able to initiate genotoxicity. While we do not yet have histopathological data on these animals, the available data clearly demonstrate that neonatal DES treatment does increase the latency for the formation of DMBA-induced mammary tumors and decreases the average number of tumors/animal as compared to females receiving DMBA and no DES pretreatment.

Our speculations as to how DES can exert this chemopreventive effect are: (1) like hormones of pregnancy, neonatal DES may be promoting the differentiation of terminal end buds to lobules (2) and hence lowering the susceptibility of normal mammary epithelial cells to future carcinogenic stimuli (2). Second, neonatal DES treatment has been shown to alter the hypothalamic-pituitary axis. Alterations in imprinting mechanisms have been associated with altered endocrine secretions, metabolism, and receptor mechanisms (4-7). These could, in turn, alter mammary cell susceptibility for biochemical insult.

References

1. McEwen BS (1976) Interactions between hormones and nerve tissue. Sci. American 235:48-58.

2. Welsch CW (1985) Host factors affecting the growth of carcinogen-induced rat mammary carcinomas: A review and tribute to Charles Brenton Huggins. Cancer Res. 45:3415-3443.

3. Prejean JD, Peckham JC, Casey AE, Griswold DP, Weisburger EK, and Weisburger JH (1973) Spontaneous tumors in Sprague-Dawley rats and Swiss mice. Cancer Res. 33:2768-2773.

4. Lamartiniere CA, Sloop CA, Clark J, Tilson HA, and Lucier, GW (1982) Organizational effects of hormones and hormonally-active xenobiotics on postnatal development. In *Proceedings of the Twelfth Conference on Environmental Toxicology*. Air Force Publication AFAMRL-TR-81-149. pp 96-121.

5. Gustafsson JA, Mode A, Norstedt G, Hohfelt T, Sonnenschein C, Eneroth P and Skett P (1980) The hypothalamic-pituitary-liver axis, a new hormonal system in control of hepatic steroid and drug metabolism. In *Biochemical Actions of Hormones* (Litwack, G. ed.) Vol. 7. Academic Press, pp 47-90.

6. Lamartiniere CA, Pardo GA (1988) Altered activation/ detoxication enzymology following neonatal diethylstilbestrol treatment. J. Biochem. Toxicol. 3:87-103.

7. Lamartiniere CA (1990) Neonatal diethylstilbestrol treatment alters aflatoxin B_1-DNA adduct concentrations in adult rats. J. Biochem. Toxicol. 5:41-46

Hormone-Dependent Uterine Adenocarcinoma Following Developmental Treatment with Diethylstilbestrol: A Murine Model for Hormonal Carcinogenesis

Retha R. Newbold, Bill C. Bullock, and John A. McLachlan

Summary

Estrogens have been associated with neoplasia in target tissues including cervix, uterus, ovary, and breast. The mechanisms underlying this association are probably varied. Recently, a model was reported for study of target organ specific hormonal carcinogenesis in which outbred newborn mice were treated with diethylstilbestrol (DES) on days 1-5 of age. Uterine tumors were observed in a time- and dose-related manner; at 18 months of age, cancers were seen in 90% of the mice exposed to 2 μg/pup/day of DES, but not in the corresponding controls. These tumors were hormone-dependent, since regression occurred when mice with established uterine tumors were ovariectomized. Estrogen treatment reestablished the growth of the lesions. In addition, when neonatally DES-treated mice were prepubertally ovariectomized, and therefore deficient in endogenous estrogen, no uterine tumors developed. Transplants of uterine tumor fragments were successfully grown and serially carried in castrated male nude mice. Like the primary tumors, these transplants required estrogen for maintenance and growth. Many of the transplanted tissues and primary lesions retained some differentiated functions such as the production of lactoferrin, an estrogen inducible uterine protein. In addition, estrogen receptor was detected by immunocytochemistry in both transplants and primary tumors. Cell lines have now been established from these DES-induced tumors, and subsequent experiments will provide the basis for studies in mechanisms of hormonal carcinogenesis, including the role of the estrogen receptor and the shift of tumors from hormone-dependent to independent status.

Introduction

Few models for hormonal carcinogenesis are constructed in which concepts such as initiation and promotion can be addressed. To do so, the model would require short or one-time exposure to the hormone, a discrete stimulus to promote or establish the lesion, a discernable progression phase, and a clearly neoplastic endpoint in a large proportion of exposed individuals. The utility of the model would be improved if, at each of the aforementioned steps or phases, the effect of estrogen on target-cell differentiation (normal or atypical) and proliferation could be studied. Finally, the model would be most useful clinically if hormonally associated neoplasia in the target cell or tissue had a human correlate.

Recently, we described a model to study target-organ-specific hormonal carcinogenesis that required short-term exposure of neonatal mice to diethylstilbestrol (DES). Uterine adenocarcinoma was observed in 90% of the mice at 18 months of age that had been exposed to 2 μg/pup/day of DES on days 1-5 of neonatal life (1). Since 17β-estradiol was also reported to induce uterine neoplasia after similar developmental treatment, although at doses three times greater than DES, the carcinogenic activity of DES was apparently not unique to DES, but may be a property of related estrogens. Therefore, this model is ideally suited to study the mechanisms of induction and expression of epithelial cancers by estrogens in their target tissues. Characterization of the hormone dependency of these lesions will aid in understanding the shift of hormone-dependent to independent growth and the mechanisms involved in this shift.

Hormone Dependency of DES-Induced Uterine Adenocarcinoma

DES-induced uterine tumors are hormone-dependent, since neonatally DES-treated mice that were prepubertally ovariectomized, and therefore deficient in endogenous estrogen, did not develop lesions (1). Further support for hormone dependency was obtained by ovariectomizing 12- to 14-month-old DES-exposed mice and observing changes in the established lesions.

At 12-14 months of age, among a group of ovariectomized mice, 13 were determined to have established uterine tumors. Although these tumors did not completely regress in nine days when the ovarian hormones were removed, 69% of the animals demonstrated evidence of regressive changes in the tumors such as desquamated cells and apoptosis. Regressive changes were characterized by cellular changes within the lesions rather than by a reduction in the extent of the lesions. In the remaining 31% of the mice, the adenocarcinomas had few regressive changes and some areas had mitotic figures. These data suggest that uterine adenocarcinomas are hormone-dependent. However, the failure of some of the lesions to show regressive changes after removal of estrogen demonstrates

Table 1. Uterine adenocarcinoma in developmentally estrogenized mice: Effects of ovariectomy on established tumors.

Neonatal Treatment[a]	Uterine Histology
Intact	
Control	No tumors
DES	Neoplastic cells form glandular structures that invade through the myometrium
Ovariectomy[b]	
Control	Quiescent uteri; no tumors
DES	Adenocarcinomas with regressive changes; adenocarcinomas with little or no regressive change 9/13 4/13

[a]Mice were given injections of DES ($2V\mu g$/pup/day) or corn oil (control) on days 1-5 of neonatal life and sacrificed 12 to 14 months later.
[b]Ovariectomy was nine days prior to sacrifice.

that either more time is necessary to show a regression after ovariectomy or a percentage of the animals have tumors or foci in the tumors that have progressed to a hormone-independent state. Both the responsive and nonresponsive tumors had estrogen-receptor positive cells. Whether there were foci of estrogen-receptor negative cells in the nonresponsive tumors remains to be determined.

Discussion

It has been shown that treatment with estrogenic compounds during critical stages of development results in long-term effects on the reproductive tract (2,3), including a high incidence of uterine adenocarcinoma (1,4). The resulting lesions are hormone-dependent, since ovariectomy before puberty blocks their growth and established tumors show regressive changes after ovarian hormone removal. We propose that DES acts to transform uterine cells during early development and that ovarian estrogens act thereafter to stimulate proliferation of the DES-transformed cells in the adult mouse. Additional studies investigating the response of established tumors to hormones will aid in understanding the shift of hormone-dependent to independent tumors.

Acknowledgment

The authors gratefully acknowledge the invaluable help of Ms. Wendy Jefferson.

References

1. Newbold RR, Bullock BC, McLachlan JA (1991) Uterine adenocarcinoma in mice following developmental treatment with estrogens: a model for hormonal carcinogenesis. Cancer Res 50: 7677-7681.
2. Ostrander P, Mills K, Bern H (1985) Long-term responses of the mouse uterus to neonatal diethylstilbestrol treatment and to later sex hormone exposure. J. Natl. Cancer Inst. 74: 121-135.
3. Forsberg JG, Kalland T (1981) Neonatal estrogen treatment and epithelial abnormalities in the cervicovaginal epithelium of adult mice. Cancer Res 41: 721-734.
4. Leavitt WW, Evans RW, Hendry WJ III (1982) Etiology of DES-induced uterine tumors in Syrian hamsters. In: WW Leavitt (ed) Hormones and Cancer, Plenum Publishing Corp., New York, p.63.

Effects of Steroidal and Stilbene Estrogens and Their Peroxidative Metabolites on Microtubular Proteins

Erika Pfeiffer and Manfred Metzler

Summary

In order to elucidate the biochemical mechanisms of estrogen-induced aneuploidy and to evaluate the role of peroxidase-mediated activation, we have studied the interaction of microtubular proteins (MTP) and the inhibitory effect on microtubule (MT) assembly in a cell-free system of various steroidal and stilbene estrogens and their peroxidative metabolites. Steroidal estrogens, e.g., estrone and estradiol, and their catechol 2- and 4-hydroxy derivatives, neither bound to MTP nor inhibited MT assembly. However, the catechol estrogens exhibited strong binding and inhibition after peroxidase-mediated activation. Binding reduced the number of free sulfhydryl groups (by one at 50% inhibition) compared with control MTP and so involved the MTP cysteines. Addition of cysteine before MTP prevented both binding and inhibition. Some stilbene estrogens, e.g., diethyl-stilbestrol and E,E-dienestrol, inhibited MT polymerization directly, whereas others, e.g., indenestrol A, needed peroxidative activation. Therefore, peroxidase-mediated metabolism appears to play a role in MTP interaction for some but not all estrogens.

Introduction

Induction of near-diploid aneuploidy in mammalian cells *in vitro* has been observed for certain estrogens, e.g., estradiol-17ß (E_2) and diethylstilbestrol (DES), and was associated with the ability of these estrogens to cause neoplastic cell transformation (1,2). We have recently proposed that covalent binding of reactive estrogen metabolites, in particular quinones, to microtubular proteins (MTP) may cause aneuploidy induction and cell transformation (3-5). To further study the structural requirements for both covalent and noncovalent interactions with MTP, we have now determined the inhibitory effect of eight different steroidal and ten stilbene estrogens on microtubule (MT) assembly under cell-free conditions. All studies were carried out with and without peroxidase-mediated oxidation in order to see whether MTP is affected by the estrogens *per se* or by their metabolic activation products. Formation of quinone metabolites and their reaction with MTP was followed by ultraviolet (UV) spectroscopy.

Results

As an example for the UV spectra and the MT polymerization assays, the results obtained with 2-hydroxy-E_2 are depicted in Fig. 1. The oxidation of the catechol estrogen by peroxidase was indicated by a pronounced change in the UV spectrum (left panel).

After addition of MTP, a new UV peak at higher wavelength was observed which is probably due to a covalent MTP adduct of the quinone. Assembly of MT (Fig. 1, right panel) was markedly inhibited by the quinone of 2-hydroxy-E_2, but not by the parent compound.

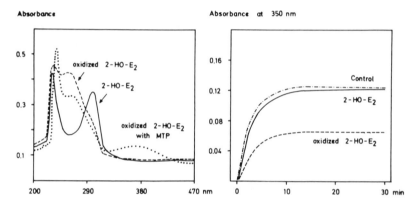

Fig. 1. UV spectra (left panel) and MT polymerization assay (right panel) of 2-hydroxy-E_2 (40 μM) before and after peroxidative oxidation.

A solution of the test compound in ethanol was added to reassembly buffer (final volume 1 mL with 50 nmol compound and 2% ethanol), followed by 13 U horseradish peroxidase and 5 μmol hydrogen peroxide. At maximum quinone concentration according to UV absorbance, 2,500 U catalase were added to stop oxidation. Two controls were performed: one without test compound and one with compound but without peroxidase.

The MT polymerization assay was carried out as previously described (4) with the following modifications: 2 min after addition of the catalase, 400 uL aliquots of the oxidized solution were incubated for 20 min at 37°C with MTP (final volume 0.5 mL with 10 μM MTP). MT assembly was then started by adding GTP (0.5 mM), and the increase in turbidity was determined at 350 nm for 30 min. The control incubation containing all components except the test compound was used as reference (100% assembly). Depolymerization at 4°C was performed to confirm MT formation and detect aggregation.

The results obtained for the steroidal estrogens are summarized in Fig. 2. Whereas estrone (E_1), E_2 and ethinylestradiol (EE_2) did not interfere with MT polymerization at all, a marked inhibition of MT assembly was observed with the 2- and 4-hydroxy derivatives of E_1 and E_2 after peroxidative oxidation, but not without such activation.

The stilbene estrogens gave a more complex result (Fig. 3). At the test concentration of 50 μM, most compounds showed 10-20% inhibition of MT assembly, but some had a markedly higher inhibitory effect, e.g., E-DES, 3,3'-DES and E,E-dienestrol (E,E-DIES) (for chemical structures see Metzler et al., this volume). The products of peroxidative oxidation, i.e., the respective quinones, did not differ significantly from the parent compounds in the case of E-DES, but were stronger inhibitors in the case of indenestrol A and also tetrafluoro-DES (Fig. 3, upper part). The inhibitory effects of those stilbene estrogens unable to form quinones (Fig. 3, lower part) were not altered after peroxidase-mediated oxidation (data not shown).

2-Hydroxy-E_2 and E-DES were chosen as typical steroidal and stilbene estrogen, respectively, to study the binding of the quinone metabolites to MTP in more detail. Incubation of MTP with oxidized 2-hydroxy-E_2 at a concentration yielding 50% inhibition of MT assembly led to a decrease in the number of free sulfhydryl groups in MTP by one per tubulin dimer, as could be determined by titration with Ellman's reagent (see Metzler et al., this volume). When the same

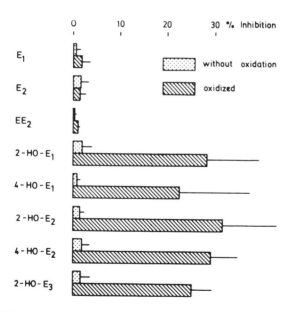

Fig. 2. Inhibition of MT assembly by various steroidal estrogens (at 40 μM concentration) without and with peroxidase-mediated oxidation. For experimental conditions, see legend to Fig. 1. Data are means of three independent experiments $\pm$ SD.

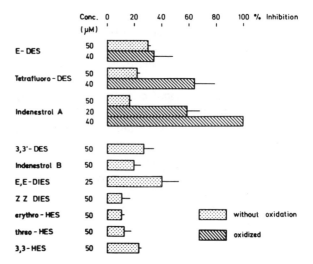

Fig. 3. Inhibition of MT assembly by various stilbene estrogens without and with peroxidase-mediated oxidation. Upper part: compounds forming quinone metabolites upon peroxidase-mediated oxidation; lower part: compounds unable to form quinones.

The chemical structures of most of the stilbene estrogens are given in the chapter by Metzler et al. (this volume). For performance of assay see legend to Fig. 1. Data are means of three independent experiments ± SD.

procedure was performed with oxidized DES, no decrease in sulfhydryl groups of MTP could be measured. This suggests that the quinone of 2-hydroxy-E_2, but not of DES, is able to covalently bind to a cysteine moiety in MTP. In accordance with this notion was the observation that addition of cysteine (at 200 μM) to the test compound after peroxidase-mediated oxidation and prior to incubation with MTP could prevent inhibition of MT assembly by 2-hydroxy-E_2 but not by DES.

Conclusion

This study has shown that both steroidal and stilbene estrogens can interfere with MT assembly in a cell-free system under appropriate conditions. Whereas steroidal estrogens were only active as inhibitors after peroxidative oxidation of the catechol form, most stilbene estrogens exhibited activity even in the absence of such metabolic activation. Thus, interaction with MTP is a conceivable mechanism of aneuploidy induction for both classes of estrogens, although a different role may be assumed for metabolic activation inasmuch as steroidal estrogens need activation, whereas some stilbene estrogens do not. As a further difference in the mechanism of interaction with MTP, activated catechol estrogens appear to involve cysteine moieties for covalent binding, whereas activated DES does not.

Acknowledgments

This study was supported by the Deutsche Forschungsgemeinschaft (Sonderforschungsbereich 172). We thank Mrs. Anita Strohauer for typing the manuscript.

References

1. Tsutsui T, Maizumi H, McLachlan JA, Barrett JC (1983) Aneuploidy induction and cell transformation by diethylstilbestrol: a possible chromosomal mechanism in carcinogenesis. Cancer Res 43:3814-3821.
2. Tsutsui T, Suzuki N, Fukuda S, Sato M, Maizumi H, McLachlan JA, Barrett JC (1987) 17ß-Estradiol-induced cell transformation and aneuploidy of Syrian hamster embryo cells in culture. Carcinogenesis 8:1715-1719.
3. Epe B, Hegler J, Metzler M (1987) Site-specific covalent binding of stilbene-type and steroidal estrogens to tubulin following metabolic activation in vitro. Carcinogenesis 8:1271-1275.
4. Epe B, Harttig UH, Schiffmann D, Metzler M (1989) Microtubular proteins as cellular targets for carcinogenic estrogens and other carcinogens. In: Mechanisms of Chromosome Distribution and Aneuploidy (Resnick MA; Vig BK, Eds) Allan R Liss Inc, New York 1989, pp 345-351.
5. Epe B, Harttig U, Stopper H, Metzler M (1990) Covalent binding of reactive estrogen metabolites to microtubular protein as a possible mechanism of aneuploidy induction and neoplastic cell transformation. Environ Health Perspect 88: 123-127.

Properties of Micronuclei Induced by Various Estrogens in Two Different Mammalian Cell Systems

Robert Schnitzler and Manfred Metzler

Summary

Diethylstilbestrol (DES) and estradiol (E_2) are know inducers of micronuclei (MN) in several cell systems. DES is able to interfere with the spindle apparatus of mitotic cells. This mechanism is discussed to be the cause of chromosomal nondisjunction and subsequently of MN formation. We have tested several steroidal and stilbene estrogens for their ability to induce MN in cultured primary fibroblasts from Syrian hamster embryos and sheep seminal vesicles. All compounds tested, i.e., E_2, 2-hydroxy-E_2, 4-hydroxy-E_2, DES, 3,4-bis-(m-hydroxyphenyl)-hex-3-ene, indenestrol A and indenestrol B gave rise to MN in both cell systems. To further elucidate the mechanism of MN induction, we have scored the MN for the presence of chromatids by CREST antikinetochore immunofluorescence staining. In both cell systems, the frequency of kinetochore-positive MN increased significantly but not uniformly for all estrogens. We conclude that the compounds tested in this study induce MN not exclusively via disturbances of the mitotic spindle apparatus. A second mechanism, possibly an interaction with the kinetochore structure could be responsible for the induction of kinetochore-negative MN.

Introduction

Diethylstilbestrol (DES) and estradiol (E_2) induce aneuploidy and cell transformation in Syrian hamster embryo (SHE) fibroblasts (1,2) as well as micronuclei (MN) in various cell systems (3,4). While DES but not E_2 disturbs the morphology of the mitotic spindle apparatus (5), misalignment of single chromosomes and cell division aberrations are typical effects of E_2 in cultured cells (6). It has been suggested that DES needs metabolism to a quinone intermediate in order to gain a high affinity to proteins such as tubulin (7). The formation of tubulin-estrogen adducts could be responsible for the formation of an altered mitotic spindle aster, which might cause chromosomal nondisjunction during mitosis. Consequently, MN induced via this mechanism should contain complete chromatids or chromosomes, and therefore, a kinetochore structure stainable by immunofluorescence. Recent studies (8) on MN induction in human peripheral lymphocytes by various spindle poisons revealed that DES-induced MN contain a high percentage of CREST serum reactive kinetochores (CRK).

We have analyzed the nature of estrogen-induced MN populations in SHE fibroblasts and sheep seminal vesicle (SSV) cells to investigate whether the frequency of CRK-positive MN is characteristic for compounds with aneuploidogenic potential.

Results

All compounds tested, i.e., E_2, 2-hydroxy-E_2, 4-hydroxy-E_2, DES, 3,4-bis-(m-hydroxyphenyl)-hex-3-ene (3,3'-DES), indenestrol A (IEA), indenestrol B (IEB) and 4-nitroquinoline oxide (4-NQO), a potent clastogenic substance widely used in short-term genotoxicity assays as positive control, induced MN in both cell systems.

Table 1. Maximum numbers of micronucleated cells (MNC) and time of maximum after removal of the test compound. All data represent the mean $\pm$ standard deviation from three experiments and are significantly different from control ($p < 0.005$) as calculated by Student's T test.

Compound, Concentration	Maximum MNC/2000 Cells			
	SHE Cells	Time (h)	SSV Cells	Time (h)
DMSO,0.1%	20 $\pm$ 1.5	1-24	31 $\pm$ 7.3	1-24
DES,50 μM	96 $\pm$ 5.0	12	74 $\pm$ 9.5	12
3,3'-DES,50 μM	115 $\pm$ 3.1	6	95 $\pm$ 10.8	3
Indenestrol A,50 μM^*	63 $\pm$ 9.6	3	62 $\pm$ 8.2	3
Indenestrol B,50 μM^*	83 $\pm$ 5.7	3	89 $\pm$ 5.5	3
E_2,50 μM	83 $\pm$ 1.5	3	112 $\pm$ 7.8	6
2-Hydroxy-E_2,5 μM	37 $\pm$ 16.0**	3	54 $\pm$ 3.1	6
4-Hydroxy-E_2,5 μM	45 $\pm$ 10.9**	3	55 $\pm$ 2.6	6
4-NQO,0.5 μM	140 $\pm$ 7.0***	24	115 $\pm$ 2.5	24

*In SHE cells indenestrol A and indenestrol B were tested at a concentration of 30 μM, because higher concentrations were cytotoxic.

**Data obtained from a different test series than the other SHE MN data. In this case, data are corrected against negative controls and represent induced MN/2000 cells

***The maximum at 24 h might not be the absolute maximum, as no measurements were performed beyond this point.

Comparison of the time dependency data from SHE and SSV cells show maxima of MN numbers at almost the same time after treatment with each compound (Table 1). Also, the absolute maxima of MN numbers were similar for each substance in both cell types.

The composition of the chemically induced MN populations shows a similar trend in SHE and SSV cells with respect to the presence of whole chromatids or chromosomes for each compound tested (Fig. 1). DES induces MN containing a high percentage of CRK-positive structures, whereas 4-NQO treatment does not lead to an increase of CRK-positive MN at all. The other estrogens used in this study gave rise to an average of approximately 50% CRK-positive MN.

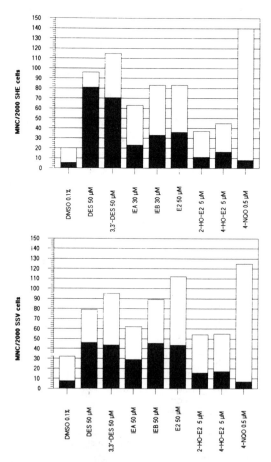

Fig. 1. Induction of micronucleated cells (MNC) and proportion of CREST serum reactive kinetochores (CRK) in SHE cells (top) and SSV cells (bottom). For standard deviations see Table 1.

All kinetochore staining data are based on the analysis of more than 250 MN per compound.

Conclusions

Our data show that several stilbene-type and steroidal estrogens induce MN in SHE and SSV cells. As the cell-cycle kinetics of these two fibroblast systems are similar (data not shown), the time dependency of the MN induction in SHE resembles that found in SSV cells.

The highest MNC frequency was observed in DES-treated cultures. Most of the other estrogens were also able to increase the number of CRK-positive MN in both cell types significantly, although they were not nearly as potent as DES. This must be regarded as clear evidence for the aneuploidogenic potential of these estrogens, because the clastogenic compound 4-NQO had no effect at all on the frequency of CRK-positive MN in SHE and SSV cells. However, the discrepancy in the percentage of CRK-positive MN between the two known aneuploidogens DES and E_2 indicates that kinetochore-staining experiments should be interpreted with caution. The comparatively lower frequency of CRK-positive MN in E_2-treated cells may have various reasons. One possibility is that the CRK-negative MN represent acentric fragments. Such fragments could be the results of a clastogenic effect of the estrogen, possibly through redox cycling and formation of activated oxygen species, as has been proposed by various investigators (9,10). Another possibility is that the CRK-negative MN contain complete chromatids or chromosomes, but their kinetochore complex has either been lost or is still present but not detectable by CREST serum antibodies, because the estrogen has masked the respective epitope. Such alterations of the kinetochore complex by the estrogen might also disturb the separation of chromosomes during mitosis and therefore represent a biochemical mechanism of aneuploidy induction. In order to distinguish these possibilities, we propose to combine immunofluorescence kinetochore staining with *in situ* hybridization of alphoid DNA probes to centromere near regions of the chromatid. The use of the probes would allow the visualization of the centromere in MN even if the kinetochore is masked, and therefore identify compounds with aneuploidogenic potential. On the other hand, clastogen-induced MN containing an acentric fragment would be characterized by the absence of both centromer and kinetochore signals. These studies are currently in progress in our laboratory.

Acknowledgments

This study was supported by the Deutsche Forschungsgemeinschaft (Sonderforschungsbereich 172). We thank Mrs. Anita Strohauer for typing the manuscript.

References

1. Tsutsui T, Maizumi H, McLachlan JA, Barrett JC (1983) Aneuploidy induction and cell transformation by diethylstilbestrol: a possible chromosomal mechanism in carcinogenesis, Cancer Res 43:3814-3821.

2. Tsutsui T, Suzuki N, Fukuda S, Sato M, Maizumi H, McLachlan JA, Barrett JC (1987) 17ß-Estradiol-induced cell transformation and aneuploidy of Syrian hamster embryo cells in culture. Carcinogenesis 8:1715-1719.

3. Schmuck G, Lieb G, Wild D, Schiffmann D, Henschler D (1988) Characterization of an *in vitro* micronucleus assay with Syrian hamster embryo fibroblasts. Mut Res 203:397-404.

4. Wheeler WJ, Cherry LM, Downs T, Hsu TC (1986) Mitotic inhibition and aneuploidy induction by naturally occurring and synthetic estrogens in Chinese hamster cells *in vitro*. Mut Res 171:31-41.

5. Tucker RW, Barrett JC (1986) Decreased number of spindle and cytoplasmic microtubules in hamster embryo cells treated with a carcinogen, diethylstilbestrol. Cancer Res 46:2088-2095.

6. Wheeler WJ, Hsu TC, Tousson A, Brinkley BR (1987) Mitotic inhibition and chromosome displacement induced by estradiol in Chinese hamster cells. Cell Motil and Cytoskel 7:235-247.

7. Epe B, Hegler J, Metzler M (1987) Site-specific covalent binding of stilbene-type and steroidal estrogens to tubulin following metabolic activation *in vitro*. Carcinogenesis 8: 1271-1275.

8. Tucker JD, Eastmond DA (1990) Use of an antikinetochore antibody to discriminate between micronuclei induced by aneuploidogens and clastogens. Mutat Environ, Part B:275-284.

9. Epe B, Schiffmann D, Metzler M (1986) Possible role of oxygen radicals in cell transformation by diethylstilbestrol and related compounds. Carcinogenesis 7:1329-1334.

10. Liehr JG, Roy D (1990) Free radical generation by redox cycling of estrogens. Free Radical Biol Med 8:415-423.

High-Performance Liquid Chromatography Method for the Separation of Potential Metabolites of Estradiol

Lisa A. Suchar, Richard L. Chang, and Allan H. Conney

Summary

A method utilizing HPLC was developed to separate estradiol (E_2), estrone (E_1), and 22 monohydroxylated and keto derivatives of these estrogens. Chromatography of a mixture of the 24 estrogen standards resulted in 19 distinct peaks. Assay conditions for metabolism studies were established so that product formation was proportional to time of incubation and microsomal protein concentration, and substrate metabolism was less than 20%. In these experiments, incubation of $4^{-14}C$-E_2 with NADPH and liver microsomes from untreated adult males rats resulted in the formation of major metabolites with the chromatographic mobilities of 16α-OH-E_2, 2-OH E_2, 2-OH E_1, and E_1. In additional studies where different assay conditions resulted in more extensive metabolism of E_2, very complex metabolic patterns were observed. The results of our studies suggest extensive metabolism of E_2 by rat liver microsomes.

Estradiol is metabolized extensively by liver microsomes. Studies on the metabolism of estradiol are often done by determination of triated water formation from [2 ^{3}H]-estradiol (1,2), [4-^{3}H]-estradiol[2], and [16α-^{3}H]-estradiol (3). An advantage of the tritium-release method is that it allows for the rapid measurement of 2-, 4- and 16α-hydroxylation. The tritium release assays, however, do not measure metabolism at other positions, and some estradiol may be metabolized to other products prior to or after hydroxylation at the 2-, 4-, or 16α-positions. Although gas chromatography/mass spectrometry (4), thin layer chromatography (5,6), and high-performance liquid chromatography (7,8) methods have been developed for studies of estradiol metabolism, there are no detailed metabolic studies with large numbers of potential metabolites as reference standards.

Estradiol, estrone, and 22 hydroxylated and keto derivatives of these estrogens were chromatographed on a Waters liquid chromatography system that was equipped with a Waters 600E solvent gradient programmer, a Waters Lambda-

Table 1. High-performance liquid chromatography of estrogen standards:[a] Relative retention times (RRT).

RRT	Compound
0.105	6α-OH E_3
0.194	2-OH E_3 / 15α-OH E_3 / 6-keto E_3
0.265	15α-OH E_2
0.276	6α-OH E_2
0.299	7α-OH E_2
0.318	14α-OH E_2
0.361	16α-OH E_2 (E_3)
0.486	16-keto E_2
0.505	6-keto E_2
0.520	16α-OH E_1
0.557	11β-OH E_2/16β-OH E_2
0.593	11β-OH E_1/12β-OH E_2/14β-OH E_2
0.666	6-keto E_1
0.743	4-OH E_2
0.792	2-OH E_2
0.879	2-OH E_1
0.913	4-OH E_1
1.000	E_2
1.018	17α-E_2 (internal standard)
1.037	E_1

[a]Estrogen standards were chromatographed as described in the text, and the compounds were detected by UV absorption at 280 nm. The retention times of the estrogen standards are given relative to estradiol (E_2). The retention time for E_2 was 50.98 minutes. Estrone and estriol (16α-OH E_2) are abbreviated E_1 and E_3, respectively.

Max Model 481 UV detector (set at 280 nm), and a solid cell radioactive flow detector from the IN/US Co. Estrogen metabolites were analyzed using a 0.5 μ ODS Ultracarb 30 column (150 x 4.6 mm). All separations were done at room temperature at a flow rate of 1.2 ml/min.

The column was eluted for 63 min with acetonitrile/methanol/water (the methanol and water both contained 0.1% acetic acid) under the following conditions: 3 min isocratic at 16/12/72; 25 min using a #3 convex gradient to 20/21/59; 10 min with a linear gradient to 24/23/53; 10 min linear gradient to 55/24/21 immediately followed by a #10 concave gradient to 92/5/3 for 15 min. The relative retention times of the hydroxylated and keto derivatives of estradiol and estrone are shown in Table 1.

Chromatography of a mixture of 24 reference compounds resulted in 19 peaks. Incubation of female rat liver microsomes with [4-^{14}C]-E_2 and NADPH resulted in the formation of metabolites with the mobilities of E_1, 2-OH E_1, and 2-OH E_2. Two metabolite peaks that were less polar than E_1 were also observed. Incubation of adult male rat liver microsomes with [4-^{14}C]-E_2 and NADPH resulted in the formation of metabolites with the mobilities of E_1, 2-OH E_1, 2-OH E_2, and 16α-OH E_2. Longer incubations resulted in the formation of at least 10 additional metabolites. Two of the metabolites were less polar than E_1 and the other metabolites were more polar than 2-OH E_2.

Acknowledgments

We thank the Schering-Plough Corporation for their support of these studies. Partial support for the studies also came from NIH grant CA-49756. We would like to thank Diana Lim and Deborah Bachorik for their help in the preparation of this manuscript.

References

1. Brueggemeier RW (1981) Kinetics of rat liver microsomal estrogen 2-hydroxylase. J Biol Chem 256:10239-10242.
2. Dannan GA, Porubek DJ, Nelson SD, et al (1986) 17β-Estradiol 2- and 4-hydroxylation catalyzed by rat hepatic cytochrome P-450: roles of individual forms, inductive effects, developmental patterns, and alterations by gonadectomy and hormone replacement. Endocrinology 118:1952-1960.
3. Fishman J, Schneider J, Hershcopf RJ, et al (1984) Increased estrogen-16α-hydroxylase activity in women with breast and endometrial cancer. J Steroid Biochem 20:1077-1081.
4. Spink DC, Lincolon II DC, Dickerman HW, et al (1990) 2,3,7,8-Tetrachlorodibenzo-p-dioxin causes an extensive alteration of 17β-estradiol metabolism in MCF-7 breast tumor cells. Proc Natl Acad Sci, USA 87:6917-6921.
5. Cheng K and Schenkman JB (1984) Metabolism of progesterone and estradiol by microsomes and purified cytochrome P-450 RLM $_3$ and RLM$_5$. Drug Metab and Disp 12:222-234.
6. Sugita O, Miyairi S, Sassa S, et al (1987) Partial purification of cytochrome P-450 from rat brain and demonstration of estradiol hydroxylation. Biochem Biophys Res Comm 147:1245-1250
7. Brueggemeier RW, Tseng K, Katlic NE, et al (1990) Estrogen metabolism in primary kidney cell cultures from Syrian hamsters. J Steroid Biochem 36:325-331.
8. Aoyama T, Korekwa K, Nagata K, et al (1990) Estradiol metabolism by complementary deoxyribonucleic acid-expressed human cytochrome P450s. Endocrinology 126:3101-3106.

Ovarian Hormones Enhance the Carcinogenic Activity of 2,3,7,8-TCDD in Rats

Angelika M. Tritscher, George C. Clark, Fu-Hsiung Lin, and George W. Lucier

Summary

2,3,7,8-Tetrachlorodibenzo-*p*-dioxin (TCDD) is a hepato-carcinogen in female rats but not male rats. Our studies, employing a two-stage model for hepatocarcinogenesis, reveal a significant difference between intact and ovariectomized (ovx) rats for the tumor-promoting activity of TCDD. In order to clarify the estrogen/TCDD interactions in this model with DEN (diethylnitrosamine) as initiating agent and TCDD as the promoting agent, we investigated two receptor systems known to be affected by TCDD-treatment and that are involved in hepatocyte proliferation. EGF-receptor binding is significantly decreased in intact but not ovx animals. Decrease in estrogen-receptor binding is also more pronounced in intact animals. Ovariectomy had no effect on the amount of induction of cytochromes P-450 1A1(c) and 1A2(d). Preneoplastic lesions (GGT-positive foci) were found at a much higher incidence in livers of intact rats than in ovx rats. TCDD markedly increased cell turnover (BrdU-labelling) only in intact rats. A long-term dose-response study showed, that the induction of P-450 1A2 correlates with the dose of TCDD. Our data suggest that ovarian hormones significantly enhance the tumor promoting activity of TCDD in the rat liver.

Introduction

TCDD is a potent hepatocarcinogen in female but not male or ovariectomized rats (1,2). It is considered to be a nongenotoxic carcinogen and is generally accepted as tumor promoter in skin and liver (3). Many of the biochemical and toxic responses to TCDD are mediated through an intracellular protein, designated the Ah receptor.

Table 1. Summary of effects of TCDD treatment on rat liver [each value represents the mean of nine rats].

	S/C	S/TCDD	DEN/C	DEN/TCDD
P450 d[1]				
Intact	35	187*	49	271*
OVX	45	236*	43	254*
EGFR[2]				
Intact	191	70*	186	72*
OVX	137	123	148	121
ER[3]				
Intact	42	17*	51	23*
OVX	50	34	67	25*
TCDD Conc.[4]				
Intact	--	16	--	18
OVX	--	35	--	34
GGT + foci[5]				
Intact	5.6	5.0	44.7*	387.5*
OVX	n.d.	n.d.	30.4*	80.7*
BRDU[6]				
Intact	0.3	6.0*	0.8	7.3*
OVX	1.1	1.0	1.1	0.7

[1]pmol per mg microsomal protein, double antibody radioimmunoassay
[2]Bmax, fmol per mg membrane protein, binding assay with $[^{125}I]$-EGF
[3]Bmax, fmol per mg cytosol protein, binding assay with $[^3H]$-17β-estradiol
[4]ppb
[5]foci per cm^3
[6]BrdU labeling index, BrdU in mini osmotic pumps implanted seven days prior to sacrifice
*Significantly different from controls (S/C) at least at $p < 0.05$
n.d., none detected

Our study used a two-stage model for hepatocarcinogenesis in rats to evaluate the influence of ovarian hormones on liver tumor promotion by TCDD. The parameters measured were preneoplastic lesions, cell proliferation, enzyme induction and binding activity of the EGFR and estrogen receptors. The rats were treated with a single initiating dose of diethylnitrosamine (DEN) followed by chronic treatment with TCDD at a dose of 100 ng/kg/day for 30 weeks (4).

Table 2. Induction of P-450d with increasing dose of TCDD (30 weeks of tumor promotion).

Dose TCDD (ng/kg/day)	P-450d (pmol/mg protein)	
	S/TCDD	DEN/TCDD
0	63.5 ± 38.4	29.9 ± 6.9
3.57	88.3 ± 22.9	87.2 ± 21.7
10.5	161.0 ± 55.7	127.9 ± 32.7
35.7	193.1 ± 60.2	233.1 ± 78.9
125.0	297.4 ± 88.3	387.5 ± 127.6

Results and Discussion

Cytochrome P-450d is induced by TCDD in hepatic but not extrahepatic tissue, and this response is considered to be Ah-receptor dependent. P-450d is very efficient in catalyzing the 2-hydroxylation of 17β-estradiol. The formation of catechol-estrogens is suggested as a critical step in the metabolic activation of estrogens that might lead to reactive intermediates and subsequent cell damage (5). We also investigated EGF and estrogen-receptor systems, which are known to be involved in hepatocyte proliferation and are affected by TCDD-treatment.

Table 1 summarizes the results of the parameters measured. TCDD induced P-450d sixfold to eightfold, although no significant difference could be seen between intact and ovariectomized animals. Decrease in EGF-receptor binding occurred only in intact animals, approximately 63% of control values. Decrease in estrogen-receptor binding was more pronounced in intact than in ovx animals.

Preneoplastic foci (foci of cellular alteration) were quantified by the phenotypic marker γ-glutamyltranspeptidase (GGT), which is considered to be a predictive marker of liver cancer in rodents (6). The livers of intact DEN/TCDD rats showed a significant increase in number of foci and the percent of liver occupied by foci. The amount of foci per cm^3 was about five times higher in DEN/TCDD-treated intact rats than in corresponding ovx rats. Ovariectomy did not significantly alter the occurrence or size of GGT-positive foci in the DEN/C groups. TCDD induced cell proliferation, quantified by the immunohistochemical detection of incorporated BrdU, occurred only in intact rats.

In a second study, we demonstrated a dose-dependent induction of P-450d by TCDD. The induction of P-450d is a very sensitive parameter for TCDD exposure. Also, this cytochrome binds TCDD and so might alter the distribution pattern of TCDD as a consequence of induction (7). The results are shown in Table 2. The induction occurred in an almost linear dose-response pattern with approximately a twofold increase at the lowest dose of 3.57 ng/kg/day. There was no significant difference between initiated and noninitiated animals. The immunolocalization of P-450d in uninduced animals showed a mainly centrilobular staining with small amounts through the midzonal to the periportal regions. Induction by TCDD increases mainly the number of cells containing detectable amounts of P-450d, in addition intensified staining could be seen in centrilobular regions as well as in single cells throughout the area.

Our data show that ovarian hormones significantly enhance biochemical and toxic effects of TCDD and may play an important role in the hepatocarcinogenic action of TCDD.

References

1. Kociba RJ, Keyes, DG, Beyer, JE, Carreon, RM, Wade CE, Dittenber, DA, Kalnins, RP, Frauson, LE, Park, CN, Barnard, SD, Hummel, RA, Humiston, CG (1978) Results of a two-year chronic toxicity and oncogenicity study of 2,3,7,8-tetrachlorodibenzo-p-dioxin in rats. Toxicol Appl Pharmacol 46:279-303.
2. National Toxicology Program (1982) Technical Report Series No. 102. Research Triangle Park, NC: National Toxicology Program.
3. Poland, A, Palen, D, Glover, E (1982) Tumor promotion by TCDD in skin of HRS/J mice. Nature (Lond) 300:271-273.
4. Lucier, GW, Tritscher, A, Goldsworthy, T, Foley, J, Clark, G, Goldstein, J, Maronpot, R (1991) Ovarian hormones enhance 2,3,7,8-tetrachlorodibenzo-p-dioxin-mediated increases in cell proliferation and preneoplastic foci in a two-stage model for rat hepatocarcinogenesis. Cancer Res 51:1391-1397.
5. Metzler, M (1984) Metabolism of stilbene estrogens and steroidal estrogens in relation to carcinogenicity. Arch Toxicol 55:104-109.
6. Popp, JA, Goldsworthy, TL (1989) Defining foci of cellular alteration in short-term and medium-term rat liver tumor models. Toxicol Pathol 17:561-568.
7. Leung, H, Poland, A, Paustenbach, DJ, Murray, FJ, Andersen, ME (1990) Pharmacokinetics of [^{125}I]-2-Iodo-3,7,8-trichlorodibenzo-p-dioxin in mice: analysis with a physiological modeling approach. Toxicol and Appl Pharmacol 103:411-419.

Index